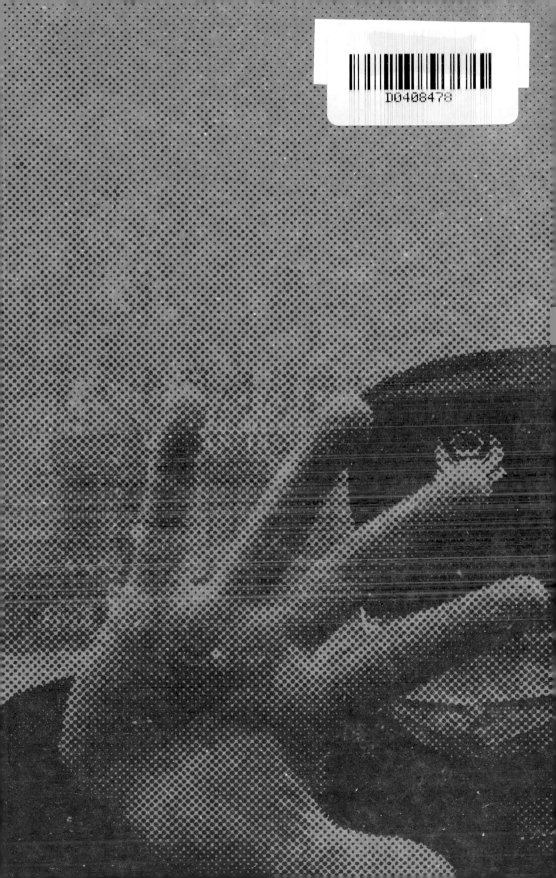

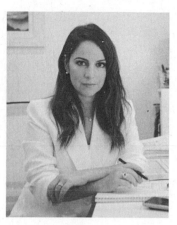

Sharri Markson is a two-time Walkley Award–winning journalist, investigations writer at *The Australian* and host of *Sharri* on Sky News Australia. She has been at the forefront of breaking news regarding the origins of the Covid-19 pandemic since early 2020. Sharri was previously national political editor at *The Daily Telegraph*, media editor at *The Australian,* editor at *Cleo* magazine, news editor at *Seven News*, and political reporter and chief of staff at *The Sunday Telegraph*. She was the recipient of the 2018 Sir Keith Murdoch Award for Excellence in Journalism, the winner of the 2020 News Award for Investigative Journalism, a winner of four Kennedy Awards – 2018 Journalist of the Year, Political Journalist of the Year and Scoop of the Year, and 2019 Columnist of the Year – and joint winner of the 2019 Press Gallery Political Journalist of the Year award.

She lives in Sydney, Australia, with her husband and child.

What really happened in Wuhan

What really happened in Wuhan

SHARRI MARKSON

HarperCollins*Publishers*

HarperCollins*Publishers*
Australia • Brazil • Canada • France • Germany • Holland • Hungary
India • Italy • Japan • Mexico • New Zealand • Poland • Spain • Sweden
Switzerland • United Kingdom • United States of America

First published in Australia in 2021
by HarperCollins*Publishers* Australia Pty Limited
Level 13, 201 Elizabeth Street, Sydney NSW 2000
ABN 36 009 913 517
harpercollins.com.au

A catalogue record for this book is available from the National Library of Australia

ISBN 978 1 4607 6108 3 (hardback)
ISBN 978 1 4607 6092 5 (paperback)
ISBN 978 1 4607 1402 7 (ebook)

Cover design by Darren Holt, HarperCollins Design Studio
Cover photograph by AP Photo/Ng Han Guan
Author photograph by Adam Yip
Typeset in Minion Pro by HarperCollins Design Studio

For every soul who has lost their life to this cruel virus,
and to their loved ones left behind

CONTENTS

CHAPTER ONE

Dimon Liu

Wrapped in a coat and scarf, Wei Jingsheng strode with purpose through an edgy Washington suburb, lowering his face from the winter chill. He managed to blend in easily among the rush-hour crowd making their way home from work at dusk. But Wei was no ordinary American. He was one of the biggest defection coups the US had pulled off from inside communist China.

Wei was on his way to dinner at the home of his old friend Dimon Liu and her husband, Bob Suettinger, the CIA agent who had secured his deportation to the United States 20 years earlier, saving him from a living hell. The Chinese Communist Party (CCP) had left him to rot away inside a cell for 18 years after catching him brazenly objecting to their regime.

Now in Washington, as Wei stepped into the warmth of Dimon and Bob's renovated red-brick townhouse near Capitol Hill, the smell of his childhood hung in the air – the Cantonese cooking for which Dimon was famous among friends. When Wei walked in, neither Dimon nor Bob had any sense of how portentous that casual Friday-evening meal would turn out to be. How they'd reflect back on it many times, turning over each sentence uttered, weighing up how they'd interpreted the information passed on to

1

them and wondering what more they could have done with this valuable intelligence.

That night they would become among the first in the world to discover a deadly new virus was spreading stealthily in Wuhan. It was November 22, 2019 – six weeks before China would reluctantly confirm to the World Health Organization (WHO) there was a mystery virus, and a full two months before they would confirm human-to-human transmission.

Dimon, with long black hair and a petite frame, has a warmth about her that draws you in. It entices the most influential players in United States politics and intelligence to her dinner table in Washington's gentrified, trendy suburb of South East Capitol Hill. She is fluent in English but still has her Cantonese accent from her formative years.

In the kitchen, Dimon stood cooking a sizzling Chinese-Western fusion of rib-eye steak and stir-fried bean curd while Bob lingered, a glass of red wine in hand. The gutsy Chinese human rights activist expertly flicked in grated ginger as she wondered what news Wei had to tell them. Having grown up inside one of the 500 founding Communist Party families from when the People's Republic of China (PRC) was established in 1949, he maintained unparalleled contacts deep inside the system.

Wei had joined the Red Guards, a student paramilitary movement under Chairman Mao Zedong, during the Cultural Revolution in 1966 when he was 16. His brother was best friends with Chinese President and Chairman of the Communist Party Xi Jinping when they were younger. Wei loved to say how the Chinese President was never that bright as a kid. He didn't think Xi was a great intellect as an adult, either.

"When you have that much power you don't have to be very bright," Dimon would comment. "The bullies in the school yard, they are never very bright but they have enough muscles to intimidate you."

Despite his pedigree and connections, the Communist Party insider was thrown into prison in 1979. He had boldly penned a manifesto advocating democracy called "The Fifth Modernization", posting it on the Democracy Wall in Beijing in 1978. In it, he called then leader Deng Xiaoping a dictator. In a move that would seal his fate, Wei signed the essay with his own name and address. Perhaps feeling invincible, he also wrote a letter denouncing the inhumane conditions in Qincheng Prison.

The Chinese Communist Party and Chinese Police moved swiftly and made an example of him. Wei was subject to a televised trial before being thrown into prison. He was brutally tortured – beaten so severely he lost many of his teeth – starved and confined to solitary isolation. He was left there, under these unbearable conditions, forgotten by the outside world, or so it felt, for 14 long years. In 1993, he was set free against the backdrop of the PRC competing for the 2000 Olympics and trying to improve its image. But it would only be a brief release.

His cruel treatment inside an assortment of China's brutal prisons only emboldened Wei to agitate harder against the Communist Party. When he was caught speaking to the visiting US Assistant Secretary of State for Human Rights, John Shattuck, the following year, he was thrust back inside a dark, isolated cell.

"Shattuck was told repeatedly not to meet with Wei, because Wei would be punished; but Shattuck wanted his headlines," Dimon says.

Wei returned to interminable days of starvation and torture. He assumed he'd spend his wasted life in there.

"I have never seen him bitter or angry about his treatment," Dimon reflects. "When I ask him he says, 'This is what I chose. I chose to resist.' I think the only thing he feels guilty about is his family. He felt he brought a lot of suffering to his brother and sisters and parents. They had their future destroyed with a famous dissident as a brother."

Bob Suettinger, a tough CIA operative, was then working in the Clinton White House as China Director of the National Security Council. In 1997, Bob sat down with the First Secretary of the Chinese Embassy in Washington DC, Liu Xiaoming (who went on to become Ambassador to the UK until 2021), and miraculously negotiated Wei's release and deportation to the United States.

Bob was renowned as a steely negotiator and had unparalleled expertise in the White House about the Chinese Communist regime. No one could pull the wool over his eyes. He knew China wanted the West to open the market and was prepared to make unprecedented concessions – including releasing a famous prisoner.

Wei's bombshell defection from China to America in 1997 made worldwide news. By the time he flew into New York City on November 16 that year, he was a celebrity.

Once in the United States, it turned out Wei made the ultimate defector. He had a flawless, photographic memory. He could recount vivid tales from inside the elite circles of the Chinese Communist Party with meticulous detail about their personalities and, crucially, their activities. The rare knowledge of an insider.

Wei once told Dimon he could remember her New York phone number from when it was passed onto him during his brief release from prison, in case he needed help. After he recounted it, Dimon had to go find an old address book to check if he was right. He was.

In his new life in America, Wei loved hunting and, quite naturally for someone who experienced starvation for two decades, eating. Sometimes he'd walk through Dimon's door proudly carrying a carved-up carcass of a wild boar he'd killed himself. Dimon would laugh and cook him a big steak, putting the rest of the meat in smaller cut-up portions in her freezer for dumplings another day.

While she usually prepared traditional Chinese food, and her cooking and conversation drew a wonderful community of China analysts and intelligence agency insiders to their home, Dimon always liked to cook a meal that Wei would love and devour. He's a red meat sort of guy.

At 70, Wei is tall with rosy cheeks and a decent head of hair. This night, they sat down to eat in the kitchen – the old friends were like family, after all.

They started chatting about Donald Trump. Naturally. Not about the impeachment trial over Ukraine that was front-page news; none of them thought he'd be convicted over that. But about his personal approach to China, how instinctive it was and how he needed good people around him. There were different camps advising him when it came to China foreign policy, and they were concerned that the "Wall Streeters" only cared about doing business with China. These advisors seemed to hold little regard for human rights violations in Xinjiang and the deprivation of basic personal freedoms throughout China. Dimon, Bob and Wei are as bipartisan as is possible in Washington DC, and had close friends on both sides of the political divide, including in Trump's administration.

It wasn't until after they'd heartily consumed the rib-eye steak, stir-fried bean curd and Chinese barley that Wei leant back and pulled out one of his cherished French cigarettes. He took his time, passing one to Bob as well.

Wei looked at Dimon and Bob. "There is a new, dangerous virus spreading in China," he said. "There is a lot of talk about people getting sick. All my friends are speaking about it," he went on. "It seems to be in Wuhan. The people who are talking about it in the chatrooms to their friends are all people from Wuhan."

Dimon was immediately concerned. "SARS was easily contained, especially in Hong Kong. It couldn't be more serious than SARS and so it's probably containable," she queried uneasily

Wei nodded but was unconvinced. This seemed different. "'There's a lot of fuss about this virus. The chatrooms are filled with it," he said.

He was paying attention to the virus and he was concerned about it, but no one knew how serious it was, or how contagious. It wasn't even clear what exactly the virus was, although there were suspicions it was another SARS outbreak.

This piece of information rattled Dimon and Bob. They mulled it over, letting it sink in from their shared perspective of knowing first-hand China's tendency for cover-up and disregard for human rights. Like Wei, Dimon knew all too well the CCP's inhumane and cruel treatment of its own people. Its brutal disregard for who would live or die – even women and children – as long as it was in the best interests of the Party.

Dimon's mother, Sun Li Shu, spent the eight years of the 1937–45 Japanese invasion running from city to city, dodging bombs that the Japanese Imperial Army dropped on the civilians, with four young children in tow, while her husband was on the front line of the Second Sino–Japanese War.

Sun Li Shu married Dimon's father, Chongzhen Liao, in 1931, but they were separated for eight years during the Japanese War and then five years during the civil war that followed. Her pregnancy with Dimon, in 1953, was a result of the intensely romantic reunion with her husband after 13 years apart. At first, she was flabbergasted by the surprise pregnancy at the age of 42, but this gave way to hand-wringing worry.

Chongzhen Liao managed to escape Communist China, moving to Hong Kong in 1938 and later to the United States in 1953, where he would spend the rest of his life. But Dimon's heavily pregnant mother stayed in the midst of "bombs and bullets", as she would describe it in a letter later on. The perilous journey would have been too strenuous and risky.

Her mother was right to worry about raising a child in 1950s China. Her daughter nearly didn't survive the Great Leap Forward, which started in 1958 when Dimon was six. During the Chinese Cultural Revolution, Mao Zedong identified five groups who were enemies of the revolution, calling them the "Five Black Categories": landlords, rich farmers, counter-revolutionaries, bad influences and rightists. Dimon's family had two strikes against them: her father had been a politician and had been educated in the West. It meant that instead of surviving on the already dire monthly ration coupons for food, her family's rations were half of everyone else's. One ounce (30 grams) of pork a month, one ounce of oil and half a pound (225 grams) of grain. Meals were often a few grains of rice and anything else they could scrape together. Tens of millions of people died of starvation. It's estimated that the number of people who died during the Great Leap Forward reached 47 million, although the true number of souls who perished may never be known. It was a fate Dimon came within a whisker's breadth of sharing.

She distinctly remembers the starvation she suffered as a child in Canton, the largest city in the province of Guangdong in southern China, describing it as a "persistent gnawing of hunger" that "felt like a sharp knife twisting and thrusting in my gut without respite. On many a night I shed silent tears until I was finally able to fall asleep – a memory so painful and vivid that it still haunts me more than half a century later," she recalls.

"Properly fed people rarely existed in China at that time, unless you belonged in the very small and exclusive club of Chinese Communist elite. Millions died needlessly and in a most painful way as the Chinese Government forcibly took the grain away from its people and shipped it overseas. Chinese Communists often extolled their system as superior to democracy because of its efficiency. It is efficient, no doubt, but also most efficient in killing its own people."

During the day, small groups of children roamed the streets searching for something to line their bellies. Dimon hunted frogs, birds and water cockroaches. She caught rats and sparrows with traps she built herself, taking them home for her mother to cook. She even scraped bark off the trees for meals, and actually ate it.

"In truth, everything was skinny, only the rats had any meat on them," she says.

Dimon's mother gave her a hard-boiled egg as a birthday present on the day she turned eight. "It was so rare and precious, I couldn't bear to eat it," she says. "I put the egg in my pocket. I took it out, looked at it and put it back into my pocket; and on and on as I wandered the streets; because staying home might mean my older brother could snatch the egg from me. Another small gang of children saw me with my egg, and ran towards me. I quickly stuffed the egg into my mouth, barely chewed it and swallowed it, eggshells and all, even as I was being jumped on and pummelled."

Dimon was so weak from starvation that when she contracted tuberculosis at seven, the viral infection took her to the brink of death. "People on our streets were dying of many infectious diseases, though no one dared to say anyone died of hunger," she says. Dimon's brother, who was working as a doctor in Canton at the time, stole antibiotics from the hospital, saving her life.

As the years dragged on, Dimon's mother knew she had to find a way to get her daughter out of Canton. When Dimon was 11, her mother begged a favour from an old friend who worked in the public security bureau. He arrived at their home with an exit visa, using a razor blade to scratch out another child's name and replace it with Dimon. To this day, her passport still has that other little girl's birthdate.

Dimon was walking skin and bones when her distraught and terrified mother put her on a train to Hong Kong, praying her youngest child would not get caught and the falsified exit visa would work.

It was 1963. At the time, China was issuing more exit visas than Hong Kong was allowing entrants. When she disembarked at Lo Wu Control Point station, Dimon watched as dozens and dozens and dozens of scrawny, malnourished people, hoping for a better life, were turned away from the Customs Office and herded into a corner. On the other side of Customs were another group of people, huddled together. They'd made it through to the chance of a better life.

Dimon, bony and famished, dropped to the floor. On her hands and knees she crawled her way through metres and metres of indistinguishable shoes, ankles and legs, holding her breath in fear, until she dared raise her head and look up. She had made it to the other side. She was through. Relief.

"When I got there, there was nobody to meet me, of course, because I left so quickly," she says. "I only had the telephone number of a woman whose husband – who had long since passed away – used to be my father's secretary, decades ago." Dimon had never seen or used a telephone before. With her heart beating, she walked into a utility store and timidly asked the man behind the counter to call the number for her. The woman was teaching in an elementary school and couldn't come collect Dimon until after work. She would have to wait.

It had been dark for untold hours when the woman finally did arrive to collect Dimon, who had been sitting all day on the pavement, patiently, anxiously waiting. Her future like a murky pond. The woman took her in and Dimon stayed in Hong Kong for two years until 1965, when her father arranged for her to fly to America for a new life. At 13, she met her father for the first time. He had led a remarkable life, attending the Ivy League school Cornell in America and then, back in China, working as Director of the Department of Sericulture, where he had bridges, irrigation canals and dams in the Guangdong province named after him. He was also an intellectual, translating religious Baha texts into Chinese. But he was unable to land a decent job in New York. He swallowed his pride and made his living as a waiter in a Chinese restaurant.

"When I came to the US things got worse. My father felt he couldn't take care of me and sent me to live with a relative in Chicago." Two years later, Dimon told her father, "Either you take me in or I'm walking away."

Dimon was 15 when she went to live with her father, and she only had two years with him before he passed away. Her sullen behaviour during those two years, when she objected to his lacklustre, basic cooking and spurned his attempts to pass on his knowledge of history and politics, still haunts her to this day. The ache of regret weighs on her heart when her wandering, restless mind takes her back to those dinner-table conversations, the memory vivid enough for her to relive and appreciate what he was trying to teach her.

After his passing, she picked herself up in this foreign country and pressed on to create a life for herself, filled with friends, two husbands and, most importantly, purpose. "I'm one of those people who is determined to survive," Dimon says defiantly.

And she was equally determined to change the oppression and cruelty of tyrannical modern China. Her life is dedicated to activism, and Dimon has testified before the US House of Representatives and Senate on human rights violations in China. She's also been an integral member of a bipartisan, global group, the Inter-Parliamentary Alliance on China, which is trying to stop its human rights abuses.

"The Chinese people shouldn't have to suffer so much. We shouldn't be forced to live in such an awful way. It's not necessary.

I don't hate the Chinese Communist Party, I just want them to stop abusing their own people," she says. "The US keeps rescuing the Chinese Communist Party, who had been systematically killing their own people. It's not tolerable."

As Dimon forged a life and career in the United States, and for a time at Hong Kong University where she had a teaching position until the horror of the Tiananmen Square massacre, her deepest heartache was the memory of her mother, whom she had left behind as a young girl. It wasn't until 1980, when Dimon was 28, that she saw her mother again. Dimon managed to get her mother out of China when Jimmy Carter "normalised" the relationship with the People's Republic.

Dimon first met Wei in 1997, the year he arrived in New York. Two years later, they formed a close friendship when they campaigned to stop the United States Congress from legislating permanent normal trade relations, known as the PNTR, with China. They spoke to 30 senators and 100 congressmen and congresswomen, their ferocious fight failing by only a few votes. "That was one of the biggest foreign policy mistakes that the US made," Dimon says regretfully.

Wei, an intellectual and defiant as ever, refused to learn English, and Dimon was his interpreter for a while. It was perhaps inevitable that their paths would cross and they would forge a solid friendship spanning decades. Dimon has always maintained strong connections with fellow Chinese activists and dissidents.

Looking at her animated face and joyous eyes, usually free of make-up, it's not remotely obvious that she celebrated her 70th birthday in September of 2020. Only when prosecuting an argument over a pivotal matter – like the best way to secure freedom for a Hong Konger cruelly imprisoned by China under their new national security law – does Dimon's forceful, combative streak swing into full flight. It's the same fiery strength that saw her survive the great famine as a child.

By the time her dinner with Wei wrapped up, Dimon went to bed with a nagging feeling about this new virus in Wuhan. If her contacts with dissidents were solid and highly respected in the United States intelligence community, Wei's were even better. Many believe he has confidential sources in very senior positions in the official Chinese apparatus. His networks are impeccable.

Yet there was nothing about this new virus on the news, nothing in the papers. No word of any virus emanating from Chinese media. It was curious and deeply disquieting.

January 2, 2020, Washington DC

Six weeks later, Wei burst through the door of Dimon and Bob's home just before lunchtime. It was the second day of the new year, a Thursday, and Wei had called only a short while before to ask if he could drop by for lunch, prompting Dimon to frantically scour her pantry and fridge to see what she could cook him. From the moment he walked in, Wei could speak about little else other than the virus spreading in Wuhan. He launched into news of it immediately.

Dimon and Bob were highly concerned. Wei told them the official line, propagated by authorities, was that the virus had emerged in the seafood wet market. "It's just not possible," Wei insisted adamantly in a raised voice. He systematically and emphatically ruled out that natural animal-to-human transmission had occurred through the wet market.

Dimon listened as she rustled up ramen noodle soup with meat and vegetables, made with stock she'd frozen for emergency situations such as this. "The only thing he spoke about at that lunch was the Wuhan disease," Dimon said later. "I was alarmed by the things he told me."

As they sat down to eat the spicy soup, what Wei said next truly shocked Dimon and Bob. With the photographic memory that can recall a long-forgotten, now defunct phone number after 30 years, he told them about top-secret, highly classified programs the Chinese Communist Party had been running for decades. "I know the PLA [People's Liberation Army] has been doing research on biological warfare since the 1960s," he said authoritatively. "The laboratories in Wuhan are very suspicious. I believe those laboratories are controlled by the military and not by civilians. The virus is from the laboratory, either through incompetence, accident, negligence, corruption or intention."

He paused, then added. "The wet market theory is only likely if the avaricious lab technicians sold the used and infected animals to the wet markets."

Dimon and Bob felt frightened. They glanced at each other again, for what felt like the fiftieth time.

Wei proceeded to tell them about Shi Zhengli – specifically mentioning her name – and said that the Wuhan Institute of Virology where she worked was the laboratory suspected of being responsible for the leak of the virus. He mentioned the uncontrollable Hong Kong protests that had been a political firestorm for the Chinese government for months and months.

Dimon asked, "Is there any possibility that Xi or Xi's political rivals released the virus?"

"Such a possibility always exists," Wei said, "because the power elite would do anything to gain advantages during power struggles. Xi would be the most likely culprit, if the virus release was indeed intentional, because Xi controls the military, and the military controls the research in biological warfare."

Dimon didn't know what to make of it. It was surreal. Unthinkable. A virus was apparently spreading and yet not a word from any official outlets? The entire matter covered up and silenced?

She asked Wei, "Are they really doing this?"

Wei said, "They have no baseline. 底线." The phrase, which has no English equivalent, is usually translated as "They have no bottom line," but more accurately means, "They can descend to a very low level."

Dimon and Bob were in shock. "This was like 'Wow'. We couldn't believe our ears," she says.

It was January 2 and Dimon had read nothing about the virus in Wuhan on the news and seen nothing about it on social media. She knew then and there she had to get the information to the White House. Specifically to Donald Trump's Deputy National Security Advisor for Asia, Matt Pottinger.

Pottinger was her good friend. Their first substantive meeting was when China-analyst Peter Mattis brought him for dinner before he started in the White House. Bob and Dimon liked him immediately. He was smart, level-headed and had expertise in the area, unlike other policy figures, whose limited understanding of Communist China meant they struggled to differentiate good advice from bad.

After dinner, she teased her husband that Matt was the best head of the China desk she had met. From that point on, Dimon would informally advise Matt and do some work for him on thorny political disputes.

He'd also already had a major impact. The National Security Strategy of 2017, which Pottinger formulated along with its primary author, former Deputy National Security Advisor Nadia Schadlow, and co-author, National Security Advisor H.R. McMaster, had reshaped the administration's position on China.

It didn't bother Dimon and Bob that Pottinger was joining the Trump administration. Having forged his career at the CIA, Bob had briefed both political parties, including George Bush Sr, George Bush Jr and Bill Clinton.

Dimon and Bob have made a great team since the pair married nine years earlier; Bob speaks the Washington policy lingo and has experience inside the White House, while Dimon maintains impeccable dissident connections and is a wealth of knowledge. Not to mention her exceptional cooking.

After Wei's visit over lunch, Dimon decided she had to let Pottinger know what was going on. She sat down to write him a memo with the crucial, valuable information she had been told. But as she put pen to paper, Wei's account seemed even more far-fetched than when she originally heard it. A contagious virus potentially leaking from a laboratory controlled by the PLA, which had been conducting biowarfare experiments since the 1960s? That hadn't been mentioned in a single news item and had already been spreading for six weeks at least?

Dimon hesitated. It sounded bizarre. There was no urgency, she reasoned. Matt had better hear it for himself from Wei, she decided.

She would put them both in touch in person at her Chinese New Year's Eve party on January 25. There was no reason to believe this situation was urgent. Not a word had been mentioned in the news and the virus had already been around since at least November 22, when Wei first told her about it.

Lest Matt think her crazy, she would make sure he spoke to Wei so he could hear first-hand the alarm and concern in this famous defector's voice. Yes, he needed to hear it from Wei directly.

CHAPTER TWO

Brave Whistleblowers

Dr Wang Lei can pinpoint the precise moment the Wuhan medical system collapsed.

It was the moment when the denial of human-to-human transmission truly became a farce. When dead bodies were piling up, left to decay for days in hospital corridors and on trucks, because Chinese health authorities refused to officially record any deaths. The bodies were for them nothing more than a logistical problem. Hospitals were at capacity and sick families were left to fend for themselves.

At the same time Dimon and Bob were first hearing about this mysterious new virus in November, Dr Wang Lei was at the chaotic epicentre of the unfolding health crisis enveloping his city. The middle-aged community doctor was on the front line of the battle against Covid-19.

He and his medical colleagues would realise very quickly that they were dealing with a new coronavirus – but they were forbidden from breathing a word about the official diagnosis. Even when they each started to fall ill from the new coronavirus, they were forced to turn up for work – with health directors refusing to acknowledge there was a problem.

It all began in early November 2019, when Dr Wang and his colleagues started seeing more and more patients walk in with fevers and respiratory problems. It would fast become an influx.

"I was treating at least double the usual number of patients with fevers," Wang says. "I have one shift starting in the morning, six or seven hours, from 8am to 3pm. I would typically see 30 patients; usually you have maybe five or six people with fevers. The others are old people, people with diabetes or hypertension or other issues. But in November, I'd easily see at least a dozen people every shift with fevers, sometimes more. They all had fevers and a cough."

Dr Wang – whose name and age I've changed to protect his life – works in a medical clinic close to the centre of Wuhan, a city of 11 million people, where he practises both traditional and Chinese medicine.

As November progressed, the virus escalated. The authorities clearly knew they had a problem on their hands this month because, Dr Wang says, a flu alert was sent out to doctors, warning them of some sort of severe influenza. But he thought something was suspicious because high school classes started shutting down in November, wherever there had been infected students. It was around the time of the mid-term exams, which went from October 29 to November 11, 2019. This made him wonder if it was something other than just the regular flu. "At that time, some students stopped going to school, it's not the school closed down but some classes [were] postponed." It's extraordinary that classes were cancelled as early as November because of a flu-like illness..

"With the flu, you also get a fever, so back in November we never thought things would develop like they did; we assumed it's just the flu," he recollects.

It soon became clear that this was definitely not the flu. Thinking back, Dr Wang says, it became apparent by the first week of December that they were dealing with a coronavirus. A coronavirus is a large family of viruses that causes respiratory illness, spreading via respiratory droplets. "We thought it was SARS again. You said that there was an official report in the [Chinese] media about detecting the spread of a coronavirus on December 27. As for us doctors, I don't remember the specific time we figured this out, but I'd say it was probably around December 8. There was discussion about this at the time; we thought this was SARS. We started referring to this illness as 'SARS PLUS'. That's what we called it when they hadn't yet given it a name."

Dr Wang and his colleagues suspected they were dealing with a coronavirus, but it was Ai Fen, at Wuhan's largest hospital, who was the first to officially confirm the horror diagnosis. Like Dr Wang, Ai Fen, the female head of emergency at Wuhan Central Hospital, had been inundated with patients suffering from pneumonia-like symptoms and chest infections. Coughing and high fever. People struggling to breathe and gasping for breath. She had never seen anything like it in the decade since she started as Director of Emergency back in 2010.

It was the chilliest month of the year, and it wasn't unusual to see people fall ill with pneumonia, but some of these patients were younger than you'd expect and weren't responding to treatment.

"Pneumonia of unknown cause" was the official term used, with chest imaging confirming the respiratory illness. But Ai Fen knew that diagnosis couldn't be accurate. When Ai Fen's patients weren't responding to any of the usual medication for pneumonia, with feverish temperatures and difficulty breathing, she sent biological samples for laboratory testing. The common bacterial and viral pathogens that can cause pneumonia weren't present.

Among her patients was a 65-year-old man who delivered goods to the Wuhan seafood market. He was admitted to the Central Hospital on December 18 suffering pneumonia. His condition deteriorated fast.

"It was a baffling high fever," Dr Ai later told Chinese magazine *Renwu* (*People*), in an interview that would be wiped from the internet within minutes. "The medicines used throughout didn't work, and his temperature didn't move."

Fluid samples from his lungs were sent on December 24 to the genomics company Vision Medicals, based in Guangdong, for testing. Usually, the test results would be sent back in a day or two. But this did not happen. There was no paperwork. Instead, they rang the head of respiratory medicine at Wuhan Central Hospital, Zhao Su, two days later.

"They just called us and said it was a new coronavirus," Zhao said of the December 26 phone call in comments to Chinese news outlet Caixin Global in February 2020.

Even though this was a result from Ai Fen's patient, it never reached her. But it did reach the Chinese Academy of Medical Sciences in Beijing. Vision Medicals has confirmed in a social media post that it was involved in early studies on the new coronavirus and contributed to an article in the *Chinese Medical Journal* about its discovery. The company shared the alarming result with the Academy of Medical Sciences after sequencing most of the virus's genome and confirming it was a coronavirus similar to SARS, according to Caixin Global.

Company executives paid a visit to Wuhan to discuss their findings with local hospital officials and disease control authorities. Even though it was a coronavirus – potentially highly infectious and deadly – the entire matter was kept secret.

And the 65-year-old delivery driver was dispensable. He was transferred to Wuhan Jinyintan Hospital, where he passed away.

On Christmas Eve, Dr Wang went out in the city with some friends. He gave each of them a mask to wear. "We knew already this was a SARS-like/abnormal virus," he said.

Some of his colleagues working at major hospitals in Wuhan were well aware it was a coronavirus but were forbidden from saying anything. In December, a senior doctor in the respiratory illness division at Tongji Hospital in Wuhan made his whole family take Tamiflu as a preventative measure.

"He didn't tell them why. His mother, daughter, wife – he didn't tell any of them why," Dr Wang says. "When he encountered patients with this illness, he self-isolated for a week. He was quarantining himself at Tongji Hospital: he knew this was a coronavirus. But then his division got so busy that he couldn't self-isolate anymore, he had to go back to work. That was very early on."

Dr Wang says Tongji Hospital was the first to take countermeasures to protect against a SARS virus. "At Tongji they knew this was a coronavirus, but they couldn't say anything. Only after the government announced this could they talk about it. Prior to that, there was a gag order," he recalls.

"In our doctors' WeChat group, someone said that they had looked at samples in their own laboratory and determined that this was a coronavirus. I can't remember if they were from Tongji Hospital or United Hospital. This news was not even shared widely on WeChat, as I remember."

Dr Wang's patients were falling sick all around him and there was little he could do to help. He felt under siege and exhausted.

"I remember one day I was seeing 25 patients and 23 of them had lung infections. I acted based on my experiences with SARS; I had been living in Beijing back then," he recalls. "Based on SARS, I assumed the virus would only be around for a month or so, so I bought a one-month supply of face masks. At that time, one mask was 0.13 yuan [a tenth of a cent]. And I warned the pharmacy at my health centre: get a few thousand face masks, just to have them here. They laughed at me: 'Oh, you're always so nervous, stop worrying. There's no virus, stop worrying.'

"A little while later, when they tried to get face masks, there were none left. I had bought 300 face masks and shared them with my family, my parents, my brother, and kept 100 for myself. On January 13, I went to buy face masks again. It was already too late. Things were even crazier than in December. I remember hearing on older lady shout: 65 yuan for one N95 mask! You used to be able to buy these masks in bulk for 3.5 yuan. Even the best N95 mask was just 5 yuan. Now they were 65 yuan each. Eventually the only N95 masks we had in our health centre were donated. If I used one of those at home, I could wear it for a week. But at work, dealing with sick people day after day, hour after hour, you have to change your mask every day."

* * *

One of Ai Fen's patients at Wuhan Central Hospital was a 41-year-old man who had no history of contact with the seafood market. After he was admitted to the hospital on December 27, his swabs were sent to a laboratory in Beijing, CapitalBio Medlab, for analysis.

On December 30, the result was sent back to her. It read: "SARS coronavirus." Ai stared at the word, re-reading it again and again, trying to comprehend the severity of the diagnosis. She broke out into a cold sweat. It was the news she had suspected and dreaded.

Acting instinctively, she circled the shock result in red and sent it with a video of a lung scan to a friend from medical school who was then working at another hospital in Wuhan. A colleague of Ai Fen's at Wuhan Central, ophthalmologist Dr Li Wenliang – who would later become the most famous whistleblower in China – quickly sent the news on WeChat to about 100 medical staff he knew from their days as medical students at university together. He wrote: "7 cases of SARS have been confirmed."

The message spread like wildfire across Weibo, particularly in medical circles. Dr Li would later face punishment for this act, detained by police and shamed on national television, along with seven other doctors who had tried to spread the word about a new coronavirus to save lives.

That night, as Ai Fen worried about the repercussions of a mysterious new coronavirus, her phone beeped with a message from her boss at Wuhan Central Hospital. It was a reprimand. Ai was told she was not to release information about the coronavirus arbitrarily, to avoid causing panic.

Knowing how infectious coronaviruses are, Ai told all of her direct reports to wear protective clothing and masks, including jackets under their medical coats. Even as she gave this directive, the official hospital policy was not to wear masks or protective clothing – again, to avoid causing any panic. CapitalBio then retracted its analysis. The company said it was a false positive for

SARS and just a "small mistake", which a gene sequencing expert told Caixin was a possibility because of a limited gene database.

"We watched more and more patients come in as the radius of the spread of infection became larger," Ai Fen later told *Renwu*. "I knew there must be human to human transmission."

Two days later, on January 1, Ai Fen was summoned to see the head of Wuhan Central Hospital's disciplinary inspection committee and officially given a reprimand for "spreading rumours" and "harming stability". She was formally told that she was forbidden from sending any form of communication to anyone about the virus, including messages or images.

In the days leading up to Ai Fen's remarkable discovery, Wuhan was already a city crippled by the virus. Health workers and specialists in hospitals and medical clinics across the city were worried and afraid to speak out.

On December 27, a respiratory doctor Zhang Jixian, from Hubei Provincial Hospital of Integrated Chinese and Western Medicine, was one of the first to officially tell China's health authorities that a new coronavirus had caused at least 180 people to fall sick. She looked at the CT scans of an elderly couple suffering from fever, coughing and fatigue, who had visited the hospital a day earlier, and saw that it looked different from common pneumonia.

The 54-year-old Dr Zhang, who had worked during the 2003 SARS pandemic, told a Chinese news outlet, Xinhuanet, that she was sensitive about a pandemic unfolding again. She insisted on doing a CT scan of the elderly couple's son.

"At first their son refused to be examined. He showed no symptoms or discomfort, and believed we were trying to cheat money out of him," Zhang told Xinhuanet. But his scan ultimately showed the same abnormalities as his parents – even though he was asymptomatic. "It is unlikely that all three members of a family caught the same disease at the same time unless it is an infectious disease," she said. The blood tests of the three, along with another patient who came to the hospital, indicated viral infections, but they all tested negative to influenza.

Dr Zhang filed a report to the hospital, which was then sent to the district-level centre for disease control and infection. "The report is about how we discovered a viral disease, probably infectious," she said.

As a result of this report, disease control authorities in Wuhan and Hubei issued an internal notice to warn of a new pneumonia in patients who had been in contact with the seafood market, asking hospitals to monitor similar cases. This notice was leaked online and was among the first official acknowledgements of an outbreak. China was still denying there was any human-to-human transmission – a denial it would steadfastly cling to for another month, backed and amplified by a gullible and complacent WHO.

One of the biggest genomics laboratories, BGI, received a sample from a hospital in Wuhan on December 26. The December 29 results found it was a previously unseen coronavirus that was 87 per cent genetically similar to the virus that caused SARS in the 2003 pandemic, Caixin reported.

Other genomics companies were inundated with samples as patients poured in to different hospitals and medical centres throughout December. But in just a few days, on January 1, these crucial early samples of the coronavirus would all be destroyed under the strict orders of the Chinese Government as it sought to cover up news of the emerging virus.

CHAPTER THREE

The News Breaks

DECEMBER 30, 2019, NEW YORK

Checking her emails after dinner in wintry New York, Marjorie Pollack, the Deputy Editor of the Program for Monitoring Emerging Diseases (ProMED), saw a message from a Chinese-speaking contact telling her there was social media chatter about a new virus in China. It was December 30, 2019. By the time her contact told her about it, the chatter on Weibo was incessant.

In the email, there were screenshots and tweets about clusters of cases in Wuhan. Attached was another picture purporting to be of a Wuhan public health commission document linking the viruses to the Huanan Seafood Market. Marjorie rang her boss, ProMED Editor Larry Madoff, straight away to warn him there might be a new SARS spreading in Wuhan.

"Marjorie called me during the day on December 30 to alert me and think about what we should say, what we should try to find out," Madoff says. "We recognised that this was significant and worrisome, though of course we didn't appreciate just how big."

Marjorie scoured Chinese media outlets and found some reporting of a new pneumonia-like virus, which Madoff says they viewed "as at least partially confirmatory".

From her more than 20 years working at ProMED, where she started as a web researcher, Marjorie, who is an epidemiologist specialising in vaccine-preventable diseases, recognised what a cluster of pneumonia-like cases could mean and understood this bore a resemblance to SARS. She had travelled to more than 50 countries working for the World Health Organization and the US Centers for Disease Control and Prevention (CDC), and this was eerily reminiscent of another alert she had been involved with 16 years earlier. On February 10, 2003, ProMED had informed the world there was a pneumonia spreading in Guangdong in China. It would turn out to be SARS.

"Having lived through and worked through the SARS outbreak, it just rang a bell. This was a déjà vu," Marjorie said in an online interview with a management consulting firm.

Her team at ProMED had only found out about the 2003 SARS because of a distant rumour. "It was a physician subscriber who said he heard from a friend who has a friend who belongs to a teacher's chatroom in Guangdong, China, reporting that hospitals are filled, people are dying everywhere, massive panic," she recalls. "Covid was a similar process. We didn't know if the picture in the Weibo post was real. So we tried looking around and found a media report saying the Wuhan Health Commission validated that the document was real."

Madoff was concerned with what they'd found out. "I shared with my wife and daughter, who I live with, that something was going on. My wife is Chinese-American – we have family in China and have travelled extensively in China and had been to Wuhan," Madoff says. "It could have been a false alarm but there were worrisome features. We worked quickly to get a post out before the end of the day."

Four hours later, just before midnight, ProMED issued an alert to its database of 80,000 doctors, epidemiologists and public health officials with the headline "Undiagnosed pneumonia – China (Hubei)".

In an indication of how the processes in place to alert global authorities to a pandemic had monumentally failed, a Florida hobby blogger got wind of the virus before the WHO. Half an hour before ProMED's report, Sharon Sanders posted a short blog about the new pneumonia. For the past 15 years, Sanders has run a blog tracking infectious diseases around the world, called FluTrackers, which is "dedicated to the public health of the world's citizens".

On December 30, 2019 at 11.35pm, she published a blog post titled: "Several suspected SARS cases in Wuhan according to China Central Television." The news moved fast. Thirty-six minutes later she published a more alarming report. Time-stamped 12.11am on December 31, 2019, it states that according to Chinese media reports, a "viral pneumonia" or "lung infection" had been confirmed in Wuhan since December 27, with most coming from "merchants in Wuhan South China Seafood City".

Every half hour or so, Sanders came across new information. She reported: "I have been trying to log onto the Wuhan Municipal Health site but it is really slow to load." By 1am, she added that there were 27 cases of viral pneumonia of which seven were critical and the other cases were under control.

It is a sad fact that China never alerted the WHO, or any government, to the coronavirus. It didn't shut down international travel or advise foreign governments to be aware that recent arrivals from Wuhan might be infected with a highly contagious and deadly new virus. It's extraordinary that a virus was taking lives for up to eight weeks before global health authorities caught wind of it. We have no idea how much longer China may have kept the virus secret had ProMED not published its report on December 30, 2019. That report set in motion a series of crucial events.

WHO officials noticed the ProMED report online the next day, December 31. That same day, Taiwanese health authorities also contacted the WHO, requesting information. WHO's Health Emergencies Programme Executive Director Dr Michael Ryan says his team in Geneva contacted the WHO China Country Office, which then made immediate inquiries of Chinese health officials, seeking verification of the media reports. This led to a reluctant – and involuntary – confirmation.

It was New Year's Eve when the WHO China Country Office was officially informed of cases of pneumonia from Wuhan. "Despite public reporting to the contrary, the PRC never notified the WHO about the outbreak in Wuhan," the United States House Foreign Affairs Committee minority staff report from 2020 states.

That same day, as China was forced to reluctantly confirm there was a pneumonia spreading in Wuhan – that it would continue to insist for weeks was not contagious – its massive cover-up of the virus began. It started with a clean sweep of Chinese social media sites, where all mentions of "unknown Wuhan pneumonia", "Wuhan Seafood Market" and other similar phrases were wiped.

As the world rang in the new year, there was no sign of the havoc that would unfold in the first year of the new decade.

It wasn't until January 6 that major newspapers around the world published reports about the new coronavirus. *The Wall Street Journal* published the story online that day with the headline: "Health Officials Work to Solve China's Mystery Virus Outbreak" and the subheading: "Viral pneumonia infects 59 in central China, triggers health alerts in Hong Kong and Singapore."

Its opening paragraphs read: "Medical authorities are racing to identify the cause of a mystery viral pneumonia that has infected 59 people in central China, seven of whom are in critical condition, and triggered health alerts in Hong Kong and Singapore. The pneumonia cases, centered in central China's Wuhan, a city of 19 million, hasn't led to any deaths, according to an update Sunday night on the website of Wuhan's Municipal Health Commission." Even this was a direct lie. Ai Fen's patients had already passed away, and Dr Wang had witnessed bodies piling up inside hospital wards.

The Times in London carried a similar story, but said SARS had been ruled out. "Health experts have not yet identified how the outbreak originated but have ruled out the deadly severe acute respiratory syndrome (SARS) virus as the cause. All patients have been isolated for treatment and 163 people who had come into contact with those infected have been placed under observation."

Again, this was utterly false information that had been provided by the Wuhan Health Commission. Health authorities had already received the lab results from genomics companies showing that it was a new type of SARS virus, which they'd been forced to destroy. In addition, the virus was already spreading like wildfire among the community at this point, and there is no evidence at all to suggest the family members of patients were in quarantine or were under observation – let alone the medical workers who had come into contact with infectious patients.

The New York Times published an online story the same day written by its correspondents in Beijing and Hong Kong. It ran on page 13 on January 7 and quotes Linfa Wang, an expert on emerging infectious diseases at Duke-NUS Medical School in Singapore, who "said he was frustrated that scientists in China were not allowed to speak to him about the outbreak". Linfa Wang has worked with Shi Zhengli and Peng Zhou from the Wuhan Institute of Virology since at least 2006.

Hong Kong had already hospitalised 21 people who had visited Wuhan in recent weeks, according to the report, and officials were installing thermal imaging systems at the international airport to monitor passengers coming in from Wuhan. Staff at the high-speed rail station were checking body temperatures. The article reported that Hong Kong's major pharmacy chains had sold out of surgical face masks. Sales for masks and hand sanitisers had increased significantly in just a week, a major chain, Watsons, confirmed.

The reports were mostly small and buried inside the newspaper. The unmitigated focus of media outlets was Trump's first Impeachment. Scant regard was paid to a new virus emerging from Wuhan.

But within the White House, by the end of that first week in January, some senior officials knew something was amiss. China was repeatedly rejecting international offers from both the United States and the WHO to help contain the virus. No one was allowed to set foot inside Wuhan.

"Did you ever watch the movie *The Sting*?" former Secretary of State Mike Pompeo boomed down the phone from Washington to me. "It's an old movie. It's a Robert Redford classic and he runs a scam and they have a whole section called the shut-out where they refuse to take this money from this guy in a bag. Anyway. We were getting the shut-out [from China].

"You could see it in the formal channels where there were formal requests for our medical team to provide support to the Chinese as they needed it and they said, 'We've got this, no problem.' Then we'd ask for data and we'd be told, 'We don't have it, we're working on it.'

"Then in the informal channels, too [it was the same story]. It became very clear. Then there was the public issues too with the doctors, all the things they were shutting down. It was pretty clear by the end of January we were going to get the shut-out."

It's an insightful analogy. In the 1973 film, nominated for 10 Oscars and starring Paul Newman and Robert Redford, the con succeeds if the mob boss doesn't realise he's been cheated until the conmen are long gone.

It's not unlike China's play on the US. America and – you could argue, although perhaps Pompeo wouldn't – some in the Trump administration were thoroughly conned by China. By the time they realised the con, the pandemic had spread around the world.

From the very first few days of January, Pompeo recalls repeated attempts to send in teams of officials, diplomats and health experts to help China fight the virus – and to find out information. But it was all in vain. Every single offer of assistance was rejected.

"We immediately began collectively, the HHS [Health and Human Services] folks, CDC, my team on the ground in China, we had multiple missions [ready to go]. We were trying to keep them safe, we were trying to support the Chinese efforts to identify where this began and we could quickly see – and then I'm speaking to the middle to the end of January – that our capacity to have visibility to what happened was going to be completely blocked at every turn," Pompeo says.

"Our inquiries through our diplomatic channels, there were efforts made by our medical authorities, everyone was trying because it was so critical to get our hands on the virus itself in its original form as close to patient zero as we could get, so that we could contain it and obviously begin the process of developing a broader solution."

Throughout January, Pompeo was on the phone constantly to an exasperated Robert Redfield. The US CDC Director was on holiday with his family at the end of 2019, about to celebrate on New Year's Eve when his mobile rang alerting him to a "cluster of 27 cases of pneumonia of unknown etiology reported in Wuhan, China". Before he could ring in the new decade, his holiday was over. The next day, January 1, the CDC started developing situation reports, which it shared with the Department of Health and Human Services.

Redfield had been appointed to the crucial role in 2018 after leading the fight against the spread of HIV and the opioid epidemic. Throughout the following days, he would have extensive discussions with his counterpart in China, George Fu Gao, the Director of the Chinese Centre for Disease Control and Prevention.

But Gao didn't reach out to Redfield to warn him about the virus or let him know there was a health crisis in Wuhan, even though Gao had been in the US just a few months earlier for a pandemic planning exercise called "Event 201" that simulated the hypothetical case of a pandemic. The recommendations from the October 18, 2019 event, hosted by the World Economic Forum and the Bill & Melinda Gates Foundation, included maintaining travel and trade during severe pandemics, developing methods to combat disinformation, as well as boosting internationally held stockpiles of medicines and vaccines. Instead, it was Redfield who emailed Dr Gao on January 3, asking to speak with him, and a call was arranged for that day. That call was particularly alarming. To Redfield's immense surprise, Gao began to cry. "I think we're too late," he reportedly said.

Gao told Redfield it was a coronavirus but it was not contagious; there was no "human-to-human transmission". Instead, he said the only people who were sick were those who had visited the wet market. He also said only people who had symptoms had the virus. Both of these crucial points were complete lies.

Redfield immediately offered US assistance, asking if he could send an American team to Wuhan. Gao said he wasn't authorised to accept such a request.

Alarmed by the phone call and the official's rare and highly unusual display of emotion, Redfield rang his boss, Health Secretary Alex Azar, who was at home sick in Washington DC with a severe head cold and laryngitis.

"It's a novel coronavirus," Redfield told Azar.

"Okay Bob, we know what this means – this is a big deal. You need to let Gao know we will send a CDC team immediately. Make the offer right away. Tell them we are here to support them. Let's make sure this is done right, unlike SARS the last time."

Azar, although he could barely speak, rang his Chief of Staff and asked him to immediately alert the National Security Council and Robert O'Brien in the White House, and make sure they were in the loop.

"Every one of my warning bells was up. A novel coronavirus was trouble," Azar has told colleagues.

Azar couldn't get his counterpart, China's head of the National Health Commission, Ma Xiaowei, on the phone – and it would be another three weeks before he was able to do so.

Redfield emailed Gao the next day, on January 4, following up on the offer, stating: "I would like to offer CDC technical experts in laboratory and epidemiology of respiratory infectious diseases to assist you and China CDC in identification of this unknown and possibly novel pathogen." On January 6, Dr Redfield once again sent an email to Gao, this time attaching a formal letter with the offer of CDC support on the ground. None of these offers – and countless others that would be made over the following weeks – were accepted by the Chinese government.

Redfield thinks that had his team been allowed into China it would have answered some of those key scientific questions on which China was not being transparent: whether it was transmissible from human to human and whether the virus causes asymptomatic illness. "I think if we had been able to get in with that team of great experts, we could have helped answer these questions probably in the month of January," he told the Council on Foreign Relations.

The CDC took China's assurance that the virus wasn't transmissible with a grain of salt and, on January 8, 2020, sent an alert to medical clinicians asking them to be "on the look-out for patients with respiratory symptoms and a history of travel to Wuhan, China". The alert said the CDC "is closely monitoring a reported cluster of pneumonia of unknown etiology (PUE) with possible epidemiologic links to a large wholesale fish and live animal market in Wuhan City, Hubei Province, China".

There was a mad scramble to develop a diagnostic test to detect the virus – something that is impossible to do without a virus sample or its genetic sequence. The virus's genetic sequence only became available on January 10, from a laboratory that the Chinese government immediately shut down, presumably in punishment. Dr Redfield's team had a workable diagnostic test by January 17 or 18. It wasn't patented, it was made freely available.

Even though the National Security Council (NSC) was officially told about the Wuhan virus by the CDC by January 3, it was another two weeks – on January 14 – before the NSC held its first meeting on Covid-19. It was chaired by Anthony Ruggiero, the NSC Senior Director for weapons of mass destruction and bio-defence. That same day, the WHO issued a tweet that there was no evidence of human-to-human transmission.

For Pompeo, China's refusal to accept help at this early stage rang immediate alarm bells and made him question whether the virus had come from the wet market at all. It was this lack of transparency as early as January that sparked the seed of doubt for Pompeo about a natural origin of Covid-19. What was China hiding?

"The reason I start my answer to your question about when did we first suspect the Wuhan Institute of Virology as the potential place that could have got a leak, we started thinking about what the possibilities were as soon as we realised they were going to have none of us [in America] figuring this out," Pompeo says. "It puts you on alert. It says goodness gracious, you would think that the global response as required by the WHO, they'd want everyone in to come help them. But they wanted the antithesis of that."

CHAPTER FOUR

Chaos

January 2020, Wuhan

Just as Ai Fen was trying to spread the word, any posts mentioning the new coronavirus started disappearing online. Chinese Communist Party censorship kicked in, alarming doctors and Chinese health authorities, who endorsed precisely the opposite approach. The hashtag #WuhanSARS was blocked, along with terms related to Wuhan pandemic and seafood market.

At work, in Wuhan's busiest hospital, it was gruelling and tragic. Ai was told there was a father who was so unwell he couldn't get out of the car by himself. Compassionately, she walked outside the hospital to help him. By the time she reached his car, he had passed away. She will never forget watching a doctor hand an elderly father the death certificate of his son, who was just 32 years old. The father stared at the doctor, not comprehending the devastating news.

The death was unrelenting. Hospitals were overwhelmed. The mounds of bodies were so high you couldn't climb them. A husband asked Ai if she could organise for his mother-in-law to be transferred to "in-patient care". As concerned as he was about his mother-in-law's state, he took the time to thank Ai for her care. By the time his mother-in-law arrived, she had passed away. "I know it was only a few seconds but that 'thank you' weighs heavily on me," Ai told

Renwu. "In the time it took to say this one sentence, could a life have been saved?"

Ai then watched, and grieved, as her colleagues fell sick, some losing their lives. Later in March, as the pandemic eased in China, Ai Fen told her story to *Renwu*. Even this interview was wiped from the internet.

Soon, Dr Wang realised this coronavirus was far more serious than the SARS outbreak in Beijing in 2003. It would not be gone in a matter of months. It was more infectious, more transmissible. Alarmingly, he and other doctors were forbidden from officially reporting any deaths as a result of the coronavirus. The government continued to claim that hardly anyone had died from the virus, but Dr Wang knew the real state of Wuhan's hospitals.

He spoke to one of his friends, whose wife's sister and sister-in-law were hospitalised with the virus. Hospital wards that would normally hold a maximum of four people had 12 sick patients squashed inside – all highly contagious, spluttering and struggling to breathe. It was diabolical.

There was a blanket refusal to report any deaths related to the virus. "One of my friend's family got sick and were treated at Wuhan Central Hospital," Dr Wang recalls. "Back then they were not reporting any deaths, but he told me that just in the room where he was treated three people had died. They didn't even take the bodies away, just left them lying there for days. He was terrified and messaged me to ask what could be done.

"I can't even begin to imagine how they could put a dozen people in a room," he adds. "It wasn't on the news, so no one knew, but we learned about this from WeChat groups for doctors and chats between doctors and patients.

"At that time, they forbade any reporting of deaths. They just said, no, no one has died. But his family of three had two people fall ill. And one of his colleagues from work also got sick. Once we got into the middle of January, it was very apparent that something was really wrong. When I shared with colleagues what my friend had told me, they all said they had heard similar things.

"Right away, I knew this was a lot worse than we thought. There were more and more people who didn't even have a fever but were going straight into respiratory failure. Taking patients' temperatures was no longer enough.

"Why wouldn't they report any of this? I remember, the head of our health centre told me there can't be any reporting on this because they don't want to create a panic. Another reason was probably just to suppress the real figures. They kept saying everything in Wuhan is under control. Before they put us in lockdown on the 23rd, we weren't even allowed to report lung issues from this illness."

It's stomach-churning to think how Chinese President Xi Jinping was praised by the World Health Organization, the United States and others for his transparency when in fact a criminal cover-up of the virus was underway.

And by January, Dr Wang began to sense that a severe crisis was developing. He was alarmed when many doctors, including his friends, started to fall ill.

As the virus spread internationally, flights out of China were still allowed. Dr Wang's director at the Community Health Centre flew to Europe in January. Dr Wang does not identify precisely which European city his director flew to, but 28 international flights from Wuhan Tianhe Airport were departing daily. Flights with hundreds of passengers went as far and wide as Paris, Tokyo, London, Dubai, New York, San Francisco and Sydney, along with regional hubs like Bangkok and Singapore.

Once Wang's director arrived in Europe, he developed a fever and respiratory problems. Instead of self-isolating straight away, he flew back to Wuhan.

"When he got to Europe, he suddenly realised he had a cough and a fever. He was terrified, worried that he wouldn't get the treatment he needed in Europe, so he hurried back to China," Dr Wang says.

In doing so, he exposed hundreds of people at the airport, on his flight and also, by being there in the first place, on the ground.

"His father specialises in respiratory medicine and advised him on what medicines to take. The problem is that he covered it up from everyone: he continued to work with us. We were on the same shift for quite a long time. His symptoms were really severe when he was in Europe," Dr Wang said.

Dr Wang was ordered by his director, once he had recovered, not to take additional precautions that might scare people and cause mass panic. This same concern about causing panic was the reason news outlets were forbidden from reporting news of the virus.

"The head of our health centre told us, and this is a direct quote: 'You can't wear masks.' This idiotic advice hung over our centre day after day until [Chinese epidemiologist] Zhong Nanshan's comments encouraging masks. I couldn't believe they would have such a dumb policy. No matter whether we are talking about the flu or a coronavirus, how could you tell doctors not to wear masks?"

Falling sick himself was inevitable. And on January 14, Dr Wang developed a cough.

"I started having this lingering pain in my chest. I thought, oh no, am I having a heart attack at such a young age? No way, it couldn't be. The next morning the pain got even worse. It was horrible," he said. "I stayed at home the entire day, checking my temperature. But I didn't have a fever. So, the next day, I went back to work and I did a chest X-ray. The lower side of my right lung showed infection. A doctor reviewing the X-ray said to me: see, this X-ray has all of the standard clinical features of this virus. Then he said to me, I've already done eight X-rays today, they all had these signs of infection in lower right lung."

Dr Wang went back home and stayed in bed, severely unwell for three days. On the fourth day he was ordered back to the clinic; his director would not allow him to take time off work. As the day progressed, Dr Wang began feeling even worse.

"I told the head of our centre that I have some vacation time, and I can't be coming in in this state and infecting our patients and all of you, so I really should take some time off. But he told me I couldn't take time off. Keep coming in until the New Year break (on January 24), he told me," Dr Wang says.

"One reason was that there was not enough staff to treat patients. Another reason was that he feared that doctors not showing up to work might create a panic. If you hadn't been officially diagnosed, you had to come in, and without a Covid-19 Nucleic Acid PCR test there was no way to be officially diagnosed.

"If you wanted to do a test back then, the line was endless. It was impossible to be confirmed with an official diagnosis because basically our entire medical system had collapsed under the pressure. In order to be treated in the hospital, you just needed a CT scan and blood work. But to be officially diagnosed you had to do a test."

By January 20, the health system was inundated with infected people. Dr Wang worried he might not survive. "I remember telling friends on WeChat: it's over for me, I got it," he said.

"One of my friends who works in internal medicine at a hospital told me, come over to our hospital, we have space for you. I said I would continue to monitor my situation. "The next day he said, 'It's too late, you should have come yesterday. Today we don't even have space to treat our own doctors.' On the 19th, he could definitely get me in, on the 20th it was getting tight, but by the 21st there was no chance. In those two days, our entire medical system collapsed."

Mayhem and anarchy were breaking out. There was no isolation in hospitals, no best-practice medical care. At a fever clinic that had been set up, a long line of hundreds of sick people stretched seemingly ever onward. Dr Wang says he watched as a woman, incredibly sick – and sick of waiting for treatment – broke out of the queue and begin spitting on the ground out of anger. Yelling that she wanted to infect everyone.

After Spring Festival, more and more doctors and nurses in Dr Wang's medical centre became infected with Covid-19-like symptoms. "We have 60 or so medical personnel at our health centre. When you add in the cleaners and the entrance guards, maybe we have 64 or 65 people altogether working here. Eventually some just stopped coming to work, they were too scared. Every day I would keep track of how many people were falling ill. It went from eight to 12 on to 20, and by that point I lost count," he said.

Parents started pressuring Dr Wang to write health certificates giving their child a clean bill of health. "There were a lot of students from middle schools and primary schools who came in. It was almost time for finals at the end of the term, and parents were eager for me to write a certificate of good health for their kids. I asked why. They said it's almost time for finals and the school is not letting our kids attend. So, we want to give the school a certificate of good health, so our kids can go to school and take their exams."

Dr Wang's first-hand account indicates that when China said on January 24 that it only had 830 confirmed cases and 26 deaths, in fact the number was far, far higher.

Months later, when the heat of the crisis passed and the days grew warmer, Dr Wang visited the home of a Wuhan academic. Sitting on the balcony, he told the academic, in intricate detail, how early the coronavirus started spreading in Wuhan, and how authorities covered it up.

A confidential source put me in touch directly with this academic, using a secure form of communication undetected by the Chinese Communist Party. He agreed to assist with my book and sent me Dr Wang's first-hand account. He asked only that I change the doctor's name and not publish the location of his medical clinic, to protect him from being arrested, tortured or killed by Chinese police. I agreed and changed any identifiable details. Monash University Chinese Studies senior lecturer Kevin Carrico kindly translated Dr Wang's words. I have since verified the doctor's identity and place of work. His first-hand testimony of how the coronavirus emerged in Wuhan shows the extent of the cover-up – and the extreme frustration and utter helplessness of medical practitioners on the front line.

While the Chinese government insists the official date for the first Covid-19 case was in December, Dr Wang makes it clear doctors were dealing with the coronavirus from November. For there to have been community transmission in November, Covid-19 likely emerged earlier, in October or potentially September.

Internal Chinese government documents also challenge the official timeline. The *South China Morning Post* reported in March 2020 that government data indicated the first known patient was a 55-year-old from Hubei province who fell ill on November 17, 2019.

China's Centre for Disease Control director, George Fu Gao, would not confirm this report, saying in an email interview with *Science* in March 2020: "There is no solid evidence to say we already had clusters in November. We are trying to better understand the origin." The journalist who wrote the article, Josephine Ma, appeared on camera on Sky News Australia to reiterate her findings, but subsequently tried to retract the information and said she'd been misquoted.

Dr Ai Fen would later go temporarily missing as punishment for her effort in alerting the world to the coronavirus. She disappeared for at least two weeks. On April 13, 2020, Ai Fen emerged publicly for the first time, posting a 30-second video to her Weibo account of her standing outside the Central Hospital of Wuhan, saying, "I hope you can rest assured that everything is fine now. Thank you."

Dali Yang, a political scientist at the University of Chicago, told Associated Press of the punishment of doctors: "It was truly intimidation of an entire profession. Doctors in Wuhan were afraid."

The true number of whistleblowers who were detained or have simply vanished may never be known. They are each brave souls who chose to risk their life to expose the truth about the pandemic that was being covered up by the Chinese government. One of those is young lawyer Chen Qiushi.

January 2020, Washington DC

A Chinese delegation arrived on US soil on January 14, 2020 to sign a historic trade deal with President Donald Trump. You can only read Trump's remarks from that day with wide-eyed incredulity, given what China was secretly covering up back home.

The formal ceremony for the signing of the trade deal was held on January 15 in the East Room – the largest room in the Executive Residence of the White House, a room of grandeur with gold draping curtains, candelabras and life-sized portraits. Against a backdrop of the American and Chinese flags, with trumpets marking the occasion, Trump, in a blue tie, heralded the signing as "a very important and remarkable occasion" and said it was a momentous step towards a future of "fair and reciprocal trade".

"It just doesn't get any bigger than this, not only in terms of a deal but really in terms of what it represents. Keeping these two giant and powerful nations together in harmony is so important for the world, not just for us but for the world," he said.

There had been incredibly tense moments in the lead-up to the deal, with shouting matches between Trump's then Acting Chief of Staff Mick Mulvaney, Trade Advisor Peter Navarro and the Chinese advisors behind the scenes. In the end, the deal included 88 joint agreements, 105 commitments from China and five from the US. China agreed to purchase a further US$200 billion of US goods over two years, along with various reforms to intellectual property protections, technology and the financial sector. The deal put an end to 18 months of trade conflict after Trump made China's unfair trade deals a central election issue.

Standing at the podium beside Vice Premier Liu He, Trump called Xi Jinping "a very, very good friend" and said China was an "incredible, incredible" nation. Vice Premier Liu read a letter from President Xi – whose absence should have raised suspicions about what was unfolding in China – which said the signing of the deal meant "our two countries have the ability to act on the basis of equality and mutual respect and work through dialogue and consultation to properly handle and effectively resolve relevant issues".

In the crowd, smiling away and applauding, was former Australian Prime Minister Kevin Rudd, a fierce Trump critic, who had been invited by the White House in his capacity as President of the Asia Society Policy Institute.

Trump's National Security Advisor, Robert O'Brien, confirmed that neither side mentioned the coronavirus during the entire two-day visit. "If the Chinese knew more about the virus, they certainly weren't letting on," he said. "They weren't raising the issue with us. They weren't coming into the White House and telling us that this is a real serious pandemic that's coming down the line. It was all about the trade deal. Covid just wasn't the focus of that visit. No one was wearing a mask." Had health officials been at the ceremony, O'Brien said, questions might have been asked, but it was a "hardcore economic trade group". "It was just really early on," he recalls. "Within 30 days, it would have been a very different environment but at the time the crisis wasn't on their agenda or our agenda for that matter."

At a lunch after the signing, Trump said the relationship with China was "the best it's ever been" and Vice Premier Liu said the deal was "conducive to world peace and prosperity". Little did the Americans know the deal would be worthless just months later, as China threatened to withhold medical equipment and other vital supplies from the United States while slapping gigantic tariffs on US allies, such as Australia. And by May, there were reports in the Chinese state media that Beijing wanted to annul the agreement or renegotiate it, which Trump firmly rejected, saying: "I'm not interested. We signed a deal."

At the signing, Vice President Mike Pence quoted a Chinese proverb: "Men see only the present but heaven sees the future, so let today be the beginning of a brighter future." Bizarrely, it was the same proverb Pence used at a 2018 conference when referencing allegations of Chinese interference in US elections and calling out their poor record on human rights. Perhaps he only knows a couple of Chinese proverbs – or perhaps he suspected something was amiss.

Two days later, the CDC started screening passengers arriving from Wuhan at San Francisco, New York and Los Angeles airports, checking their temperature. The move was based on advice from the NSC. At the time, there were multiple pressing issues on the administration's agenda demanding President Trump's focus. Top of the list was his upcoming impeachment trial, set to begin the following Tuesday. Trump had just unveiled his legal team of eight, led by Harvard law professor Alan Dershowitz and Florida Attorney-General Pam Bondi. It was major, front-page news.

Lev Parnas, a close associate of Trump's lawyer Rudy Giuliani, had gone on television claiming Trump knew about efforts to pressure Ukraine into investigating Joe Biden's son. Damning documents released overnight were said to include evidence obtained by the FBI alleging that Trump had previously met with Parnas. Television breakfast shows across America splashed new photographs of Trump and Parnas. Also making news that day were thousands taking part in the fourth annual Women's March coinciding with the third anniversary of Trump's inauguration. A coast-to-coast storm was causing havoc, while the Royal Family announced Harry and Meghan were stepping aside from royal duties. The coronavirus was not a story that was anywhere near the top of most news bulletins.

Escaping from the pressure and chill of Washington, the President repeatedly fist-pumped the air as he arrived in West Palm Beach, Florida, that weekend, alongside his wife, Melania, and their son. On January 18, he was enjoying the balmy 26 degrees Celsius (79 degrees Fahrenheit) at his upmarket, exclusive golf resort, Mar-a-Lago when Health Secretary Alex Azar asked to speak to him about the coronavirus. Cases were spiking in China and Azar wanted to make sure the President understood the potential threat.

Trump and Mulvaney were understood to be on the golf course when Azar rang around 11am and it was close to dinner before the President returned his call.

Not realising why Azar had phoned him, Trump launched into a diatribe about how the Health Secretary had been wrong to get him to ban flavoured e-cigarettes. They then had a back and forth about replacing Obamacare. Trump felt the call was finished and was about to hang up when Azar interrupted, "Hold on, Mr President, I have to tell you about this new virus that's a real problem in China."

Azar told him about prior SARS and MERS outbreaks and why this was a significant issue. Only a few months earlier, Azar had briefed Trump on pandemic flus and explained how China is a mixing bowl for new virus strains, so Trump already had some understanding of what they were dealing with. Azar told Trump they had begun screening passengers from Wuhan the previous day and said the US was on alert and had stood up its CDC incident management centre. He also said there were no known cases in America, to the best of his knowledge.

"We have new viruses in China all the time and new strains of flu that are potentially a pandemic all the time," Azar told him, but the tone of Azar's call was that this was a potentially serious issue and he was briefing Trump on a weekend for a reason. "We're on alert as this could be serious. I don't want you to be surprised if someone asks you about this in the media."

The President listened and took it all in but did not ask any questions. The call lasted between 8 to 10 minutes.

Azar then put in a call to Robert O'Brien, a UC Berkeley School of Law graduate and founding partner at a boutique law firm, who had joined the Trump administration in 2017 and served as the Special Presidential Envoy for Hostage Affairs from 2018. When Trump demanded John Bolton's resignation, O'Brien was promoted as the President's fourth and final National Security Advisor.

In an interview for this book, O'Brien said that, in early to mid January 2020, there was no sense the coronavirus was going to be a major global issue. "It was being monitored as a potential public health issue. It seemed like it was more of a regional issue and we were keeping our eye on it," he said. "We weren't getting a lot from China and we weren't getting much from the WHO either. The WHO was, as it turns out, the instrumentality of the Chinese Communist Party, in our view, and were simply a mouthpiece for whatever China was saying. There was no independence whatsoever."

The first confirmed case to be reported in the United States came a few days later, on January 21. A 35-year-old man from Washington state had returned from visiting his family in Wuhan on January 15. Although he had not been to the seafood market and had no known contact with anyone who was unwell during his trip, when he developed a cough and fever for four days after his trip, he went to an urgent care clinic in Snohomish County, Washington, on January 19.

He wore a mask while he sat in the waiting room and, after 20 minutes, was taken into a doctor's private examination room.

Based on the man's travel history, the doctor took a nasal swab and sent it off for testing. Two days later, the results confirmed it was the new coronavirus.

The CDC press release issued that day stated: "While originally thought to be spreading from animal-to-person, there are growing indications that limited person-to-person spread is happening. It's unclear how easily this virus is spreading between people." The release went on to urge calm, saying there was no reason for the American public to be worried. "The confirmation that some limited person-to-person spread with this virus is occurring in Asia raises the level of concern about this virus, but CDC continues to believe the risk of 2019-nCoV to the American public at large remains low at this time." Of course, the reality was that the virus had likely spread throughout America by this point – this was simply the first laboratory-confirmed case.

In Australia, the first recorded case came three days later, January 24, at Monash Medical Centre in Melbourne. At 9.30am, a man in his late 50s arrived in the emergency department struggling to breathe, with flu-like symptoms. On-call doctors would have dismissed the case, except the man said he had recently returned from Wuhan. Professor Rhonda Stuart told *The Australian* newspaper they tested him for coronavirus, with a positive result arriving the next day.

Retired travel agent James Kwan, aged 78, who contracted the virus on the *Diamond Princess* cruise ship in Japan, was the first Australian to pass away from the virus, on March 1. Australian Health Minister Greg Hunt issued a statement that day assuring the public that "the WHO is working with Chinese authorities to learn more about the virus, such as its origins, incubation period and severity, which ranges from very mild to severe".

One week after the first confirmed case in Australia, the UK announced a university student and his parents, who had flown in from Hubei province, had tested positive. The 23-year-old student's mother started developing symptoms a few days after arriving in York, west of Manchester. That very day, a Boeing 747 chartered rescue flight arrived near London carrying 83 British passengers who had been evacuated from the by-now locked-down city of Wuhan. An unprecedented national health crisis had just hit the UK.

After his weekend at Mar-a-Lago, Trump flew to Davos, Switzerland, for the World Economic Forum, taking off from Andrews Air Force Base at 6.30pm on Monday night. On this trip, President Trump spoke about the virus publicly for the first time. His remarks came when he sat down for a one-on-one interview with CNBC journalist Joe Kernen on January 22.

Kernen asked him at the start of the 20-minute sit-down about the case of coronavirus identified by the CDC in the US. "Are there any worries about a pandemic at this point?" Kernen wanted to know.

Trump replied: "No. Not at all. And we have it totally under control. It's one person coming in from China, and we have it under control. It's going to be just fine."

Kernen followed up with a question about the transparency of Chinese President Xi Jinping. "Do you trust that we're going to know everything we need to know?"

Trump said he completely trusted the Chinese President to be transparent. "I do, I do, I have a great relationship with President Xi. We've just signed probably the biggest deal ever made. I do, I think the relationship is very good."

Azar was pissed off at how the President downplayed the threat and praised China during the media interview. On Air Force One on the flight home from Davos, O'Brien took a call from the Health Secretary. "Robert, this is serious, he can't say it's under control. That's a term of art in public health and it isn't accurate," Azar said. "The President can't keep saying what he said on CNBC.

"We're devoting some more resources to it," he added. "We are taking steps to try to control this, we're doing health screenings."

When he got off the phone, O'Brien went to see the President during the flight. He told him they were monitoring the situation but were not getting any cooperation from the Chinese government. O'Brien says no one had a "good feel for it" at that point.

Back at the White House, on January 24, Azar briefed the President in the Oval Office on the escalating situation.

"How is China doing?" Trump asked.

"It seems pretty bad over there," Azar replied.

"Are they being transparent?" the President wanted to know.

"Well, they're being more transparent than they were with SARS, but that's a very low bar, and with China you just don't know what you don't know," Azar said.

"I need to get the CDC in there on the ground to help them," Azar went on, "I've offered that. I need samples from China because we've got to do the infectious-disease tracing to figure out how this came about – what the origin is – and we need to get the original generation-one samples that they aren't sharing."

Trump said, "Well I'm going to tweet a statement that praises them for being transparent" as he called in his aid, Dan Scavino Jr, who wrote the first drafts of many of his official tweets.

Azar said, "Please don't do that," to no avail as Trump began to dictate to Scavino.

For some official tweets during the day, Trump would have Scavino write the tweet down and bring it back into the Oval Office printed and blown-up in gigantic letters so the President could see any errors clearly. He'd make edits with a black sharpie and then say to Dan, "Let it rip."

Azar implored Trump not to send the tweet. "If you give any praise to President Xi that's a big win for him domestically," he said. "He's in trouble domestically because he's clearly mismanaged this. There's turmoil in China and if you pat him on the back and praise him, that's validation, so please don't do that."

Azar felt Trump was quite set in what he wanted to do and continued on with Scavino. Frustrated, Azar walked out of the Oval Office in the middle of their meeting and strode across the lobby to O'Brien's office.

"Robert, the President is about to send this tweet … We really can't have him giving praise to China because we don't know what we don't know with China. We've got to stop him, and I'm not able to stop him," he said.

O'Brien went into the Oval Office and Pompeo was due to arrive in the West Wing shortly. Azar hoped the pair would be able to talk Trump down from praising China publicly, assuming that if Trump didn't value advice on China from his Health Secretary, he might listen to his National Security Advisor and the Secretary of State.

But Trump went on to send the tweet on January 24, assuring the public that China was cooperating with the United States: "China has been working very hard to contain the Coronavirus. The United States greatly appreciates their efforts and transparency. It will all work out well. In particular, on behalf of the American People, I want to thank President Xi!"

At the time, the media spotlight was entirely on the US Senate for Trump's impeachment trial. That same day, Mulvancy organised an hour-long coronavirus briefing – the very first for congressional members – at 10.30am. It was held in the Health, Education, Labor and Pensions Committee hearing room. "The novel coronavirus is an emerging public health threat. Senators will have the opportunity to hear directly from senior government health officials regarding what we know about this virus so far, and how our country is prepared to respond as the situation develops," Senate Health Committee Chairman Lamar Alexander and Democrat Patty Murray said in a joint statement the day before the hearing.

Mulvaney took Azar, Redfield from the CDC, Anthony Fauci from the Infectious Disease Operation at the National Institutes of Health and a couple of other sub-cabinet members to brief America's politicians. Fauci spoke to reporters before the meeting, extraordinarily telling them he believed China was acting in a more transparent manner than in previous outbreaks. He said he could not see the United States shutting down major cities, even though it was 45 hours after Wuhan had gone into lockdown.

Hardly anyone showed up to the briefing. "It was notoriously poorly attended. I mean, there's 100 senators and only five show up," Mulvaney said. Only a handful of journalists arrived to hear

Azar's briefing for the media on the coronavirus and, according to Mulvaney, "none of the big names were there. They were all on impeachment. So it was hard to get anybody to pay attention to it outside of the White House."

The New Yorker later reported that the health authorities were reassuring and that Redfield told the small group gathered: "We are prepared for this." Nothing could have been further from the truth.

This confidence from Fauci and Redfield was unusual given the day before, January 23, China had announced a lockdown of Wuhan. Why would China be nailing people into their homes for a virus that was not infectious? This should have raised alarm bells about the lack of transparency from China. Instead, the top medical officials in the Trump administration seemed blindsided by Xi's lies and cover-up over the disaster unfolding inside China.

With the repeated public assurances from the CDC, Fauci and Trump, people all over the world were misled into believing there was no impending threat to their health or livelihoods.

CHAPTER FIVE

Chinese New Year

January 25, 2020, Washington DC

The rhythmic notes of Canadian pianist Glenn Gould's rendition of Bach were playing in Dimon's home on January 25, 2020 as guests began to filter through her door for her annual Chinese New Year soiree. For the best part of 30 years, Dimon had thrown an annual Chinese New Year party. There was always a jovial atmosphere, as people who don't usually socialise would come together: spies from different agencies and countries, government officials, journalists and dissidents all mingled, finding corners for quiet conversations. At the largest one, she'd had 140 guests; her house was heaving and it took weeks to return to normal post celebration. Chinese Lunar New Year in January 2020 would prove to be an auspicious day. It was the day two influential figures in the Trump administration would make startling discoveries relating to the pandemic that was about to sweep the globe: Mike Pompeo's China advisor Miles Yu and Trump's Deputy National Security Advisor Matt Pottinger.

Dimon was soon to be 70, and preparing food for more than 100 people took a toll behind the scenes. She personally cooked 32 dishes over three days. Kale with tea-smoked bacon, sautéed pork with dried bean curd, sesame chicken, edamame with xuelihong, shrimp wontons, salt and pepper shrimp and Chinese-Russian oxtail stew. And for dessert, tangerine pie, chocolate-covered strawberries, lemon pie, and cold-pressed apple, date and apricot cake with honey. Her tables groaned with mouth-watering plates of food, as her guests ate and mingled throughout the downstairs rooms of her house.

Dimon lives in a red-brick townhouse originally built in 1882, that she renovated to ensure the rooms flow into each other, using her architectural skill to create a space perfectly suited to socialising. When she moved to Washington DC in 1995, people told her to buy in Georgetown, but the homes were twice the price of those in Capitol Hill and there was no parking. South East Capitol Hill was dangerous back then. Now, it's gentrified. The back room of her townhouse opens out into the garden, but in the chill of January, no one dared go outside.

Dimon's home is adorned with beautiful, unique artefacts from her travels: Chinese calligraphy on one wall; a large, ornate wall-hanging from an ancestral hall on another; a portrait of her by a famous artist in return for paying his rent; antique peasant bowls from a couple of hundred years ago that Dimon literally, on her hands and knees, dug up from the abandoned Islands of Hong Kong.

Her New Year's party was important this year. It was where she would make sure Matt Pottinger heard first-hand from famous Chinese dissident Wei Jingsheng the true state of the virus in Wuhan. And not just the virus, but the virology laboratories and China's classified research program all the chilling information she had been carrying around like a heavy burden for weeks. The pair *had* to speak that night. She would make sure of it.

As she poured drinks and chatted to her guests, Dimon kept glancing at the door to see whether Pottinger had arrived. Naturally, most of her 100 guests had all walked in before he did. It was close to 9pm when Pottinger finally appeared. Dimon immediately took him by the arm and led him through to the back room, where Wei was holding court standing beside the sofa. She left the pair of them to speak, surrounded by other dissidents holding plates of food and eating.

Luckily, Pottinger's spoken Chinese is very good from his time in Beijing where he worked as a journalist. So much so that he would go on to give an entire speech in Mandarin months later, in May – a speech written with the help of Miles Yu, Pompeo's advisor.

And so, standing there in Dimon's Washington home on Lunar New Year, Pottinger heard first-hand from Wei – who came from one of the Communist Party's founding families – about the contagion and how it was spreading throughout China. It was eye-opening, a revelation. The conversation would change the course of history.

Pottinger knew he had to warn the President. And fast. "I will never forget that dinner," he said to Dimon afterwards. It was a crucial turning point in how the White House would investigate and understand the nature of the outbreak.

In any other year, Miles Yu would have been at Dimon Liu's place all night for Chinese New Year. The principal China policy advisor to US Secretary of State Mike Pompeo had begun life, like Dimon, in rural China, in the Sichuan province, under the communism, cruelty and famine of Mao Zedong's Cultural Revolution. Outspoken and passionate, Yu was a regular at Dimon's parties over the years.

She lauds his book *OSS in China: Prelude to Cold War* on the intelligence activities of the Office of Strategic Services in China during World War II, for which he relied upon formerly classified material from the US National Archives. "He didn't pull any punches," she says. "I bought 20 copies to give to all my friends. He's a very good writer."

But on January 25, 2020, Yu was swamped with work for Pompeo and could only pop in briefly to Dimon's party. While others were preparing for a glass or two of bubbles that night, Yu, then 57, was in his office in the State Department in front of his two computers – one strictly for classified documents.

Yu looked up at the Chinese-published world map on his wall. It was no ordinary map of the world. This map had China at the centre. The very word China, or Zhongguo, is comprised of the Chinese characters for "middle" and "country". The Middle Kingdom.

Chinese philosophy since at least 1000 BCE holds that their empire is at the centre of the earth, and many maps in Chinese classrooms still place China in that position. This giant map hung on Yu's wall to remind him on a daily basis of the nature of the tyranny he was facing. It was the first thing anyone noticed when they walked in. He liked it that way. It separated him from the 1600 other employees.

Yu had joined the ranks of the State Department on the Policy Planning team in late 2018. The unit occupies a powerful place on the seventh floor of the State Department headquarters in Washington. For 26 years, Yu had been a professor of modern China and military history at the United States Naval Academy in Annapolis, Maryland. At the State Department, he was the only native Chinese-speaker with a devoted academic focus on the CCP, who could read, absorb and analyse documents very quickly. His unique skills would frustrate him at times, as he was overwhelmed with demands from senior figures across the US government for advice and translation requests.

Yu's story is remarkable. Born in 1962, he moved to the United States in 1985 as a student, where he won awards for excellence at Pennsylvania and California universities. He says his move to the US was prompted by his admiration for President Ronald Reagan, whose speeches he listened to in secret via the Chinese service Voice of America.

"Although I was too young to fully experience the political madness, my childhood innocence was brutally upended by the radical revolution's violence, absurdity, ideological shriek, destruction of life, social trust and public mores, and utter hatred for anything Western or 'bourgeois'," Yu said in a profile piece for *The Washington Times*, for which he wrote a column called "Inside China" over several years. "Having grown up in communist China and now living my American dream, I think the world should be incalculably grateful to America, because, as Reagan said, America represents 'the last best hope of man on Earth.' And I truly believe that."

In the US, Yu supported the pro-democracy protests that led to the Tiananmen Square massacre, and helped refugees from Tiananmen settle in San Francisco. He gave a voice to Chinese dissidents by hosting a lecture series called the China Forum. Yu doesn't like to speak about it, and changes the subject when you ask him, but I'm told his suffering at the hands of the CCP was immense. His fight against the Communist Party is deeply personal. Back in his country of birth, Yu was dubbed a "traitor of the Han race" by Chinese government mouthpiece the *Global Times* for the work he did for Pompeo.

Yu came to Pompeo's attention very quickly; his perspective grew to be influential and was embraced by the Secretary. The pair often enjoyed one-on-one conversations about the best US policy approach to the CCP, and Yu had accompanied Pompeo to foreign international meets, such as the Quad in Tokyo.

In *The Washington Times* profile piece, Pompeo said his chief China advisor was "a central part of my team advising me with respect [to] how to ensure that we protect Americans and secure our freedoms in the face of challenges from the CCP." Former Assistant Secretary of State for East Asia and Pacific Affairs David Stilwell also contributed to the piece, describing Yu as a "national treasure [who] understands the difference between democratic and authoritarian governance and can explain it better than anyone I know."

On joining the State Department, Yu made his presence felt by holding a China policy boot camp for senior officials with China-related portfolios. He was also given final clearance power for all memos to Pompeo relating to the Asia-Pacific, acting as a gatekeeper. His growing influence sparked internal jealousy and met with some bureaucratic resistance. While his analytical and policy notes could go directly to Pompeo through legitimate Policy Planning channels without anyone's approval, at times his memos for specific action recommendations were unusually slow to make it to the Secretary. On a couple of occasions, they were even blocked in the chain of command. Yu developed an ally in Pompeo's right-hand woman, Senior Policy Advisor Mary Kissel, who ensured his papers made it directly onto the Secretary's desk.

In a policy sense, Yu's biggest gripe is the misunderstanding in the United States of the true nature of the CCP and President

Xi Jinping. "We have unwillingly succumbed to the CCP's often blistering bluffs," Yu said in 2020. "For decades, our China policy was carried out based upon an 'anger management' mode – that is, we formulated our China policy by calculating how mad the CCP might be at us, not what suits the best to American national interest."

On January 25, in those very early days of the pandemic, when Yu glanced up at his map, it reminded him the CCP would always put its own interests first – over and above any commitments to international health obligations. It's like Pompeo had always reminded him. "The best way to deal with the Chinese Communist Party is distrust and verify. You have to have a suspicious mind first, don't trust them in the first place, and then you try to prove yourself wrong," Pompeo had told him. "This was Pompeo's policy and we all follow him," Yu said.

Pompeo's phrase is clearly an appropriation of President Ronald Raegan's attitude to dealing with the Soviet Union towards the end of the Cold War. It was an approach Pompeo would articulate in public six months later when he gave a hard-hitting speech at the Richard Nixon Presidential Library that excoriated America's "blind engagement" with China.

Yu sat at his desk and thought about the widespread Chinese social media chatter on this new coronavirus while the CCP had kept quiet. He thought about a report he'd read on Chinese media that mentioned every institute and hospital involved in the handling of the virus but strangely omitted the Wuhan Institute of Virology. Knowing how the Communist Party operates, this was suspicious, Yu felt. It set off alarm bells. Turning to his unclassified computer, Yu typed into Google "Wuhan Institute of Virology" and started reading through its entire website. He voraciously devoured its coronavirus research projects, noted its extensive international cooperation, absorbed the staff lists and the official announcements, copying the pages and taking screenshots as he went.

Yu realised the gravity of what he was reading – the world's premiere coronavirus laboratory was in the same city as the outbreak of a novel coronavirus – and he knew instinctively what it could mean. The very city where the outbreak began is home to a Biosafety Level 4 (BSL-4) virology laboratory genetically manipulating coronaviruses in a dangerous way. Yu found the Wuhan Institute of Virology was one of only two BSL-4 laboratories in China. The second is the Harbin Institute of Veterinary Research, where work on animal viruses is conducted.

Alarmed by what he was reading, Yu saved essential pages from the Wuhan Institute of Virology's website. When he opened those same links just a few weeks later, they had all been wiped. Deleted.

Yu whipped up a report with his findings, which included the discovery of a collection of virus-carrying bats by Chinese scientists in Wuhan, and emailed it to the National Security Agency (NSA) and Pottinger at the NSC, who was, generally speaking, on the same page when it came to China policy. Little did he know Pottinger was, at close to that very moment, obtaining equally alarming information from dissidents in Washington.

The next day Yu told Pompeo what he'd found. "I don't want you to make any public statement yet about any possible connection between the Wuhan Institute of Virology and the virus but I'm very suspicious," Yu said. Pompeo took the matter seriously and asked Yu to keep him informed of any new developments. "Keep an eye on this for me, Miles," he said.

Over the coming days, Yu continued his research at an intense pace. He investigated Shi Zhengli, the Wuhan Institute of Virology scientist who would become known as "bat-woman", and a second coronavirus facility near the wet market. He found that the Chinese Academy of Social Sciences claimed in the past 12 years to have discovered 2000 viruses known to mankind, while it had taken the past 200 years for the rest of the world to discover that many.

Aside from Pompeo, Yu was disappointed by the reaction to his crucial discoveries inside the State Department and in other agencies. Some were incredulous at his claim the Wuhan laboratories could be linked to the outbreak. He felt that no serious action was taking place to investigate a potential link. "It was very frustrating to me that I sent the documents out and had no reaction back from the NSC," Yu says. "Nobody knew what the Wuhan Institute of Virology was."

Yu suggested to Pompeo, "Before our principals can make any public statement, I would like the NSC to compel the intelligence community to verify this." Pompeo agreed with him and asked the intelligence agencies to corroborate the information Yu had uncovered.

Pompeo also asked Yu to compile a document on whether there was enough circumstantial evidence that the virus may have emerged from a Wuhan laboratory, in order to launch an official investigation. Yu set to work, night and day, investigating the laboratories, China's bioweapons programs and the early whistleblowers, and scouring Chinese-language news sites.

"This was a time when everyone was busy responding to the Covid outbreak," Yu recalls. "Very few people were looking at the reason for the outbreak, let alone to establish the culpability of the CCP on this. I knew we had to find out the origin of this, we had to find out who is responsible for the spread of this virus. The overarching point was, we have to find out if China is responsible enough to keep bio-research safe."

It would be a several-months-long effort that Yu would finally present to Pompeo in April, with a long list of strong circumstantial evidence against the Wuhan Institute of Virology and an emphasis on the Chinese lab's substandard and negligent biosafety practices.

And so it was that Miles Yu became the first person in the United States government to sound the alarm on the Wuhan Institute of Virology. But the American public weren't to learn about the concerning laboratories in Wuhan just yet. It would be another two months before any senior figure in the Trump administration publicly confirmed a suspicion that the coronavirus had originated in the Wuhan Institute of Virology. It would be decried as a conspiracy theory.

CHAPTER SIX

The Last Train to Wuhan

JANUARY 24, 2020: WUHAN

It is a very different Chinese New Year across the other side of the world for young lawyer Chen Qiushi. Standing outside Wuhan station, it's six degrees Celsius (43 degrees Fahrenheit), light rain is falling and Qiushi shakes in the 10pm chill. His adrenaline is pumping. Wearing his leather jacket and grey skivvy, the handsome lawyer speaks fast and passionately. He knows the gravity of the risk he is taking, but he feels compelled. It is his duty.

The 34-year-old has just caught the train from Beijing, where he works and lives, leaving at 3.20pm for the five and a half hour trip. It is the last train into Wuhan. When he boards, the train driver warns him the service will be suspended for at least the next month and he'll be hard placed to find accommodation. Roads into the city are blocked; flights are cancelled indefinitely. A citywide lockdown is in place. There is no transport out of Wuhan; no exit route.

"I don't expect to leave Wuhan in the next month," Qiushi tells the driver.

When he arrives that night, on January 24, he is nervous about what he is getting himself into. Qiushi didn't dare tell his parents he was headed to Wuhan, at the centre of a terrifying outbreak. He was aware Chinese authorities were watching him. His WeChat account had been permanently closed a month before, on Christmas Eve, as a result of his reporting on the Hong Kong protests back in August 2019. On the front line of the protests, filming with his phone, he had suffered burns to his skin and been immersed in teargas.

Qiushi was banned from flying to Japan in December. He'd organised a trip for 40 friends and family and had looked forward to taking his mother, a primary school teacher, outside of China for the first time in her life. But as he was about to fly out, on December 10, 2019, Qiushi took a phone call from police summoning him to the station and advising him he was not permitted to leave the country. He farewelled friends and family at the airport, with police watching him closely to ensure he did not board the plane. Qiushi later wrote on Twitter that he knew this wasn't a legal issue – it was a political one.

Living under police surveillance, Qiushi's courage was admirable. His public commentary saw him come under pressure at his law firm and his contract was not renewed on December 31, 2019. But he wouldn't be silenced. On social media he called for a boycott of Huawei after an employee was locked up for 18 months.

It is with his freedoms and liberties curtailed, even his livelihood taken away from him, that Qiushi makes his way to Wuhan amid the coronavirus outbreak. As he crosses the road outside Wuhan's Hankou train station, there is not another soul on the street. Normally, in a city of 11 million people at one of the three main stations, on Chinese New Year's Eve of all nights, there is celebration, excitement, colour, music, food, lights, happiness and good fortune.

Across other parts of China, families and friends are starting to celebrate at parties and on the streets. But Qiushi is entering a city no one wants to be in. A dead zone. Empty streets, people dying, too many bodies, hospitals overcrowded. A city in fear.

"Why do I come here?" he asks, staring directly down the camera. "My duty is a reporter for citizens. As a reporter, if you don't dare to come to the front line at the first moment when there is a catastrophe, how can you be called a real reporter? Therefore I took the last high-speed train to Wuhan."

The day before Qiushi arrives, Wuhan went into a brutal lockdown. Residents were ordered to shut their windows while cleaners in hazmat suits disinfected the streets. Videos spread on social media of Chinese police boarding up apartments, nailing wooden slats across the doors to permanently lock residents inside. Qiushi tweets this is "illegal detention".

It is estimated that up to 300,000 people fled the city by train in the hours before the lockdown began. Qiushi is diving headfirst into the heart of the pandemic that would later paralyse the world. There is no word to describe his actions other than brave.

"If, unfortunately, I become infected, I will accept my fate," he says into the camera. "I'd rather die in the city than flee from Wuhan." He rails against Chinese President Xi Jinping for not travelling to Wuhan and says the truth about the virus must be told. "The current outbreak is comparable to the SARS outbreak in 2003," he says. "In the two outbreaks, it is the cover-up of the truth and the block of the information that leads to both of the outbreaks. We cannot make the same mistakes over and over again. At least we can [and should] allow the news and information [about the coronavirus outbreak] to be spoken out and spread. If we spread the news and information faster than the virus does, then we can win this war."

His video has now been viewed more than 1.5 million times.

Despite the late hour, a determined Qiushi starts work straight away, reasoning that doctors would have more time at night to speak. As he arrives at Wuhan Central Hospital's fever clinic, an ambulance pulls up at the emergency entrance, its lights flashing. Masks and protective equipment are strewn across the footpath. Qiushi puts on a mask, gloves and white swimming goggles as he walks into the hospital's waiting room. Even in the waiting room, people are sitting with IV drips attached to their arms. There is vomit on the ground, and it remains there for an hour and a half. No one notices him filming – they are all too busy dealing with the influx of sick patients. He uploads a video of his visit in the early hours of the morning.

At 5am, Qiushi emerges from Wuhan Central Hospital into the darkness before dawn. He has nowhere to stay. Kindly, many locals had sent him messages saying he'd be more than welcome to sleep at their homes, but he wisely does not take them up on the offer, not wanting to risk spreading infection. Others offered to send him money but he asked for their donations to go towards the pandemic. The Chinese government has banned hotels from accepting reservations, but a small hotel relents and lets him stay the night. He's the only guest and he isn't safe there for more than one or two nights.

His next visit is to the severely overcrowded Eleventh Hospital, full of the new form of pneumonia. Qiushi reports hearing people yelling they are out of medicine, while bodies lie on stretchers. He finds it hard to tell who is alive and who has already died. "Initially I thought it was someone lying there receiving intravenous injection," he says of one body. "Then I looked from the other side. I realised that the patient's face was covered by white cloth, without breath. That must be a corpse."

A nurse tells Qiushi that just a few days ago "the entire hallway was stuffed with patients". "Couldn't even move," he quotes her as saying. "Must have been more than a thousand people. We were so nervous then. That was great pressure. We were crying all the time during those days."

"The government is doing nothing," the nurse laments.

Later that day, Qiushi's parents realise he is in Wuhan and send him a video message expressing their grave concerns for his safety. "We were not prepared mentally and psychologically," his father speaks from a couch, with his mother closely watching on. "Why didn't you tell us ahead of time? We worry about your safety."

They seem to understand his mission and his drive. "You should help the Wuhan people, do your best, you should report objective and fair news ... Protect yourself," Qiushi's mother pleads. "We say three times when something is important. Safety! Safety! Safety! We wait for you."

With these encouraging words from his parents ringing in his ears, Qiushi heads out again into Wuhan, visiting the Huanan

Seafood Market, which had been closed since January 1. "New equipment," he tweets alongside a photo of himself wearing blue reflective swimming goggles and a white mask. The market's large iron gates are shut. There are no signs of life in the narrow lanes where live and dead animals would usually be bought from 1000 stalls. "It's ghostly inside, suitable for a horror scene," he describes. A security guard walking past laughs as Qiushi comments on how the dead could be coming back to haunt the market.

As the days roll on, Qiushi becomes aware the authorities are onto him. He visits hospitals and speaks to doctors and nurses. He even helps deliver 30,000 masks to the Huoshenshan Hospital.

In what will be one of his last videos, an emotional Qiushi sits on a bed in a small hotel room, with ruffled hair, wearing just a singlet with the sunlight streaming in and stares down the Communist Party. The authorities have made several calls, asking why he is in Wuhan – they want to know where he is staying. "I am scared," he says. "I have the virus in front of me. Behind me is China's law enforcement. If I am still alive in this city, I will continue my report." Fighting back tears, his fist clenched with one finger pointing at the camera, he says: "Fuck you, I'm not even scared of death. You think I'm scared of you, Chinese Communist Party?"

Less than a week later, Qiushi disappears. He had told friends and family he planned to visit Fangcang shelter hospital, one of the large-scale makeshift hospitals. But they don't hear from him again. The next day, his mother makes a desperate appeal to Wuhan citizens to help find her son. "From around 7 or 8pm this evening until now, 2am, in the morning, Qiushi has been out of contact," she says in a recorded video. "I am here to urge all netizens, especially netizens in Wuhan, to do me a favour and help find Qiushi. Please help, thank you," she pleads.

One Wuhan supporter who watches this video tracks down Qiushi's hotel room and knocks on the door. Silence. No one is there. Millions of people who viewed Qiushi and his mum's videos wonder what fate has met him. Where is he now? Is he dead or alive?

FEBRUARY 2020

Chinese journalist Li Zehua had closely watched Qiushi's video reports from Wuhan. The 25-year-old had worked at China's state television as an on-air host. But when he sees Qiushi has gone missing, Zehua speaks to his producer, quits his job and plans to follow the young lawyer into Wuhan to investigate what was going on. Zehua does not intend to go in alone, but his friend's parents discover their plans and lock Zehua's friend at home.

Zehua sneaks into Wuhan by buying a train ticket to the stop after the city but persuades the conductor to let him off early. He checks into the hotel next to the where Qiushi was staying, but he can only stay one night, with police warning the hotel owner they will search every room to ensure the premises is empty.

In a video, Zehua says he's more scared about filming in Wuhan than he was reporting from North Korea. Like Qiushi, he is determined to discover the truth about the coronavirus. "Now all the bad news about the epidemic has been collected by the central government. The local media can only report on good news," he says in a video posted on February 12. "They don't want us to know what we want to know."

Sitting on his bed wearing an LA Lakers jumper and a baseball cap, Li speaks to the camera. "This is why I'm here. I have to use my eyes and ears to catch information, and make the judgement."

With a Sony camera and GoPro rolling, Zehua sets out in Wuhan and speaks to locals, raising the prospect that authorities are covering up the real number of infections and deaths. He visits funeral homes and learns Wuhan morgues are so busy they are desperately trying to recruit more staff, cremating more bodies than the official death toll declared by the government. "When I left, the boiler in this funeral home seems to be still working. The boom is loud," he says of his 11pm visit.

But in a move that will seal his fate, Zehua decides to investigate the Wuhan Institute of Virology. He drives there in a two-door Volkswagen on February 26 and lingers outside. Unable to get in, he starts to drive away, but as he does a white unmarked SUV with plain-clothed officers inside signals for him to pull over. Instead of abiding by their demands, Zehua, petrified, speeds away and a car chase ensues. He starts filming the SUV chasing him. While driving he manages to post a 30-second "SOS" video to YouTube.

Visibly distressed, Zehua, shaking and speaking fast, says he is being pursued by a gang of men. "They are chasing me, help!" The police pull up alongside him on the opposite side of the road, but Zehua doesn't stop, putting his foot down on the accelerator, he somehow manages to get away.

Back in the temporary safety of his hotel room, Zehua streams live to YouTube – with the lights off. The footage is black. He is silent. Thousands of viewers watch this dramatic vlog live, their hearts in their mouths, anxiously praying for his safety but knowing this will not end well. Eventually, amid the blackness, there is loud banging on the hotel room door. *Bang, bang, bang.* They're trying to figure out if Zehua is in this particular hotel room. He is silent and the knocking continues.

"God, please bless him, he did nothing wrong," a person comments under his livestream as this unfolds.

"Keep silent," someone else says.

The authorities finally leave – only to return four hours after Zehua started his livestream. Four hours of terror. Forty minutes later, he realises he has no choice. There is no point in hiding. "There's no chance to run away, and this is not what I planned to do," he says. Presuming the worst, Li says this could be his "final speech". "It would be absolutely false if I say I'm not scared now. But what does it matter whether [I feel] fear or not? If they want to get me arrested they will do. Before coming here, I had expected that I would eventually end up like him [Chen Qiushi], but I didn't see it would come so fast."

The Chinese police tell Zehua to open the door, that there won't be any problems. Finally, he opens the door. Four police officers slowly walk in. Zehua is arrested and taken away. Another disappearance. Another cover-up. Another young life on the line.

Chen Qiushi and Li Zehua are sadly not alone. Many more would go missing amid their valiant attempts to alert the world to Beijing's cover-up of the deadly new virus crippling Wuhan.

Fang Bin was a businessman trading textiles in Wuhan. Like Qiushi, he felt compelled to tell the world what was happening in his own city. His first video report, dated January 25, is devastating and graphic. Its 41 minutes show bodies of coronavirus victims inside buses that have been converted into improvised hearses. Fang counts: "Five, six, seven, eight, eight bodies in five minutes. So many dead."

Wearing just a mask, he bravely ventures inside a hospital – into the overcrowded wards – and films coronavirus victims, doctors in full protective gear, family members crying. On February 2, he reports in a video that police have confiscated his laptop and he has been interrogated. Two days later, he reports in a live video from his Wuhan home that he is surrounded by police. The harassment and surveillance continue for days.

His last video lasts just 12 seconds – and it's hard not to cry when watching it. He shows a roll of paper where eight characters were calligraphed. They read: "Let all citizens resist! Power to the people!" Nothing has been heard of Fang since.

Civil rights activist and former Beijing University lecturer Xu Zhiyong, then 47, published an essay calling on Xi Jinping to resign for his failure to govern in early February. He said he was "clueless". "You didn't authorise the truth to be released and the outbreak turned into a national disaster," Xu wrote, "Please step down." While in hiding in the home of a friend of his, he was arrested and detained.

A similar fate met distinguished Professor Xu Zhangrun who, at 57 years old, published an essay called "Viral Alarm: When Fury Overcomes Fear" condemning Beijing's censorship of information and suppression of freedom of speech. After his essay was published, Xu disappeared, his WeChat account was suspended and his name wiped from Weibo. It later emerged that he was under house detention, with security agents on 24-hour guard around his house monitoring his movements and cutting off his internet access. In July 2020, he was released from custody but was later fired from his job at Tsinghua University.

Seventy-year-old real estate tycoon and political commentator Ren Zhiquiang, with an extraordinary 37 million followers on Weibo, disappeared after criticising Xi Jinping over his handling of the pandemic. He was then sentenced to 18 years in prison on charges of corruption, bribery and embezzlement after a single-day trial in September 2020.

Three youths, Cai Wei, 28, Chen Mei, 27, and Cai's girlfriend, Tang Hongbo, all disappeared in April and May 2020 after being caught saving information the CCP was wiping from the internet. Their families were belatedly told that they were under "residential surveillance" and would face a trial.

On April 19, Beijing police arrested Chen Mei and took him to an undisclosed location, only notifying his panicked mother by letter almost a month later. I spoke to Chen Mei's brother, Chen Kun, who was living outside China, shortly afterwards. He told me he feared his brother was being tortured and held in a secret location. "It has been months since he has been arrested but we still don't know where he is," he said. "I'm worried about my parents and security and my family, my wife, my daughter and me, our security."

Chen Kun told me his message to Western governments is: "Don't forget them. [The] more and more people know about them, the more and more people call on the Chinese government to release them."

Citizen journalist and lawyer Zhang Zhan, 37, was reportedly tortured for three months by police before being sentenced to four years' imprisonment for live-streaming from Wuhan. She is reported to have staged a hunger strike for seven months, with authorities handcuffing her arms and legs and keeping her alive by feeding her through a tube. She was charged with "picking quarrels and provoking trouble".

Chinese Human Rights Defenders documented 897 cases between January and April 2020 of people being punished for challenging "the official propaganda that President Xi Jinping handled the outbreak with transparency and expertise". Another organisation, Reporters Without Borders (RSF), has kept a careful record of those who have disappeared or been subjected to detention. They say China "is the biggest prison in the world for journalists, with at least 120 detained or missing according to the most recent count made by RSF".

CHAPTER SEVEN

The White House in Disarray

JANUARY 27, 2020: WASHINGTON DC

Pottinger didn't take the information he'd gleaned from Wei and the other dissidents he'd spoken to at Dimon Liu's New Year's soiree lightly. He knew the breadth of Wei's on-the-ground contacts, and knew it would be a mistake to dismiss this valuable human intelligence. "Wei and others who were there had shared their impressions from their conversations with people in China that the epidemic was much worse than was being reported and that it was in many more places than just in Wuhan, and that it was also a crisis in Beijing," Pottinger tells me.

After the party, acting out of instinct from his decades as a journalist, he hit the phones, contacting confidential sources from when he'd worked for *The Wall Street Journal* and covered the SARS outbreak in 2003. He confirmed what Wei had told him, and his body of on-the-ground human intelligence grew. He also spoke at length to his brother, Paul, who is an infectious disease specialist, and his wife, Dr Yen Pottinger, a virologist and former CDC official.

By the end of that Sunday, he knew he needed to raise the alarm inside the White House. From what he'd gleaned in just 24 hours, he was now acutely aware that the administration was not taking this seriously enough. Back at work on the Monday, he called a Deputies

Committee meeting for the following day, Tuesday the 28th. He invited several cabinet secretaries and agency heads to attend. It was, perhaps, slightly presumptuous given he was a Deputy National Security Advisor and principals usually only attended meetings chaired by the National Security Advisor, but it was done with his boss Robert O'Brien's approval and support. "Matt worked for me as my deputy. He was starting to get information out of the region from Taiwan, from China and from Hong Kong. The sources were doctors who were saying this virus is a real problem and it's going to be worse than SARS," O'Brien says.

Pottinger asked O'Brien's assent to invite several public health officials. The meeting was attended by Alex Azar, Robert Redfield, Anthony Fauci, Deputy Secretary of State Stephen Biegun and others. Pottinger passed on the information he had gleaned and reminded those gathered about China's cover-up during the SARS epidemic in 2003. He raised the idea of shutting down travel from China, but no one supported his suggestion, dismissing it as absurd. The public health officials said a travel ban from China would be counterproductive, arguing it would stop the flow of medical equipment, create hysteria and inspire covert travel that would lead to disease spread.

One senior figure recalls he responded, "You've got the world's leading infectious disease expert sitting next to you who says this isn't a serious problem, that we don't need to stop flights from China. Why should we believe you over Fauci?"

The condescending reaction from another senior Trump official was, "Okay, Matt, that's great, what's your basis for that? Your time at *The Wall Street Journal*?" They thought his rhetoric was alarmist and they saw no reason to listen to him. It was patronising. Ignoring Pottinger's sage advice was a decision those present may now live to regret. Somehow Pottinger kept his cool. He did not react angrily.

After the meeting, Trump's senior advisors were scathing about Pottinger. He was considered a "serious guy" by Trump's close aides but they didn't consider him an "expert", and they didn't take his warnings as seriously as they would have had they come from someone else. "We worried about his credibility, because his wife worked at the CDC in infectious diseases and he was relying heavily on word-of-mouth reports from China because he used to be a journalist there," one aide says. "Matt is not a scientist, Matt's a journalist. He's a talented journalist and really good on national security issues, but he's not a doctor, he's not a physician, he's not an infectious diseases expert. We were just not comfortable, you know, going with that type of basis for a policy."

Over the coming days, Pottinger continued campaigning for a travel ban. "The public health sector was trapped by dogma," he told me. "The century-old orthodoxy was that you never shut down travel in response to a pandemic."

The same day that Pottinger told the health officials to ban travel from China, the WHO's Director-General Tedros Adhanom Ghebreyesus met with Xi Jinping for the first time since the outbreak, and Azar finally spoke on the phone with his counterpart in China, Ma Xiaowei. Azar and Tedros had a late-night call on the evening of the 26th to plan ahead. Tedros, who had just arrived in Beijing, was dog-tired. "Listen, Tedros, I've got CDC people waiting on standby to fly to China right away. We need the first-generation viral samples they're not providing us," Azar said.

Tedros replied, "I think it would be better if it's a WHO team."

"I don't care, we just have to get people in there," Azar pushed. "I'm ready to support you fully. You have to be hard with Xi because they do not want a repeat of SARS where they appeared non-transparent." Tedros seemed agreeable. Azar forged on, "You have to hit him hard and I'm going to hit Minister Ma hard." Azar hung up the phone feeling like they were on the same page and had teamed up to force China to cooperate.

Azar and Ma did not have a close relationship by any stretch. They had met before, in Geneva at the World Health Assembly the previous year, and had sat down for a bilateral meeting. But Azar was a well-known Taiwan advocate and had loudly campaigned for Taiwan to have representative status at the World Health Assembly, which meant any meeting with Ma began by him reading out a

Communist Party diatribe attacking him and the United States for interference in domestic policy.

In their call on Tuesday the 28th, Ma apologised profusely for taking so long to phone Azar back and said he had been on the ground in Wuhan. Azar reiterated strongly the request to send a team into China. "Minister Ma, we are here to help you in any way we can. I can get a team from the CDC deployed immediately or, if you prefer this be a vehicle through the WHO, we'll fully support that," he said. "The key is we have to get outside experts on the ground so we can learn about this virus and the best way to take care of people; the best infection and epidemiological control. We all need to work together on this." It was all platitudes back from Ma and he would not make any firm commitments. It would be another three weeks before China allowed WHO investigators into China, and even then only three of them were allowed into Wuhan for just 48 hours.

Amid the debate about banning travel, US Senator Tom Cotton sent a letter to Secretary of State Mike Pompeo, Azar and Acting Secretary of Homeland Security, Chad Wolf, saying the virus may have come from a laboratory. He was the first Republican figure to publicly raise the possibility – and he was ridiculed for it. "If the virus didn't originate in the seafood market, it's critical to determine where it did – especially, I must add, since Wuhan is also home to a biosafety-level-4 super-laboratory that engages in the study of coronavirus, among other deadly pathogens," he wrote. He was mocked by most media outlets, which labelled the laboratory theory "debunked".

Assistant to the President, Director of Trade and Manufacturing Policy Peter Navarro, a loud, opinionated economist and environmental activist, had authored a book six years earlier that predicted a worldwide pandemic. He was alert to the possibility of an outbreak originating in China. Navarro had a bolshier and more direct approach than Pottinger. He waltzed straight into the Oval Office and spoke to Trump about banning travel from China. Other big issues were preoccupying the President at the time: impeachment, for starters; and the killing of Iranian military leader Qasem Soleimani. But he seemed to be on the same page as his Trade

Advisor and told Navarro to go make the case to the Coronavirus Task Force. He did that on Wednesday January 29.

"He sent me basically to bring the task force onside in favour of the travel ban," Navarro recalls. But perhaps he wasn't the best person to send to persuade the health officials. No one could describe Navarro as a natural negotiator or peacemaker. Navarro had an almighty blow-up with Anthony Fauci in the Situation Room over whether to shut down travel from China.

Navarro sat down at the table with Fauci opposite him. He had never met Fauci before. Truth be told, he didn't even know who he was when he sat across from him. Their first meeting did not go well. "My impression of him was an arrogant, smug airhead. Very full of himself. He spoke with such authority but it was like, 'You don't know what you're talking about, dude,'" Navarro says.

Navarro, confident of the President's support, stated the case for a travel ban in no uncertain terms. "We need to shut down travel from China now before millions of people are infected in the United States," Navarro said, before outlining how this needed to take effect as soon as possible.

Fauci immediately took the opposing side of the argument: "Travel bans don't work," the health official said authoritatively.

Navarro hit back, "What evidence do you have for saying that?"

"In my experience, travel bans don't work," Fauci replied, although what experience he had of implementing a travel ban during a pandemic was left unsaid.

"You mean to say that if China brings 20,000 people a day with some of them likely infected with the coronavirus, that's not going to spread the virus?" Navarro bellowed.

Fauci's irritatingly repetitive reply was, "Travel bans don't work."

Navarro blew up. "He was like this dumb parrot rather than a human being," he told me. "Mulvaney was just as bad. Azar and Redfield all agreed with Fauci not to ban travel from China."

Pottinger was in the meeting, but Navarro said he was not given a say against the more senior officials. "He was there but he's not a high-ranking official. He's a deputy at the NSC, big deal," he said.

Fuming, Navarro stormed out of the room and decided to put pen to paper. He would warn them all, in writing, of what would unfold if they didn't heed his sage advice. He started crafting a memo putting them on notice that millions of people could die and there would be trillions of dollars in damages if they didn't stop flights from China immediately.

That same day, Pottinger spoke with a doctor in China who gave him a warning far more grave than any other he had heard to date. This would not be a repeat of 2003 SARS, the doctor said. It would be a repeat of the 1918 Spanish influenza. He also claimed there was asymptomatic spread of the virus – something that the WHO and US health officials were insisting was extremely unlikely.

The significance of this message spurred Pottinger to take more drastic action. This was potentially not only a health crisis but a national security one as well, yet his warnings to senior health officials were falling on deaf ears. Within hours, Pottinger would have a chance to make his appeal directly to the President. He explained to O'Brien what he had learned and O'Brien said, "Come with me."

Washington DC: The Oval Office

O'Brien had a previously scheduled Oval Office intelligence briefing for the President. Knowing that Covid-19 was on the agenda and aware of Pottinger's new information, he asked his deputy to join him. Over the preceding days, O'Brien developed a strong gut feeling the virus was going to turn out to be bad, very bad – although he couldn't have known half a million Americans would lose their lives in the next 12 months. What he did know was that there was a massive cover-up underway in China.

O'Brien's warning left the President with no question over the magnitude of what America could be facing. In a commanding voice, O'Brien said, "Mr President, this has all the hallmarks of a Chernobyl situation. The WHO is not being forthcoming. The Chinese aren't being forthcoming. This could be the biggest national security threat you'll face during your administration."

Trump said, "Wow, that's a pretty big statement."

"We are dealing with a different type of Communist government in China," O'Brien went on. "It's much more like a Soviet-style government than maybe earlier iterations of the Deng Xiaoping, Hu Jintao model. I just have a feeling that Chernobyl is going to happen all over again."

O'Brien then asked Pottinger, who was sitting behind the Intelligence Committee briefers on the Oval Office couch, to relay to the President some of the information he had received through informal channels. Pottinger went on to detail what they were learning from doctors and what was unfolding in not just Wuhan but Beijing as well. "The 1918 Spanish flu is how serious a pandemic can be. These things can get out of control," Pottinger said.

Trump took their message seriously. "He was very attentive, listening and asking questions about it," Pottinger recalls.

It was Trump, fresh from his conversation with Navarro, who then asked the pair what they thought about a travel ban.

O'Brien replied, "Yes." Pottinger strongly seconded his opinion.

O'Brien told the President, "A travel ban is wise until we get our arms around what's happening. We need to pause and figure out what's happening."

Trump listened to their arguments, but did not make a decision at that point. Or if he did, he didn't voice it. "He took it seriously," O'Brien said. "He trusted me and he moved pretty quickly after that."

Navarro then fired off his memo to all and sundry. The President, the Chief of Staff, the economic advisors, the leadership team, the NSC. In it, he warned, "The lack of immune protection or an existing cure or vaccine would leave Americans defenceless in the case of a full-blown coronavirus outbreak on US soil." Navarro's memo went on, "This lack of protection elevates the risk of the coronavirus evolving into a full-blown pandemic, imperilling the lives of millions of Americans." He also specifically called for a travel ban: "If the probability of a pandemic is greater than roughly 1 per cent, a game-theoretic analysis of the coronavirus indicates the clear dominant strategy is an immediate travel ban on China."

The memo quickly leaked to the media. Navarro says someone else leaked it.

Navarro's reputation meant his advice was ridiculed. Some White House senior officials saw him as "crazy" and "notoriously unreliable." "Peter is one of the least reliable sources in the West Wing and everybody knew it," one senior official says. They mocked a character he allegedly invented to cite his academic research, calling it his imaginary friend or his alter ego. It was "Ron Varra", an anagram of his surname, and the character even had a CV. When questioned by a journalist on it in October 2019, Navarro said it was a "whimsical device and pen name I've used throughout the years for opinions and purely entertainment value, not as a source of fact."

Navarro, who was not included in the Coronavirus Task Force, told the President, "Two million people are going to die this year."

"We looked at him like, we're trying not to start a panic and you're sitting here making up bullshit numbers," Mulvaney tells me.

Another senior official who was present for various Oval Office conversations says, "We did have people running around with their hair on fire, but they were not credible."

If Navarro and Pottinger made an unlikely alliance on the one side, there was Fauci and Redfield on the other, advocating a far softer position. They said there was no need for travel bans. Mulvaney and Larry Kudlow, Director of the National Economic Council, agreed with the health officials and were more concerned about the economic impact of a shutdown than the health pandemic at that time. They warned Trump against any overreaction, while Navarro's message to the President was that this could be, effectively, the end of the world.

There was firm evidence of community transmission in the United States by Thursday January 30. There was also corroborating information that asymptomatic people could spread the virus, with a case in Germany confirming asymptomatic spread. This coincided with reports about a substantial increase in new cases in China. All of these elements led to a complete backflip from the public health officials during their morning meeting, with senior CDC official Nancy Messonnier reversing the recommendation from just a day earlier to now support a travel ban from China.

At the Coronavirus Task Force meeting held afterwards, Azar lobbed the grenade in that the CDC had overnight changed its recommendation. "We believe we should stop travel from China and enforce a quarantine on any Americans who have been in Hubei province," he said. It was a radical change, but the Task Force accepted it.

Mulvaney said, "We need to talk to the President. He's flying to Iowa for an event this afternoon. We're not going to brief him on this on the phone, so let's do it tomorrow." It gave the team time overnight for operational planning.

The rampant asymptomatic spread of the virus was one of the contentions Pottinger had made early in the week, based on his information from doctors in China. "As the gravity of the outbreak in China became clearer, the logic of using a travel ban to slow, not stop, the spread to our shores became clear to everyone," Pottinger told me.

That afternoon Trump, who had flown to Michigan to visit a manufacturing plant, gave a speech downplaying the threat of the virus. He said there would be a "good ending" for the US and that he was working "very closely with China". "We think we have it very well under control. We have very little problem in this country at this moment – five – and those people are all recuperating successfully," he said in the speech. Trump also tweeted: "Working closely with China and others on Coronavirus outbreak. Only 5 people in US, all in good recovery."

That same day, the United States' Permanent Representative to the United Nations in Geneva, Andrew Bremberg, spoke with China's ambassador, Zhang Jun. Bremberg wanted to make sure Jun wasn't going to block a move at the WHO to declare a Public Health Emergency of International Concern (PHEIC). "You can not block this PHEIC determination," Bremberg said.

The Chinese ambassador said, "Xi Jinping has taken control of the situation in China. We don't think it's appropriate for the world to be second guessing what is happening domestically. It would show a lack of confidence."

Bremberg looked at the ambassador in amazement. "He could tell I was looking at him very strangely," he says. "What are you talking about? This has nothing to do with China's domestic response," Bremberg retorted. "This has to do with issuing a warning to the rest of the world that there's a potential pandemic pathogen out there. If there's a PHEIC declared, the US is not going to say China has done a bad job responding domestically to the virus. However, if the PHEIC is not declared, we are absolutely going to say that the Chinese have blocked and opposed the recommendation."

Jun said, "That's very interesting."

Bremberg succeeded and a Public Health Emergency was declared at the WHO. The formal WHO statement said that the declaration "should be seen in the spirit of support and appreciation for China, its people, and the actions China has taken on the front lines of this outbreak, with transparency, and, it is to be hoped, with success."

On the Friday afternoon, the President consulted his advisors, calling a meeting in the Oval Office. He hadn't made a final decision on banning travel from China. There were only a handful of cases in the United States. In the Oval Office, Trump's acting Chief of Staff, Mick Mulvaney, sat in the gold chair by the fireplace, directly opposite the President, with Pottinger on the chair by his side. Mulvaney ran the meetings, tapping Pottinger on the shoulder to speak or nodding at Redfield on the couch to voice his opinion, making sure the President heard all perspectives – even ones he personally didn't agree with.

Azar briefed the President and said a travel ban was a sensible precautionary measure. Fauci never fully advocated for the travel ban, while the economic hardheads, like Mulvaney, Senior Counselor Kellyanne Conway and Acting Chairman of the Council of Economic Advisers Tomas Philipson still did not change their minds.

But the President did. He could not ignore the advice of his health officials.

Navarro thinks it was his leaked memo that forced them to change their tune. None of the officials who had opposed the travel ban could afford to ignore a warning like this in writing that had appeared in the media, he says. "I wrote that memo and they had no option other than to reverse their position now that the memo was out," Navarro tells me. "I can tell you that they would not have reversed that position if not for what I did. I like Matt, but he didn't have the juice, as they say, to move anybody in that room. What moved the needle was that game-theory memo I did, which predicted millions would die." Health officials deny his memo made them change their minds. "I don't think Navarro's memo had the least bit to do with career people at CDC and NIH changing their views overnight as they saw cases exploding in China and more spreading around the world in other countries," one official said.

And so it was that five days after Pottinger had first begged cabinet officials to ban travel from China, the Trump administration announced the drastic move, effective from that Sunday at 5pm.

While Trump agreed to ban travel from China, he did not want to take ownership of the decision. "Why don't you go to the podium here in the White House and announce it?" the President said to Azar. This was not Trump's usual style, to delegate a major press conference. "I suspect this was a case of 'Let's let Azar get out there, hang him out there a bit and see how it goes,'" one official says.

Azar walked across from the Oval Office to the Roosevelt Room to prepare for the big press conference and to sign the national declaration of a Public Health Emergency. The White House staff refused to photograph it, so Azar's Chief of Staff Brian Harrison recorded the historic moment on his iPhone.

The announcement was made at 5pm. US citizens who had been in China's Hubei province in the past fortnight would have to quarantine for 14 days if they travelled back to the US. It was the first quarantine order in 50 years. But it was the travel ban that sent shockwaves. "Foreign nationals other than immediate family of US citizens and permanent residents who have travelled in China in the last 14 days will be denied entry into United States," Azar said.

Eight hours later, Australia announced a similar travel ban on Saturday, February 1 at 5pm local time. Australian Health Minister Greg Hunt was watching his son play cricket that morning when Australia's Chief Medical Officer, Brendan Murphy, rang him with some bold advice. Murphy told him it was time to shut our borders to China to prevent coronavirus from reaching the shores.

Hunt immediately phoned Prime Minister Scott Morrison and said, "Boss, you're not going to like this."

They patched in Murphy and spoke about the unprecedented step of banning flights entirely from one of Australia's largest trading partners. At the time, this was a radical move that was strongly rebuffed by major universities and the tourism sector. For two and a half hours, Hunt walked around the cricket oval making phone calls, watching the game and occasionally cheering for his son. By 9pm that night, the borders were closed to all of China.

Australia would later go a step further and ban all international travel, with the exception of returning citizens who were subject to quarantine. This succeeded in keeping the country relatively free of the virus. "Australia has taken unprecedented steps at a far earlier time in the progression of the virus than almost anyone in the world," Hunt said. Amid the decision to shut down travel from China, Morrison and New Zealand Prime Minister Jacinda Ardern had an unscheduled call on Saturday February 1. In the course of that call, Ardern allegedly asked Morrison what he was going to say about the origins of the virus and whether it came from a laboratory. Virologists advising the governments at that point were split 50/50 on whether Covid-19 had been genetically manipulated.

Morrison, fresh from the call with Ardern, relayed the conversation to Cabinet ministers. "Ardern was the first world leader to raise the possibility it had come from a lab," a senior Australian Government source said. A Cabinet Minister confirmed their initial advice stated there was a 50 per cent chance the coronavirus leaked from a laboratory, but this was later downgraded substantially to 5 per cent before rising again.

Morrison doesn't recall the nature of the conversation with Ardern, although his advisors confirmed the call took place. Ardern's spokesman said "details of her conversations with Prime Minister Morrison are confidential".

The day after this conversation between Morrison and Ardern, New Zealand followed Australia, announcing a travel ban from China in the afternoon of Sunday, February 2. The UK did not introduce a travel ban, and neither did Europe. Only Italy, South Africa, the Czech Republic and North Korea introduced flight suspensions from China.

O'Brien encouraged his European counterparts to similarly ban travel from China – but they refused. "I said you should do the same thing. Unfortunately, the Europeans demurred and said, 'Oh, it's a Brussels issue, we don't have enough information'," O'Brien tells me. "Ultimately, what happened is the Chinese banned travel internally but they continued to allow folks from Wuhan and Hubei to go to Europe and ultimately most of the infection that took place in the United States came from Europe through JFK, because the Europeans allowed in massive numbers of Chinese travellers. Had the Europeans taken the same approach as the US, Australia and New Zealand on the travel ban, this thing could have been contained in a much more aggressive fashion."

After Trump banned travel from China, then Presidential hopeful Joe Biden sent a tweet he would likely live to regret. "We are in the midst of a crisis with the coronavirus. We need to lead the way with science – not Donald Trump's record of hysteria, xenophobia, and fear-mongering. He is the worst possible person to lead our country through a global health emergency," he tweeted on February 1.

Biden's press team later claimed he wasn't specifically referring to the travel ban when he accused the President of racism. His campaign spokesman Andrew Bates said that Biden "has decried

Trump's xenophobia for years, and was saying that it shouldn't influence the US approach to this outbreak. This was not in reference to coronavirus travel restrictions."

This is a stretch, given Biden sent the tweet the day after Trump announced the travel ban from China – and this was the only big move he had made in relation to China at that point. Remember, Trump was still praising Xi Jinping.

The move to shut down flights from China was also rebuffed by the WHO, whose medical advice did not recommend travel restrictions and claimed China was on top of the unfolding health crisis. "First, there is no reason for measures that unnecessarily interfere with international travel and trade. WHO doesn't recommend limiting trade and movement," Tedros said on January 30. "We call on all countries to implement decisions that are evidence-based and consistent. WHO stands ready to provide advice to any country that is considering which measures to take."

Australia had declared that this was a global pandemic 10 days before the WHO did.

As the US election year rolled on, the early travel ban was one of the only things Trump could point to that he had got right when it came to the pandemic. Looking back now, Mulvaney is somewhat defensive. He doesn't accept the criticism that the administration didn't do enough in those early days. "People say we underreacted? Well, in hindsight, I actually think we overreacted with the lockdown, because the disease turned out not to be nearly as fatal as we thought that it would be. It was less than 2 per cent fatal in this country, as opposed to the 15 to 35 per cent that we were worried about," he said. "We never should have locked down. We should have left the economy open and protected the most at-risk populations."

When they implemented the travel ban, the recent experience with two coronaviruses, MERS and SARS, led senior Trump administration to believe that the fatality rate would be high but transmission easily contained.

"We knew that coronaviruses generally could be very, very deadly, and we knew that SARS and MERS were sort of hard to transmit, not as easy to transmit as the flu," Mulvaney explains. "We've focused exclusively at the outset on what's called containment, to try to keep people who might be infected out of the United States. That's what gave rise to the cessation of all travel from Wuhan, and then from Greater China, and the funnelling of international travellers through various airports."

China's reaction to the travel ban was fiery. Foreign Ministry spokeswoman Hua Chunying said Trump's travel ban was "certainly not a gesture of goodwill". "A friend in need is a friend indeed. Many countries have offered China support in various means. In sharp contrast, certain US officials' words and actions are neither factual nor appropriate. Just as the WHO recommended against travel restrictions, the US rushed to go in the opposite way," she said.

China's Ministry of Foreign Affairs' issued a Tweet noting Chinese Foreign Minister Wang Yi's remarks that a "certain country has turned a blind eye to WHO recommendations" by imposing "sweeping travel restrictions against China". China also expressed its "deep regret and dissatisfaction over the Australian government's announcement on the extension of travel restrictions over foreign nationals from Chinese mainland".

In what can only be described as pure chutzpah, China's Deputy Head of the Chinese Embassy in Australia, Wang Xining, called for Chinese students who could no longer travel to Australia to be financially compensated. "We are very concerned about the interests of the Chinese students who will not be able to come to Australia over the next 12 days," he said. "We hope their rights and interests will be safeguarded, including proper expansion of visas and also maybe proper compensation for some of the financial losses during this period." He called the travel ban "a vicious cycle of panic and [overreaction]."

China's response to Israel was equally outrageous. On Thursday, January 30, Israeli Health Minister Yaakov Litzman announced that

Israel had banned all incoming flights from China, and the following day Interior Minister Aryeh Deri barred foreign nationals who had recently been in China from entering Israel.

China's Acting Ambassador to Israel, Dai Yuming, referencing the Holocaust, said in a press conference, "In the darkest days of the Jewish people, we didn't close the door on them. I hope Israel will not close the door on the Chinese."

CHAPTER EIGHT

Transparency

America's Ambassador to Geneva, Andrew Bremberg, pulled Tedros aside outside a WHO meeting in Geneva. Tedros had just returned from his one-on-one with Xi Jinping in Beijing. The pair had shaken hands, smiled and posed for photographs. Tedros had then assured the world how truly transparent and cooperative China was being, lavishing praise on Xi Jinping for his handling of the outbreak. "China identified the pathogen in record time and shared it immediately, which led to the rapid development of diagnostic tools," he said on January 29. "They are completely committed to transparency, both internally and externally. And they have agreed to work with other countries who need their support."

Listening carefully to every word, Bremberg was highly concerned. The reality was China had not been forthcoming. It was a month since the WHO had discovered the virus existed, but despite repeated US efforts, virus samples had not been obtained and no health officials were allowed to set foot in Wuhan.

As he stood downstairs in the modern WHO building, Bremberg's tone was concerned. "Be very careful in what you're saying. I fear you are saying things we hope are true but may not be," he warned Tedros.

Tedros insisted everything was fine. He was proud of his recent visit and was content with the commitments he'd received from Xi Jinping to allow a team into China.

"You're getting out over your skis, and if it doesn't turn out this way your institutional and personal credibility will be at risk," Bremberg implored Tedros.

The WHO chief insisted everything was fine. "Don't worry, I'm not over my skis, everything is good," he soothed.

This made Bremberg even more nervous. In the 10 days that followed, it became clear Xi Jinping's commitments were worth little. The daily conversations between Tedros and Bremberg grew tense as the US Ambassador pushed for a plane of experts to depart for Wuhan. "If they're slow-rolling you, you need to say this, because then we won't blame you, it's not your fault," Bremberg said.

Eventually, Bremberg issued a threat of his own to Tedros, without the express permission of the President. "We are going to cut off funding all together if you don't get this trip together," Bremberg told Tedros. Tedros was deeply unhappy, but the ultimatum worked. A few days later, the WHO trip to China was approved.

Twenty-five health officials from nine countries flew into China for a fact-finding mission from February 10 to 24. Towards the end of the inspection, it became apparent there was a major problem. Bremberg discovered that the WHO had struck a side agreement with China to change the terms of reference, taking the origins of the virus off the table. The inspectors would simply be learning from China about how to respond to an outbreak. "They had totally caved on the terms of reference, that was supposed to examine the origins as soon as possible," Bremberg says.

Instead, China only allowed three WHO officials to visit Wuhan and only for two days. They were Bruce Aylward, Chikwe Ihekweazu and Tim Eckmanns – none were American. They did not visit the wet market or the Wuhan laboratories. Instead, their visit included trips to hospitals and they had meetings with officials. The WHO's excuse is that it was too difficult to visit Wuhan. "They didn't get any real information," Bremberg says.

When I questioned the WHO's spokeswoman Margaret Harris on why officials did not even visit the wet market or the laboratory, she was defensive. "The focus of the mission was on learning from the response, not looking at the origin, so the wet market, lab, etc. were not on the agenda," she told me in a May 2020 interview. "The mission was not even going to go to Wuhan because there was such intense transmission at that time and the hospitals were actually overwhelmed. The people our experts needed to speak to were their counterparts, and at that point the infection prevention and control experts in Wuhan were flat out dealing with a very large outbreak."

There was no access to the earliest virus samples that the US felt were critical to obtain. These samples were something the Chinese government had gone to great lengths to hide. The day after China was forced to admit to the WHO it had an unknown pneumonia spreading, on December 30, 2019, authorities ordered that all viral samples be destroyed from genomics laboratories, according to investigative Chinese media outlet Caixin Global. Genomics companies were also told to stop testing samples linked to the outbreak, and were banned from releasing any results to patients or medical staff – they could only be sent to authorities. The Wuhan Institute of Virology was also blocked from sharing sample isolates with its partner laboratory, the University of Texas Biocontainment Laboratory.

The samples were crucial. "I spent weeks talking with Tedros, saying you need to ask China to share samples. We are getting ready to do not just the current diagnostics and next therapeutics, but vaccines are going to be critical. We need earliest known virus sample strains to test and pressure, to figure out the right approach," Bremberg says.

China never shared the samples.

"I shook my end at the beginning of 2021, when the reason we had pushed so hard was in the daily news. Everyone was realising we've got these new variants coming out and the biggest question was: are the new vaccines going to be efficacious against the new variants. That's exactly why we wanted the samples in the first place," he says.

* * *

China's cover-up at every stage of the outbreak exasperated its international counterparts. China's official line in the early days was that the virus originated in the wet market, and only coronavirus cases linked to the wet market could be recorded, but evidence that could have proved or disproved this was eradicated. On January 1 – the day after the WHO was informed of the virus – the Huanan Seafood Market was shut. Teams of cleaners went in sanitising, disinfecting and spraying the market, destroying any forensic evidence that could have been collected.

On the same day the brave doctors like Ai Fen shared news of the virus over WeChat and the WHO became aware of a coronavirus in Wuhan, Chinese authorities started systematically removing any mention of the virus online. This began on December 31, when technology services in China censored key words linked to the pandemic. The live-streaming platform YY censored words including "unknown Wuhan pneumonia" and "Wuhan Seafood Market". WeChat censored phrases related to the pandemic, banned both speculative and factual information related to the outbreak, and removed even "neutral references to Chinese government efforts to handle the outbreak that had been reported on state media", according to the Citizen Lab's March 2020 report. The CCP censorship alarmed doctors and Chinese health authorities, who knew the precise opposite approach should be taken in order to save lives. This crucial point clearly shows China's deliberate, intentional and clear-eyed decision to cover up the virus; to stop their own people and those internationally from finding out about it.

The censorship order came right from the top. Xi Jinping, in a speech on February 3 published by state media, issued a directive to promote "positive energy" and "strengthen online media control to maintain social stability". Families were left fuming as their conversations online about the deaths of loved ones were deleted, according to media reports. Images from funeral homes were censored and families in mourning were assigned minders, *The New York Times* found.

The most egregious of China's cover-ups, which directly led to the spread of coronavirus globally, centred on the denial of human-to-human transmission. China had evidence the coronavirus was infectious as early as December 6, when a woman fell sick five days after her husband. She had no history of visiting the market. Yet China refused to admit there was human-to-human transmission of what has turned out to be one of the most infectious diseases in human history for another six and a half weeks.

On January 6, Xu Jianguo, the Beijing director of an expert team sent into Wuhan, said, "China has many years of disease control, there's absolutely no chance that this will spread widely because of Spring Festival travel." He insisted, "there is no evidence of human-to-human transmission" in comments he gave to Hong Kong news outlet Takungpao. The message was repeated just a few days later by prominent PRC government expert Wang Guangfa, who said, in an interview with state broadcaster CCTV, the outbreak was "under control" and mostly a "mild condition". He added that there was no sign of human-to-human transmission.

But Chinese officials knew the virus was infectious. PRC National Health Commission chief Ma Xiaowei reportedly made serious admissions about the outbreak in a confidential teleconference with provincial health officials, according to Associated Press. He said that the novel virus is "the most severe challenge since SARS in 2003, and is likely to develop into a major public health event", adding that "clustered cases suggest that human-to-human transmission is possible". He also sounded the alarm about the spread of the virus among those travelling for the Lunar New Year. That same day, the WHO Emerging Diseases Unit stated, "It is very clear right now that we have no sustained human-to-human transmission."

It wasn't until January 20 – six and a half weeks after they had firm evidence, with the wet market seller's wife falling sick – that China officially admitted there was human-to-human transmission.

In the meantime, China allowed millions of people to travel both domestically and internationally for Chinese New Year.

Authorities also deliberately downplayed the number of cases, not letting foreign governments know the true nature of the spread. The CCP only began recording cases in late December 2019, when the virus had been spreading throughout Wuhan since at least November and likely October. On January 3, the Wuhan Health Commission said a case could be counted as part of the outbreak if a patient had ties to the Huanan Seafood Market. And even then, cases were only recorded if an official laboratory test confirmed the diagnosis of Covid-19 and if the patient was symptomatic. The trouble was, it was very difficult to get such a test.

"Prior to mid-February, the CCP only reported cases that were symptomatic, clinically diagnosed and confirmed by laboratory tests," the United States House Foreign Affairs Committee Minority Staff Report (aka the McCaul report) said, referencing an NPR media report. Only on March 31 did the CCP policy change to allow asymptomatic cases to be included in the official number of confirmed Covid-19 cases. There was an uptick of 14,840 cases in a single day. Classified CCP data obtained by Josephine Ma at the *South China Morning Post* showed that 43,000 asymptomatic people had tested positive by the end of February. This was about one-third of all cases.

In late March, China's official death toll was 2500. The McCaul report pointed out that these figures could not be true, given the Hankou Funeral Home in Wuhan received a shipment of 5000 new urns from a supplier in a single day. The report also quoted Wuhan residents who gave an interview to Radio Free Asia as saying that the true death toll may have been higher than 40,000 by the end of March – a far cry from the 2500 reported.

The local media, meanwhile, were silenced, with police detaining journalists reporting from Wuhan Jinyintan Hospital in mid-January, compelling them to delete their footage and inspecting their phones, according to Hong Kong news outlet TVB. TVB said its reporter was "taken to the police room in the hospital for questioning, and asked to delete the materials shot in the hospital". Another journalist was threatened with arrest at the Huanan Seafood Market.

There was even secrecy around the genome of SARS-CoV-2. Chinese scientists had mapped the genome at the Wuhan Institute of Virology by January 2 and had known it was a coronavirus since at least late December, when genomics companies returned test results to Ai Fen. There was a delay of three days until researchers at the Shanghai Public Health Clinical Centre told Chinese authorities on January 5 that the genome had been mapped. Instead of openly releasing these results immediately, the Chinese government censored them and stopped the centre from publicly sharing it.

And it wasn't until January 8 – after *The Wall Street Journal* had already reported that there was a new coronavirus – that the Chinese government officially provided it to the WHO. China's Centre for Disease Control Director, George Fu Gao, told *Science* in an email interview in March 2020 that it was "a very good guess from *The Wall Street Journal*". He insisted that the information was shared with scientific colleagues "promptly, but this involved public health and we had to wait for policymakers to announce it publicly".

His excuse for not sharing the genetic sequence immediately was that they didn't want to cause alarm. "You don't want the public to panic, right? And no one in any country could have predicted that the virus would cause a pandemic. This is the first non-influenza pandemic ever."

Finally, on January 10 US-time, the genome was uploaded to virological.org by a scientist in Sydney, Australia with ties to the Shanghai Public Health Clinical Centre. As punishment for alerting the world to the genetic sequence, the Centre was closed temporarily for "rectification".

On January 15, China's Centre for Disease Control implemented the highest-level emergency response inside China, but its instructions on how to identify cases were marked "internal" and "not to be publicly disclosed", according to an Associated Press article.

While China was downplaying the virus, the number of infected patients and the number of dead, it was quietly buying up medical equipment and protective personal equipment from around the world. It simultaneously dropped its exports of medical supplies. Associated Press cited a Department of Homeland Security intelligence report, which stated that in early January 2020 the Chinese government "intentionally concealed the severity" of the pandemic in order to allow for its own stockpiling of medical supplies. According to the US House Minority Report, China "nationalised the supply chains and manufacturing capacity of foreign companies like General Motors and 3M to produce medical supplies while denying export licenses for their products".

All the while, China was requesting – at times demanding – public praise for its handling of the pandemic from the international community. CCP officials contacted the President of the Wisconsin Senate, Senator Roger Roth, asking that the Senate "pass a resolution praising the PRC's response to the pandemic", *The New York Times* reported. Chinese diplomats made similar requests to German officials. China then punished countries that questioned the outbreak or its handling of the pandemic with economic coercion.

Despite the CCP's clear obfuscation and suppression of data, Chinese President Xi Jinping succeeded in only receiving commendations from world leaders and health authorities in early 2020. Instead of acknowledging there was a coronavirus outbreak and responsibly alerting global health authorities and foreign governments, in an effort to contain the virus, the CCP did the precise opposite. Every action Beijing took had the effect of spreading the virus and making more people ill globally. It deprived foreign governments of the critical information needed to protect their own populations. While shutting down domestic travel on January 23, it still allowed international flights to leave China.

"The Chinese authorities have gone to great lengths to destroy evidence and silence anyone in China who might be in a position to provide evidence on the origins of Covid-19," says former White House official in the Clinton administration Jamie Metzl. "In the critical first weeks after the outbreak, Wuhan authorities worked aggressively to silence the whistleblowers and destroy evidence that could prove incriminating."

This wasn't even China's first cover-up of a coronavirus. Global health authorities and world leaders should have, from the very get-go, been more alert to the possibility of a cover-up of the contagion from China, given immediate past experience from SARS in late 2002 and 2003. Back then, China had faced international condemnation for covering up the virus outbreak and failing to alert global health authorities. In China, public health information is classed as a "state secret" until the Ministry of Health approves its release. The virus originated in China's Guangdong province, where it is believed to have spread from bats to a palm civet and then to humans. The outbreak took eight months to contain.

"The SARS epidemic delivered a political shock to the Communist Party, which was widely condemned for mismanaging the outbreak, covering up cases and smothering news reports," *The Washington Post* reported in January 2020. This should have instantly encouraged suspicion and inquiries about what information China was sharing and whether it was being transparent. But everyone was ready to give China the benefit of the doubt. None more so than the WHO.

The WHO's culpability in kowtowing to the CCP and thus allowing the spread of the virus globally cannot be understated. The WHO's role in spreading China's disinformation and the cover-up was crucial. WHO Director-General Tedros repeatedly praised China for its "transparency". It's extraordinary now to read the WHO press release from January 5. "WHO advises against the application of travel or trade restrictions on China. WHO does not recommend any specific measures for travellers," it states.

Their subsequent praise of the January 23 Wuhan lockdown made America's Ambassador to Geneva's blood boil. "China put in place the most draconian travel restrictions of any country ever by locking down all of the Hubei province in January. The WHO endorses and praises these efforts, while objecting to complementary international travel restrictions," Bremberg tells me.

The WHO released a statement on January 9 praising Beijing: "Preliminary identification of a novel virus in a short period of time is a notable achievement and demonstrates China's increased capacity to manage new outbreaks." On January 22, Tedros chose not to declare the coronavirus a "public health emergency of international concern".

Wuhan was literally under siege, its hospitals crippled by the pandemic, but Xi Jinping was resisting a visit from the WHO. Tedros was still misleading the world even in March, when he said that "Covid-19 does not transmit as efficiently as influenza", to Bremberg's great despair.

It was not until March 11 – three months after Chinese officials knew there was an outbreak – that the WHO declared the novel coronavirus a "pandemic". The official recorded infections were 118,000 people in 114 countries.

Despite the public embarrassment, the WHO refused to admit its advice on the travel bans had been wrong.

The excessive control China exercised over the WHO would continue, even to the point of having a say in which scientists and academics from the international community could investigate the origins of the virus, according to a report in the *Daily Mail*. The outcome was that the CCP, with the help of the WHO, deliberately hid news of Covid-19 and the nature of the highly contagious virus. It's why the United States grew so frustrated and eventually withdrew funding from the body.

"It is beyond doubt that the CCP actively engaged in a cover-up designed to obfuscate data, hide relevant public health information, and suppress doctors and journalists who attempted to warn the world," the House Foreign Affairs Committee Minority Staff Report in 2020 states. "Senior CCP leaders, including CCP General Secretary Xi Jinping, knew a pandemic was ongoing weeks before it was announced. By responding in a transparent and responsible manner, the CCP could have supported the global public health response and shared information with the world about how to handle the virus. It is likely the ongoing pandemic could have been prevented had they done so."

The Chinese Communist Party's culpability in deliberately covering up the virus instead of alerting the world is a crime as shameful and abhorrent as the Tiananmen Square massacre. Millions of lives have been lost, and counting, with families in every corner of the earth struck by tragedy, while economies have been decimated, livelihoods lost and people thrown into poverty.

The question is, why did they act like this and what were they covering up?

CHAPTER NINE

Don't Panic the Markets

It's against the backdrop of China's cover-up that President Trump and President Xi had a phone hook-up to discuss the coronavirus on February 6. It was their first interaction after the convivial trade-agreement signing just a fortnight earlier. In that call, Xi told Trump he would be very forthcoming and would pave the way for doctors to visit China, senior sources familiar with the call tell me. Trump hung up in a positive, upbeat mood.

During the conversation, Xi made some astonishing claims about the virus. He told Trump it would disappear in the warmer summer months and even said that Chinese medicine was successful in preventing Covid-19, as first reported by journalist Josh Rogin in his book *Chaos Under Heaven*. The sentiment was echoed in a tweet from Trump the next day. He praised Xi as "strong, sharp and powerfully focused" on containing the virus. "He will be successful, especially as the weather starts to warm and the virus hopefully becomes weaker, and then gone," Trump tweeted. "Great discipline is taking place in China, as President Xi strongly leads what will be a very successful operation. We are working closely with China to help."

On February 19, Trump was still praising President Xi Jinping's handling of the virus. "I'm confident that they're trying very hard," he told Fox 10 in Phoenix. "They're working it – they built, they built a hospital in seven days, and now they're building another one. I think it's going to work out fine."

Those close to Trump deny he genuinely believed China was handling the pandemic well, insisting it was a conciliatory tactic the President used to try to extract information out of Xi Jinping and encourage him to cooperate with America and the WHO. "It's human nature. Sometimes you get better results with honey than with vinegar. The President might have been saying nice things about China in an effort to try and get them to cooperate. It's a business negotiation. Why start the negotiation by calling the other guy a bunch of names?" Trump's Chief of Staff at the time, Mick Mulvaney, says. "The President had a feel for President Xi and how he might be able to get him to work more closely with us, that he might respond better to flattery than to insults. I think that's right. The Chinese don't work very well when you insult them."

Another senior Trump official familiar with the call and strategy agrees with this. "I don't know that the President really thought that Xi was being transparent, but he was doing what the WHO was doing in the sense he was trying to encourage China to be transparent and to open up and to let us in, so he was trying to be supportive and positive," the official says. "I don't think it was for any other reason than he was trying to get them to cooperate."

Australia's former Ambassador to Washington Joe Hockey thinks it was more a case of Trump having an affinity with the "strong man". "He liked strong leaders, people he saw as alpha-males, like Putin, Kim Jong-un – and Xi Jinping," he says.

Another senior Trump administration official, who does not wish to be named, says Trump's praise was likely to keep Xi Jinping onside while the US administration figured out how to get Americans safely out of Wuhan. "We were scrambling at the State Department to figure out how we were going to get Americans out of Wuhan, that's what we were focused on," the source says. "We got 100,000 Americans home in an unprecedented operation that we stood up from zero, in cooperation with private airlines. So part of it might be the President was thinking: How big is this problem? How do we contain it? And how do we keep them all safe?"

Yet another senior Trump official tells me the President's attitude was also designed to protect the trade deal that had just been signed. "The President was sitting up above providing a halo of nice talk to them as an inducement," they say, "while Pompeo, Azar and Pottinger were being the bad cops criticising China, and Navarro was being the super-bad cop".

Before the phone call with Xi, Trump was briefed, as he always was, by his National Security Advisor Robert O'Brien and Secretary of State Pompeo. The appeasing tactic the President took with Xi was a deliberate one that had been agreed on with these advisors. The conversation before the call canvassed whether it was possible that the Chinese leadership and the Chinese President might not actually be aware of the full extent of what was being hidden from them as well.

"What Chinese official wants to go deliver the bad news to Xi? You could end up being Rosencrantz and Guildenstern, right, you don't leave the room after delivering the message," O'Brien said referring to the situation in *Hamlet* where the messengers are killed. "So we didn't know if Xi actually had the information, if it was coming through his bureaucracy. It was still early on in the process. One of the reasons for that phone call was to try and encourage China to allow CDC doctors, WHO doctors and experts to get into China to figure out what was happening and how we could respond to the pandemic," he explained.

This strategy of trying to encourage cooperation from China continued for some time. Trump couldn't afford to create a hostile relationship given China had a stranglehold on America's supply chain for personal protective equipment (PPE), advanced pharmaceutical ingredients, parts needed for ventilators and masks. Lives were at stake.

"It was a huge wake-up call for folks in our government to realise how dependent we had become on China for critical items," O'Brien says. "Almost everyone realised how much we needed to bring our supply chain home or to have a trusted supply chain with our allies for key products. There was real concern as the pandemic arose that we wouldn't get access to the data we needed to find out the origins and the nature of the pandemic and how to stop it. There was also a concern that China would cut off the supply chain for PPE, pharmaceuticals and other essential products."

Ultimately, China's attempt to leverage its superior position with "wolf warrior" PPE diplomacy around the world backfired, O'Brien believes. "Covid has accelerated the bipartisan consensus that's developed around China, that China can't be trusted as a provider of 5G services, for medical equipment, advanced pharmaceuticals and chips. We can't be as dependent on China as we had become for essential products. Other nations have come to the same conclusion."

The decision to play nice with Xi Jinping wouldn't last long, and within a month the US–China relationship would deteriorate to new lows. Despite Trump dismissing the gravity of the virus publicly, sources close to the President say he was acutely aware of the danger of the virus. He sat in the security briefings and heard the dire warnings. They were impossible to ignore.

But there was one thing Trump was even more concerned about than the spread of the virus through the United States – and that was creating panic in the population, sparking an economic collapse. "We worried about a panic, no question, 100 per cent. We were absolutely worried about a panic," Mulvaney says. "It never bothered me that the President tried not to create a panic. The President was very concerned about creating a panic, and the President believes in the power of positive thinking. He would much rather focus on the positive than the negative. And I think that came across in how he handled the Covid crisis. It was very difficult for him to go out there and give a worst-case scenario.

"When he goes out and says the disease will be gone by springtime, that was not entirely baseless. But it was certainly against the overwhelming evidence that was presented to him. Was there a chance that the disease would have gone away as the temperatures went up? And the days got longer? Yes. He would take little kernels, and then magnify them in order to put the best face forward. In hindsight, obviously, it turns out to be something that hamstrung the administration's response to the crisis."

Azar asked Mulvaney to pull together a working group with regular meetings on the coronavirus, formalising a group Pottinger had first created two weeks earlier. Mulvaney ran it but it was considered Azar's group. It kicked off on January 29 and became the "Coronavirus Task Force". Its first mission was to evacuate American diplomats and their families from Wuhan and shut down international travel from China to the US. Azar, Mulvaney, Deputy Secretary of State Stephen Biegun, Redfield, Kadlec, Fauci and others were gathered in the Situation Room, with Mulvaney at the head of the table. One agency head updated the room that the hundreds of Americans from Wuhan had been evacuated and the two 747s were on their way back to the States. "Great news, the planes are in the air."

There was backslapping around the room before someone asked a prescient question, "Where are they going?" Each agency head, the most senior leaders in the Trump administration, looked around the room, waiting for another to speak. There was silence as the realisation dawned that there was no intended location yet. The planes, carrying hundreds of passengers from China, all potentially infected with coronavirus, had no place to go, no health procedures to follow. Considerable planning had gone into the refueling stop in Alaska, but the final destination was less settled. The working plan was the planes were going to land at a commercial airport, probably LAX, then the passengers would be put on buses and taken to a nearby hotel for two weeks. "Can you imagine what kind of outcry that will create?" one official said. "Everybody sort of looked around the table and said, 'How did that happen?'"

After this initial panic, the Department of Defence official left and went out in the hallway, tapping at his mobile phone. About 15 minutes later he walked back in with the solution to take the hundreds of potentially infected Americans to an air force base in southern California. It was remote and had housing for hundreds of people.

The chaotic situation shocked many members of that group. "It was classic bureaucracy," one participant tells me. "Too many agencies involved. Nobody in charge. Those planes took off without us knowing exactly where they were going to land. Unbelievable."

Trump was, by the start of February, getting almost daily briefings on the virus. Staff from 10 different agencies would meet at 10am; the working group, co-chaired by Azar and Mulvaney, would meet at 3pm; and Trump would be briefed at 6pm by the Coronavirus Task Force.

Those nightly briefing sessions with the Coronavirus Task Force would grow tense and argumentative. The President was surrounded by big personalities who had major differences of opinion on how to respond to the virus. The meetings were large, with 15 to 20 people crammed into the Oval Office at 6pm daily; there was standing room only. With Trump permanently ensconced behind the presidential desk, the back-and-forth arguments erupted around him.

"This is how the President functioned. He liked big meetings," says one attendee.

The way the President preferred to consume his information was to listen to a verbal briefing. There were no data or policy recommendations or briefing notes or analysis for him to consume and think about overnight. If there was a document of sorts – perhaps a graphic representation showing a spike in Italy's cases or some raw data – it was at most one page, never even three pages. It was all verbal, a fresh flow of information. That's how Trump worked. The nightly press conferences arose from this, following his 6pm briefing.

Partly because of the decision to pull US diplomats out of Wuhan, there were few Americans on the ground in the city. Information was limited and the Trump administration was overly reliant on Chinese authorities for intel about the severity of the virus and its properties. "We knew it was a coronavirus and we knew it was centred in Wuhan, that's about all that we knew, keeping in mind the Chinese had restricted the World Health Organization access," Mulvaney says.

Navarro was furious that the administration still was not taking the virus seriously enough. His point of view was dismissed so regularly that he continued writing memos in the paperless White House, to ensure his advice would be recorded. The White House was paperless because senior members of Trump's senior team were not allowed to communicate via text or WhatsApp under the Presidential Records Act. Not allowing paper also suited Trump's paranoia about people leaking information about him. The official mobile phones belonging to some senior figures even had text messaging and cameras blocked.

"My government-issued phone was not capable of taking pictures and not capable of texting," one source says. "We were not allowed to communicate like that. We were heavily restricted in what we could text in the White House. There was no way, at least early in the administration, to guarantee that text messages could be preserved by law." Meeting arrangements and administrative matters could be communicated via email.

But Navarro ignored the directive. "I papered the shit out of them," he tells me. "I think in February there was a dozen memos. They knew their arse was on the line. That was the power I had."

Navarro sent a memo, on February 23, to the President, copying in the National Security Advisor, the Chief of Staff and the Covid-19 Task Force, warning of mass deaths and insisting that resources needed to be thrown toward vaccine development. "There is an increasing probability of a full-blown Covid-19 pandemic that could infect as many as 100 million Americans, with a loss of life as many as 1–2 million souls," Navarro wrote in the memo that was later leaked to news website Axios. "We CAN develop a vaccine and treatment therapeutics in half the usual time. We must get appropriate protective gear and point of care diagnostics." He hit back at "any member of the Task Force who wants to be cautious about appropriating funds for a crisis that could inflict trillions of dollars in economic damage". This was a not-so-subtle dig at Mulvaney and his Deputy Chief of Staff, Chris Liddell.

Senior figures in the CDC, however, were starting to come to terms with just how severe the virus could be. "I got my first projection of the impact of the pandemic in late February and it was a difficult evening that evening because it projected up to 2.2 million people would be dead by September. This pathogen was going to be a big problem," Robert Redfield said in a conversation with the Council on Foreign Relations after he left the role. Two days later, senior CDC official Nancy Messonnier warned Americans that Covid-19 was likely to spread throughout the United States and the disruption to daily life would be "severe". She warned about the possibility of a pandemic. Her press briefing had followed a decision by the Coronavirus Task Force to escalate the pandemic threat plan. But Messonnier, under the instruction of Redfield, jumped the gun and announced it before the President had been informed.

Trump, on his way back from India following a 36-hour trip with his family, rang Health Secretary Alex Azar from Air Force One to praise him for his performance at a hearing that day answering coronavirus questions. Trump hadn't caught up with the comments made by Messonnier but had been informed by Louisiana Senator John Kennedy that Azar had done a stellar job while then Acting Homeland Security Secretary Chad Wolf had been "terrible". Trump asked Azar to start a daily Covid-19 press conference. It was a surprisingly positive call, seeing as just the month earlier Trump had called Azar "panicky" in front of witnesses, with the conversation leaking to the media.

In the morning, Azar took an early call from the President, who had just landed and was back at the White House. Trump was fuming about Messonnier's comments, which he was now across. "What the hell is she doing out there scaring the markets?" he wanted to know.

The Dow Jones had fallen nearly 900 points in the worst week since the Global Financial Crisis in 2008. "Mr President, what she said is factually correct, in fact, we are coming to brief you this afternoon on precisely this. She just got ahead of her skis. But it's completely correct and it's what we need to be saying," Azar replied.

Trump said, "I want to have a press conference this afternoon to settle things down, we need to explain all of this to the public because it's out of control. The market is overreacting."

Azar deliberately chose to defend Messonnier, who he had worked alongside in the Bush administration. But it would cost him.

By 8.45am, a story had popped on Politico that said Trump was considering appointing as coronavirus czar Scott Gottlieb – a doctor and the former Commissioner of the Food and Drug Administration (FDA), who had been informally advising the White House. The FDA was part of HHS, which was run by Azar.

Though it was Mulvaney who had been running the Coronavirus Task Force, this appointment was seen as a move that would replace Azar.

Azar was giving evidence at a House Appropriations Committee hearing when the story broke, and the chairwoman Rosa DeLauro quizzed him on it. He hadn't read it.

Trump phoned Azar during a break, "Hey, should I appoint Scott Gottlieb as coronavirus czar?"

"Scott is great. I love Scott but he's not going to do it," Azar replied, explaining Gottlieb had deliberately left the White House to move to Connecticut with his family and was also unlikely to leave his board position at Pfizer. Trump then also raised Deborah Birx as a possibility. Azar told Trump he would see him for their pre-planned meeting at 5pm.

Mulvaney, unaware that this conversation had taken place, caught up with Trump in the Oval Office. "We need to make a change," Trump told him. "We need to put somebody big at the head of this thing." It wasn't only because of Messonnier's comments. In late February, as the situation grew grave in Italy and alarm and anxiety began to consume the American public, Trump wanted someone serious at the head of the Task Force. It would be good for optics and to indicate the "seriousness of the group" by putting someone big in at the helm of the multi-agency initiative.

"Mr President, no problem with that, that makes perfect sense. Who do you want?" Mulvaney replied. Trump wanted Gottlieb. "We can't have Scott Gottlieb," Mulvaney reasoned. "He used to work for Azar, and if you put him in charge of the Task Force, Azar will quit, because he will deem it to be a personal affront. And he'd be right to do so, because this would be putting his subordinate above him. He would almost be forced to quit."

The President considered this and Mulvaney pressed on, imploring the President not to make a decision that could erupt in yet another scandal. "Mr President, we cannot afford to have the [Health Secretary] quitting in the midst of what could be an international worldwide pandemic," Mulvaney pleaded.

By 5pm, Trump had come up with the idea of putting Mike Pence in charge, who was automatically senior to the cabinet secretaries. Pence would end up running the entire coronavirus strategy, but he kept a relatively low profile and managed to escape scrutiny and blame, which fell on the President's shoulders.

That evening of Wednesday, February 26, Trump addressed the nation for the first time on the coronavirus. Flanked by Pence, his newly-announced coronavirus czar, and half a dozen senior officials, Trump, in a bright pink tie, reassured Americans only 15 people in the US had coronavirus and were "getting better". "The risk to the American people remains very low and we have the greatest experts in the world right here," he said. The naive, relaxed attitude to a deadly virus that was quickly spreading around the globe worried Azar, Navarro and Pottinger, among others.

While the CDC was highly concerned about the virus, Trump's senior officials continued with their strategy of downplaying the virus in order to save the markets. Mulvaney went on television and urged Americans not to wear a mask. The interview was at the direction of Fauci. Fauci later defended his position on masks by saying there was a shortage of them in the United States at the time, and he wanted to preserve the limited supply for medical professionals, but Mulvaney denies this was the explanation given to him by America's top doctor at the time.

"That's not what he told me or the team. He said, 'Tell people not to wear masks, because wearing masks can actually make things worse. If you're not trained on how to properly use a surgical mask, it can actually create a circumstance where you're touching your face more often, and could increase transmission of the virus. Please,

please, please tell people not to wear masks.' And I went on national television and said exactly that in February," Mulvaney recalls.

Another senior health official confirmed to me this was, in fact, Fauci's advice. "His view was that wearing a mask could be counterproductive because you fiddle with it and your unclean hands could actually introduce disease into your respiratory channel." The health official says there was also a shortage of masks at the time and they needed to be kept for hospital frontline workers, rather than a rush on them by the American people.

Fauci's contradictory advice on masks was later laid bare for all to see in an email he sent on February 5, 2020 that was released under the *Freedom of Information Act* to Buzzfeed in June 2021. "Masks are really for infected people to prevent them from spreading infection to people who are not infected rather than protecting uninfected people from acquiring infection," he wrote. "The typical mask you buy in the drug store is not really effective in keeping out [the] virus, which is small enough to pass through the material. I do not recommend that you wear a mask, particularly since you are going to a very low risk location."

The tensions between the two camps advising Trump came to the fore when Mulvaney gave an interview to Stephen Moore at the Conservative Political Action Conference in Maryland, where he appeared to call the virus the "hoax of the day". In the February 28 interview he certainly downplayed the virus, saying "this is not Ebola … it's not SARS, it's not MERS". "We sit there and watch the markets and there's this huge panic and it's like, why isn't there this huge panic every single year over flu?" Mulvaney said the media was focusing on the virus because "they think this is going to be what brings down the President". "Why didn't you hear about it? What was still going on four or five weeks ago? Impeachment, and that's all the press wanted to talk about … That's what this is all about."

On message, Trump repeated the claim the virus was a hoax at a campaign rally 700 kilometres (400 miles) away in South Carolina. "The Democrats are politicizing the coronavirus," he declared. "One of my people came up to me and said 'Mr. President they tried to beat you on Russia, Russia, Russia. That didn't work out too well.' They couldn't do it. They tried the impeachment hoax. This is their new hoax."

At that time, the virus had killed 2800 people globally and infected about 80,000. It didn't seem to some in the Trump administration that it was a real and major threat. Between the hoax line and Navarro telling Fox News host Maria Bartiromo in an interview that the virus may have come from a biowarfare laboratory, the messages emanating from the Trump administration couldn't have been more inconsistent.

CHAPTER TEN

Pompeo

It might have seemed like President Xi Jinping was pulling the wool over Trump's eyes, but this certainly wasn't the case with Secretary of State Mike Pompeo. He came to the State Department in April 2018 from the CIA. He already intimately understood the serious strategic threat China posed from his time as CIA director. "Nobody had to tell him that, that wasn't a revelation to the secretary," an insider says.

Much of Pompeo's first six months was focused on the Trump administration's withdrawal from the Iran deal, Obama's signature foreign policy agreement, in the month after he started. Pompeo had a particular interest in Iran. Alongside US Senator Tom Cotton, he unearthed the secret nuclear side deals between Iran and the International Atomic Energy Agency when he was a congressman in 2015.

In late 2018, Pompeo turned his attention to China. Under his stewardship, there would be a monumental reset in the relationship and foreign policies between the United States and China. The long-held position on China from both Republican and Democrat administrations in the United States was to view China as a partner, an equal collaborator and an opportunity to get rich. Under Pompeo in particular, this changed dramatically and irrevocably. This China pivot cannot be overstated.

Trump had already opened Americans' eyes to the unequal trade terms with China, but Pompeo sought to expand it beyond the economic remit to human rights, the exposure of influence operations, intellectual property theft and China's other malign actions that sought to disadvantage America. "The question was how was Pompeo going to handle it because the President had taken the lead on it," an insider said. But Trump had not shown an appetite for tackling China beyond the "unfair trade deal", a hallmark of his election campaign in 2016.

Pompeo and Trump were more often than not in lock step. Pompeo was careful not to make a move without Trump's blessing, unlike his predecessor, Rex Tillerson. Tillerson reportedly said Trump was a moron at a private function, with the President calling him to demand answers three hours later. The rifts in their partnership extended from policy on North Korea to Russian strategy, along with whether to pull out of the Paris Climate Change Agreement.

Pompeo was a far better ideological fit for Trump. The former soldier, businessman and conservative congressman was elected to the House in 2010 as part of the Tea Party wave; Trump believed they were on the same wavelength. Raised in California, straight-talking and affable, Pompeo patrolled the Iron Curtain before the fall of the Berlin Wall and then went on to graduate from Harvard Law School.

Pompeo was a strong critic of US foreign policy under Obama, especially with Iran, and has expressed scepticism on climate change and human responsibility for it. Unlike Tillerson, Pompeo applauded the decision to pull out of the Paris Agreement, to withdraw from Obama's Iran deal and to bring troops home from Afghanistan.

Pompeo remained loyal to Trump throughout and after his presidency, while still managing to emerge from the Trump era with his credibility intact.

While bizarre stories emanated from the White House about the President watching television late into the night, tweeting his opinions on prime-time programs to his millions of followers,

Pompeo's work ethic couldn't have been more different. Up at 5am, Pompeo was typically in the office between 6.15 and 7am. His diary was scheduled in 15-minute increments from that moment, often featuring calls with foreign leaders, until 5pm. He'd have dinner with his family and then retreat to his home office to work until late in the evening.

He followed this gruelling schedule every day of his life from April 2018 until January 2021, when the administration ended. One White House insider describes it as "a very, very brutal schedule". "Here was a guy who went to West Point [Military Academy], who served the country from the time he was 18," the insider said. "It's how they're made. He was a very unusual Secretary. I really doubt any other Secretary worked like that guy worked. It was completely insane." His senior staff often kept the same work hours as their boss.

Pompeo's focus on China coincided with his decision to hire *The Wall Street Journal* editorial board member Mary Kissel, whose illustrious career includes a Harvard pedigree, and time as a Goldman Sachs investment banker and as a financial columnist for *The Wall Street Journal*'s Hong Kong bureau. Her editorials critical of Singapore's lack of judicial independence saw WSJ Asia sued by the Singapore government in the High Court. Kissel was also a regular critic of the CCP, its human rights record and its encroachment on Hong Kong's freedoms when she edited the Asia opinion pages.

The headlines around her hiring focused on her criticism of Trump's foreign policy from her time as a *Wall Street Journal* editorial writer. The media took delight in reliving Trump's Twitter response to her criticism on American television program *Morning Joe* that he had no policies. Trump had retweeted someone who commented, "Major loser." When Pompeo hired Kissel, news site Politico reported a former official saying, "Trump would lose his mind if he knew about this."

But her conservative credentials were well established through her contributions on Fox News and her time as host of Foreign Edition, a foreign-policy podcast where she often focused on the ideological battle of the 21st century with China. She has famously interviewed the Dalai Lama, which she described at the time as "like meeting the divine. Truly extraordinary", and she called out Australia's former Prime Minister Malcolm Turnbull as "conservative in name only" years before many others cottoned on.

While her hiring confounded some ardent Trump supporters, Pompeo recognised her foreign policy expertise, in particular her knowledge of China, where she had lived and developed an extensive network. And so she moved from *The Wall Street Journal*'s headquarters in midtown Manhattan to Washington DC as his Senior Policy Advisor in late 2018, to advise him on policy and messaging on the threats America faced, but especially those from China.

It was a Herculean effort to re-craft how Americans viewed China and to change the narrative after successive administrations had encouraged ties with China for so long, oblivious to the pernicious effects of the relationship. The message had been: China is a partner, invest with China. Never mind the threat of CCP recruitment programs, intellectual property theft, espionage, cyber attack and misuse of American research and technology for military modernisation.

Success has many fathers, but Kissel's role in shaping the United States' shift on China foreign policy was significant. She made her mark on the State Department, helping Pompeo execute his broader China strategy, driving the public arguments about the CCP. "It is widely recognised in the China world that Mary was an absolute dynamo within Pompeo's State Department on the China issue," the Inter-Parliamentary Alliance on China's Luke de Pulford says. "Having lived and worked in Hong Kong, she is resolutely committed to the rights of Hong Kong people, and that shone through in much of the work of the department. It would be unfair to call her the 'power behind the throne', as Pompeo himself was clearly no slouch on China, but it would be foolish to doubt her influence and efficacy in shaping US–China policy."

Miles Yu says he and Kissel are like brother and sister. "She is a feisty lady, oh my goodness," he says with a laugh. An Australian official says she has a "significant intellect", while Pete Navarro says, "You don't want to get on the wrong side of Mary."

From late 2018, Pompeo began to substantially change long-held aspects of America's foreign policy approach to China, starting with formulating a strategy around the persecuted Uighur people in Xinjiang and on China more broadly. The administration's language immediately shifted. Instead of calling Xi Jinping Chinese President, Pompeo called him the "General Secretary of the Communist Party of China", and China was described as the "Party State". Pompeo also sought to reframe the conversation around China by speaking about the national security concerns with 5G and device manufacturer Huawei. "We watched Australia very closely," a senior administration source said. "Australia was years ahead of us in influence operations on campus and on buying politicians."

From January 2019, Pompeo often spoke about Huawei and the plight of the Uighurs in public, clearly framing the problem in the broader strategic context. With Kissel, he devised the "empty promises" campaign, which was originally the "broken promises" campaign, to highlight China's lies about Hong Kong's sovereignty. The message was, if the CCP can do it in Hong Kong, it can break its promise to others as well. How can its word ever be trusted?

The central reason for Pompeo's visit to Britain in May 2019 was to lobby the then May government to cut off Huawei from the UK's 5G network over national security concerns, which the UK ultimately did, albeit a year later. He also campaigned on the treatment of Uighurs at the United Nations.

In a statement on June 4, 2019, Pompeo called for accountability for the victims of the Tiananmen Square massacre for the first time ever. He looked back to the horror in 1989, when 1 million pro-democracy advocates in Beijing's Tiananmen Square called for an end to authoritarian dictatorship but were gunned down by Chinese troops in an early morning attack. Up to 10,000 innocent Chinese citizens were killed. The CCP now tries to deny it ever took place.

On the 30th anniversary of the June 4 bloodbath, Pompeo urged "the Chinese government to make a full, public accounting of those killed or missing to give comfort to the many victims of this dark chapter of history". It sent shockwaves in Beijing, which had grown accustomed to the US avoiding inflammatory remarks. Chinese officials called Pompeo "arrogant" and said anyone who patronises and bullics them "will only end up in the ash heap of history".

"I made sure our statement was released at 12.01am Beijing time, just to make a point to the CCP that we were marking it on China time, to recognise the suffering of the Chinese people," Kissel says.

Behind the scenes, Kissel arranged for Pompeo to meet with Hong Kong businessman and media mogul Jimmy Lai in July 2019 in Washington. "We were pushing very hard on the human rights abuses in Xinjiang, removing unnecessary bureaucratic constraints on Taiwan interactions, exposing influence ops on American college campuses, expanding Clean Network, getting UN campaigns up to full speed to blunt CCP influence, cementing the Quad, exposing China's environmental record. Those were Pompeo's priorities on China in his final year," Kissel says.

Pompeo's landmark speech where he articulated the challenge Communist China posed and his vision for the pivot in foreign policy took place at the Hudson Institute on October 30, 2019. He had been wanting to deliver a major address on China for months, and had been waiting for the right moment.

Yu stood beside Kissel as they pulled together the ideas for that speech with Chief Speechwriter David Wilezol, who had a beautiful way with words. "That speech didn't come out of nowhere. We had planted this idea there was a broader problem," Kissel says. "The Hudson Institute speech was the China speech, the big coming-out for Pompeo where we explained the nature of the party and why it had taken us so long to wake up."

In the speech, Pompeo said, "We've been slow to see the risk China poses to American national security because we wanted friendship with the People's Republic from the very start. But, in our efforts to achieve this goal, we accommodated and encouraged China's rise for decades – even at the expense of American values, and security, and good sense. We did everything we could to accommodate China's rise, in the hope that Communist China would become more free, market-driven, and ultimately, hopefully, more democratic. It is no longer realistic to ignore the fundamental differences between our two systems, and the impact that these differences may have on the United States. Above all, we as Americans must engage China as it is, not as we wish it to be."

Pompeo's speech led to a broader strategy to have key figures in the Trump administration each deliver an oration each to enlighten Americans about the true nature of Communist China. The concept was nutted out in a meeting in Pompeo's office with Attorney-General Bill Barr, FBI Director Chris Wray and O'Brien to map out the plan of attack, so to speak. "It was an effort to educate and mobilise the American people as to the challenges that we're facing from China, aside from the coronavirus," O'Brien says.

In the room, O'Brien raised the "X Article", written by George F. Kennan under the pseudonym "X" and published in *Foreign Affairs* magazine in 1947, which outlined the Soviet Union under Joseph Stalin's hostile view of the West. The team discussed laying out the case against China for Americans in this new era. "We looked at the situation as if it was a trial and we needed to put our case to the American people about the threat that we were facing," O'Brien recalls. "We had four lawyers who had significant legal practice experience and training, and I think we instinctively thought, let's divide up the case. We would each take a portion of the argument and let the American people know what we're facing and how serious this challenge is."

The four speeches amounted to a strategic exposition of the Chinese threat. O'Brien delivered the first speech in June 2020 in Phoenix, Arizona, focusing on the Communist Party's ideology and its insidious effect on American life. He highlighted cases like the Houston Rockets basketball team, whose general manager tweeted support for the Hong Kong protestors, and in response the CCP announced that the team's games would not be shown on Chinese TV. "Together with our allies and partners, we will resist the Chinese Communist Party's efforts to manipulate our people and our governments, damage our economies and undermine our sovereignty. The days of American passivity and naivety regarding the People's Republic of China are over," he said.

FBI Director Chris Wray spoke about economic coercion, malign foreign influence and CCP recruitment programs that are responsible for stealing American intellectual property, patenting it in China and selling it back to the US. He also spoke about the threat to academia. "China is engaged in a highly sophisticated malign foreign influence campaign, and its methods include bribery, blackmail and covert deals," he said. "Chinese diplomats also use both open, naked economic pressure and seemingly independent middlemen to push China's preferences on American officials."

Attorney-General Bill Barr's speech, later in July 2020, demonstrated how China has emerged not only as a rival to the United States but one that has a stranglehold on supply. "The ultimate ambition of China's rulers isn't to trade with the United States. It is to raid the United States. If you are an American business leader, appeasing the PRC may bring short-term rewards. But in the end, the PRC's goal is to replace you," he said.

Finally, Pompeo ended the series with a speech at the Richard Nixon Presidential Library in California on July 23, 2020, where he said "the free world must triumph over this new tyranny" and the "old paradigm of blind engagement with China" would no longer suffice. "The kind of engagement we have been pursuing has not brought the kind of change in China that President Nixon hoped to induce. The truth is that our policies – and those of other free nations – resurrected China's failing economy, only to see Beijing bite the international hands that fed it." Pompeo's rhetoric escalated as well. He called Chinese President Xi Jinping a "true believer in a bankrupt totalitarian ideology".

The speech was particularly poignant for one member of the audience. Watching Pompeo's historic address was China's "father of the democracy movement" Wei Jingsheng, the defector who had first sounded the alarm about the new coronavirus months earlier.

Pompeo, Pottinger, Navarro, O'Brien and 24 others, along with their immediate family members, would all be sanctioned by China when Biden won office, banning them from entering the mainland, Hong Kong or Macao, and their companies restricted from doing business with China.

Pompeo even made an indelible mark on foreign policy in Australia. On May 24, 2020, he gave an interview with conservative host Rowan Dean on Sky News Australia, where he warned America might "simply disconnect" from Australia under the intelligence-sharing agreement because of Victoria's Belt and Road deal with China. "We will not take any risks to our telecommunications infrastructure, any risk to the national security elements of what we need to do with our Five Eyes partners," he said.

When he gave the interview, Victorian Premier Daniel Andrews was finalising an agreement with China, blatantly ignoring national security advice from the federal government. Pompeo's remarks shook the intelligence community and were a major news story. Within hours, the US Embassy in Canberra released a statement trying to hose down the situation. Then US Ambassador to Australia Arthur B. Culvahouse Jr, said the Secretary had been answering "a very remote hypothetical" question. "We are not aware that Victoria has engaged in any concrete projects under BRI [the Belt and Road Initiative], let alone projects impinging on telecommunications networks, which we understand are a federal matter," his statement said. "If there were telecommunications initiatives that we thought put the integrity of our networks at risk, of course, we would have to take a close look at that, as the Secretary suggested."

But the Secretary had not slipped up in his words. And he had made his point. Within a year, the Morrison Government would introduce legislation to Parliament allowing it to tear up Victoria's deal.

Pompeo laughs as he remembers the havoc his brazen comments unleashed. "It was really quite something. I mentioned it just that one time, it created a bit of a firestorm and it was good stuff," he says.

The Biden administration has not, as of the time of writing, backed away from Pompeo's pivot on China. Unlike with Iran, there has been continuity on China under the Democrat presidency. Aside from the confrontational first meeting between new State Secretary Antony Blinken and new National Security Advisor Jake Sullivan, the temperature has mostly been dialled down. The Biden administration often uses the term "without going the full Pompeo" when speaking about how to handle China. As in, "Let's not go the full Pompeo here." The Biden view, as of early 2021, is to avoid turning the China issue into a civilisation clash between the traditionally Christian West and atheist Communists. They are continuing Pompeo's focus on strengthening the like-minded coalition of the Quad in the Asia-Pacific. China's sights on Taiwan could change all this, of course.

And so it was that while Trump praised Xi Jinping for his transparency, Pompeo was alive to the reality of China's cover-up of the virus. On a weekly, and sometimes daily basis, he kept abreast of the conversations of Chinese whistleblowers and activists on WeChat, thanks to Yu. Many posts vanished just minutes after they were published. Pompeo understood there would only be a cover-up if there was something nefarious to keep quiet. It's why he started to seriously examine the possibility that the virus did not have a natural origin.

"We began to look for alternative ways [it started] and everybody heard the wet market bat story, the pangolin story and you saw scientists saying this couldn't have been man-made because we've looked at this thing, which was a bit of a straw man," Pompeo tells me. "Man-made belies the reality of what could have been done in a laboratory even if it was a natural source. In any event, you saw the Chinese begin to push that story [of the wet market and pangolins].

"Of course we knew the history of the lab because there had been Western connections to it. We knew a great deal about the laboratory. The French built it, designed it, we had provided scientists there that had partnered with them on research so we knew a good deal about what was taking place. And so it didn't take us long after January before we had as a working hypothesis this possibility."

While he was careful to never disagree with the President in public, it's understood that Pompeo made his views known to Trump about China's cover-up and responsibility for the global outbreak. If his message was getting through to the President, it certainly wasn't to his most senior advisors.

The question remained: When was it time to tell the American public and the world about China's activities at the Wuhan laboratories?

MARCH 2020, WASHINGTON DC

Within weeks the virus had begun its march around the globe, and the first devastating outbreak was in Italy. When Bob Redfield was told of the prevalence of asymptomatic transmission in Italy Mulvaney recalls the words spilled out of his mouth: "Oh shit."

Redfield relayed the news to Mulvaney and other White House officials that his international counterparts had called to confirm the grim news. Asymptomatic transmission was something China had been denying.

It's fair to say that when the virus crippled Italy, senior officials in the Trump administration were shell-shocked. Their entire containment strategy to protect the United States was built on the premise the virus was not transmissible if someone was asymptomatic. That incorrect working assumption alone, based on medical advice from health officials, would cost the United States hundreds of thousands of lives.

"It meant that everything we'd done on containment is pretty much useless," Mulvaney says. "It meant people with the disease could walk right through the airports and out into the greater population, which we expect is probably what happened."

On March 1, Trump's Deputy Chief of Staff, Chris Liddell, threw a small dinner party at his home in Washington DC. It was a Sunday evening and still chilly in the nation's capital. Gathered around the elegant dinner table were the upper echelons of the Trump administration: Chief of Staff Mick Mulvaney and his wife, Pamela

West, and National Economic Council Chair director Larry Kudlow and his wife, Judith.

Liddell, Trump's Deputy Chief of Staff – one of the few to remain in the job until the end of the Trump Presidency – had led an illustrious business career before joining the administration. He was the Chief Financial Officer for Microsoft, a Vice Chairman at General Motors, the Chairman of Xero Corporation and CEO of Carter Holt Harvey in his former Wall Street career. He then took charge of Trump's strategic initiatives at the White House before being promoted to Deputy Chief of Staff. Unquestionably, Liddell, originally from New Zealand, is a smart guy.

To get the conversation rolling as they ate, Liddell posed a question to his guests, for each to answer around the table. "What is the big issue of 2020?" he asked. And one by one, the guests ticked off various topics. The soaring economy, Liddell himself nominated. The election that Trump was going to romp home, said Mulvaney. And so it went, around the table. Extraordinarily, not one of the six Americans nominated Covid-19 as the defining issue of 2020. None of them.

The four Australians present – one of them, a doctor – were astounded. They all said the coronavirus would be the defining issue of the year. Australian Ambassador Joe Hockey suggested to the group that perhaps it would be a good idea to tell the American public to wear masks. "Maybe everyone should be wearing masks, because you remember SARS in Asia, that's how they managed it. With masks," he said to the men who had become his friends since he moved to Washington four years earlier. But he was shouted down, told that masks were "useless". "You'd never get Americans to wear masks," Mulvaney said.

Hockey, who remains close friends with Mulvaney and Liddell, couldn't believe what he was hearing. They all thought it would pass, it was like a bad flu season. "None of them had ever managed a crisis because none of them had ever been in government before – at least not a crisis they didn't manufacture themselves," he said. "They were in denial, total denial. They thought it would be like Singapore, come the summer, it'll pass. They were saying, 'We've got it under control.

It's a mild flu.' They had all the excuses. I don't blame them. They were receiving confusing advice and they were following confusing leadership. They could see it potentially undermining Trump's re-election strategy."

Trump made the comparison with the flu himself days later on March 9. In a tweet he said, "So last year 37,000 Americans died from the common Flu. It averages between 27,000 and 70,000 per year. Nothing is shut down, life & the economy go on. At this moment there are 546 confirmed cases of CoronaVirus, with 22 deaths. Think about that!" The next day he said, "And it hit the world. And we're prepared, and we're doing a great job with it. And it will go away. Just stay calm. It will go away."

Puzzled, Hockey wondered whether the same intelligence that was warning Australia about the impending gravity of the situation was reaching the President and his most senior advisors. The Americans were so relaxed about the situation, Hockey questioned if maybe Australia was heading into lockdown unnecessarily. "At times I thought Australia was overreacting because I was in an environment where everyone was saying 'Don't overreact'," he recalls. "Washington is the centre of the universe and if something is happening on the other side of the world, it doesn't seem real."

Australia's Defence Minister Peter Dutton, who at the time was Minister for Home Affairs, says that in the United States "there was a belief that this wasn't going to hit their shores at that point in time. Australia had seen the intelligence. The predictions for us at that point were fairly dire. The initial advice to us was quite confronting, that we were going to run out of capacity within ICUs [intensive care units]. Fortunately, that didn't transpire."

The White House's dismissive approach to the coronavirus also alarmed Fox News's top-rating host, Tucker Carlson. He made his first ever trip to Mar-a-Lago on March 7, 2020 to warn the President the situation could get really serious. He was particularly concerned the US may not have the medical capacity to deal with a pandemic.

Carlson had intended to keep his trip a secret, and even asked the Secret Service to help him sneak in undetected, but unbeknown to him, former Fox News host Kimberly Guilfoyle was holding her birthday party there. He was spotted instantly and news of his mission quickly leaked.

Carlson told Trump "this could be really bad" and expressed his view the United States had "missed the point where we can control it".

"My concern was that we may not have the capacity to take all these patients and that we may not have the drugs to treat them," Carlson said in an interview with *Vanity Fair* 10 days later.

"I think Trump has a really finely calibrated sense of danger and I think it served him well. I think a lot of the people around him, and I mean broadly around him – particularly Republican members on Capitol Hill, in leadership too – were determined to pretend this wasn't happening. I kept reading pieces about how easy it was to transmit the virus and I just became obsessed with reading about it, and there was actually a lot of publicly available information, a lot of it speculative, but it was informed speculation in my view. And it led me to think that this could be a massive problem in the United States."

Carlson said he felt embarrassed about giving advice to the President of the United States, but trying to ensure the Trump Administration took Covid-19 more seriously drove him to make the visit.

"I'm just a talk show host. But I felt – and my wife strongly felt – that I had a moral obligation to try and be helpful in whatever way possible," he told *Vanity Fair*.

Mulvaney concedes that he didn't understand the coronavirus would emerge as the primary problem of 2020 back in early March. "The mood in February, March was that the president would win between 40 and 42 states." Mulvaney told me. "We were extraordinarily confident of re-election in February and March of 2020. If you had asked me in February what the defining event of 2020 would end up being I would have said the election."

Pottinger was wearing a mask in the White House by March, He even moved out of the West Wing and into the Eisenhower executive office building, west of the White House, he was so concerned. But Fauci still insisted it wasn't necessary. Not only that, he actively said masks would make the public health situation worse.

Azar and HHS Assistant Secretary Robert Kadlec worked with Hanes – a company that manufactures clothing for Bonds and other brands – to develop enough cloth masks for every American. They proposed sending a pack of five masks to every postal service mailing address in the entire United States, pitching the idea to the Pence-led Coronavirus Task Force in the third week of March. But it was shut down by Pence and his team.

"They thought it was an overreaction and thought it would create hysteria sending it to everyone in the country," one insider says. "They didn't like the look of them and said they looked like training bras."

Fauci's strong advice against masks suited Trump. Trump's closest aides reveal there was a big reason the President resisted the growing calls in the media to wear a mask. "This will have to absolutely be on background," confides one senior Trump official conspiratorially, preparing to divulge what sounded like it would be a state secret. "The President was against the mask for visual purposes. He thought he looked bad in them. He did not like the masks. It had nothing to do with science, nothing to do with health and everything to do with the fact it didn't fit his brand. It didn't look right. That's why he fought it for as long as he did."

Another senior official confirms this. "The President did not like mask wearing. He thought he looked weak wearing a mask. He physically said that, 'Masks make you look weak.'"

The official claims Trump also insisted military leaders, in particular, not wear masks because it made them look weak, along with health officials. "Before we would go on stage he would say, 'Take those damn things off' or 'If you are going to wear that, don't stand at the podium with me.'"

Later, in September, Azar briefed the President on a Japanese study that showed when two people wear a surgical mask at one metre distance it cuts down viral spread by 72 per cent. "We need to wear masks, they work," Azar said.

"That's your call, that's good for you," Trump allegedly replied. Pictures from the Republican National Convention in August on the South Lawn show Azar is a lone figure in the front row wearing a mask. It was a deeply uncomfortable moment for him, and senior figures expressed their displeasure in no uncertain terms.

Finally, on March 11, the WHO declared the coronavirus a pandemic, and Trump declared a national emergency two days later after coming to the realisation the US was going to be impacted in a major way. But still there seemed to be a denial about the extent to which the United States would be hit. On March 12, Trump said, "It's going to go away. The United States, because of what I did and what the administration did with China, we have 32 deaths at this point … when you look at the kind of numbers that you're seeing coming out of other countries, it's pretty amazing when you think of it."

Five days later, on March 16, Trump finally seemed to wake up to the reality of China's cover-up. He changed his tune and referred to the "China virus". O'Brien says the reason for the shift was twofold. Firstly, it became clear that China was never going to cooperate; and secondly, not only were they not helping but they were using the virus to their strategic advantage.

"The cover up was gaining steam and not losing steam," he says. "The idea that maybe the local and regional officials were covering things up from Xi, and he didn't know any better, and once he got to the bottom of it, China would open up … We realised this cover-up was going all the way to the top. There would be no cooperation. Then there was the fact that the Chinese Communist Party weaponised Covid and tried to use it to gain an advantage over the US and its allies by trading masks and PPE, and eventually vaccines, for access for Huawei to countries that were otherwise concerned about turning over their 5G backbone to the Chinese. It became pretty aggressive; the whole wolf-warrior diplomacy effort of the Chinese started taking real shape."

The attitude shifted significantly inside the White House, O'Brien recalls. "At that point, folks in our government started to realise there's not going to be any goodwill or cooperation from Beijing.

The Chinese are going to use this virus that they allowed to spread around the world to increase their power and dominion."

The other reason for the change in language was that the spreading coronavirus in the United States was fast becoming a major political problem for Trump. Shifting the blame back onto China was a political decision.

The economic hard-heads, like Kudlow and Secretary of the Treasury Steven Mnuchin, were reluctantly coming to terms with the fact their treasured trade deal with China had effectively been rendered meaningless. "It became a management issue very quickly. Trump had to create an enemy, that's why he called it the China virus. He didn't want to have a fight with Xi Jinping, he likes a strong man, he likes winners, that's Trump's headspace," Hockey says. "Pompeo was the one driving China, China, China. And Pompeo, don't forget, was the director of the CIA. He sees it all, so he's a crucial guy. And then Trump realised that he couldn't dismiss it."

By April, Pompeo finally had the preliminary results of Miles Yu's investigation, which involved multiple agencies. Yu had dedicated a significant amount of time canvassing a large quantity of Chinese publications, digging into the Wuhan Institute of Virology and the other virology laboratories in Wuhan, and the research they were conducting. The result was a report called "The PRC's Biosafety Negligence and Circumstantial Evidence Against the Wuhan Institute of Virology".

Carrying a two-inch-thick binder, Yu walked to Pompeo's office, near his own on the highly secure seventh floor of the State Department. The report within was concise, but the documentation supporting it was hundreds and hundreds of pages. He placed it on Pompeo's desk and the Secretary immediately started to read through it, commenting, "This is incredible."

The dossier begins, "China is a country obsessed with dangerous viruses. State-run media outlets often tout China's great discoveries of a phenomenal number of new viruses heretofore unknown to mankind. Over the past 12 years, China's army of virologists have discovered close to 2000 new viruses while over the past 200 years, the rest of the world has only discovered 2284. In its rush to greatness and dominance in virus studies, China often neglects biosafety, with catastrophic consequences."

Yu's report, dated April 26, 2020, which I obtained during my investigation for this book, states it is most likely the virus originated in a Wuhan laboratory. "The labs in Wuhan and the chain of physical contact related to the capture and study of coronaviruses in bats are the most likely vectors of original infection for the Covid-19 virus, and any credible investigation into the origin must start there," it states. "Only after this likely source has been completely ruled out should we move our investigation on to other potential sources."

His report states, "There is no direct, smoking gun evidence to prove that a leak from Wuhan Institute of Virology caused the pandemic, but there is persuasive circumstantial evidence to link China's pervasive biosafety negligence to such a possible leak from WIV." He adds that his evidence is "descriptive" and is "not meant to promote the lab leak theory".

His report goes on to detail Xi Jinping's own comments around biosafety concerns, along with how the French government, US officials and the international community were worried about safety problems at the Wuhan Institute of Virology. Yu's report also raised the bombshell possibility that China may have invented a Covid-19 vaccine prior to the outbreak. "It may seem likely that WIV has been researching a vaccine *before* the outbreak," he wrote. He explained the unusual case of Remdesivir. In mid-January 2020, Fauci donated free Remdesivir samples to China for an experimental clinical trial to save Chinese lives, to see if it was effective against Covid-19. Remdesivir was an American invention, developed by scientists at USAMRIID in conjunction with the American pharmaceutical company Gilead Sciences, using taxpayer funds. After Fauci donated the samples, the Wuhan Institute of Virology compiled a commercial patent for the treatment on January 19 in a case of intellectual property theft.

Yu wrote of this, "Yet days later, on January 19th, even before the Chinese government admitted the virus could be transmitted from human to human and before Beijing locked down Wuhan, WIV finished compiling a 'user patent' application for Gilead's Remdesivir and filed it on January 21st to Chinese patent authorities in Beijing."

Yu wrote that this "may give credence to the following possibility: prior to the surprise outbreak in its close vicinity, WIV had possessed the novel coronavirus in its lab and had known of its lethality and pathogenicity for a while. It had been actively researching a vaccine before anyone else could succeed, thus giving China the sole patent right."

He went on to say, "It raises the possibility that WIV has been researching a Covid-19 (treatment) of its own all along, and would like to prevent Gilead's Remdesivir from entering the Chinese market. Filing a patent requires lengthy documentation, clinical statistics, and international and national legal opinions. It normally would take months or even years to prepare and compile the application, rather than a few days."

The dossier also detailed China's bioweapons research, claims from scientists Covid-19 had been genetically engineered and presented evidence of Shi Zhengli's own work genetically manipulating viruses, including warnings from a paper she co-authored nine months before the pandemic that there would be a future SARS- or MERS-like outbreak originating in China.

He also claimed that the Wuhan Institute of Virology's own laboratory level-4 director Yuan Zhiming "harbored doubts about biosafety at WIV and other high BSL labs in China before WIV was accredited in 2017 and went operational in 2018".

Reflecting back on his dossier, Yu says, "The most important thing about that paper I wrote was not necessarily the conclusions or the suggestions or the loopholes I found. It is really the original sources. I documented every single thing.

"Of course the ultimate smoking-gun evidence has to be found inside China, but the overwhelming sort of evidence I gave him, pages and pages of this circumstantial evidence including many of the statements by the Chinese government officials including by Xi Jinping himself, they all admit China had this viral safety problem.

There were shortcomings in that the Chinese biological system was not safe, that's the overwhelming admission by the Chinese themselves.

"The report also reveals really bizarre Chinese government behaviour manifested directly from the very top of the Chinese public health authorities to the Wuhan Institute of Virology leadership team. The entire Chinese government system, including all agencies of public security, public health, state media and science research institutions, all acted as if they were hiding something big and became absolutely knee-jerk about any mention of possible lab leaks.

"Secretary Pompeo took a great interest in this. I produced a lot of evidence, all the possible things I could find, so the discovery of that Chinese CDC documentary [that showed scientists becoming infected with blood from bats] as well as the peculiar behaviour of the WIV raised my suspicion."

In addition to the open-source and Chinese-language material Yu had unearthed, Pompeo had access to classified information and top-secret documents from intelligence agencies. Eventually, towards the end of April, Pompeo felt there was enough circumstantial evidence to warrant a discussion about whether the American public should be informed that the Wuhan laboratory was a possible origin of the virus.

It was a careful line between not withholding information from America, and not forerunning any investigation. Yu was cautious. "That's why when he [Pompeo] went on air, he made a statement urging the Chinese government to open up, to find out what the truth is. He's been saying that all along," Yu says.

One senior official credits the Secretary of State for leading the way in pushing for an investigation into the Wuhan laboratories when there was so much resistance to it. "Pompeo deserves an enormous amount of credit. No advice, no dossier matters if he doesn't follow through," one advisor said. "If you didn't have a Secretary of State who was willing to put himself out there, none of it would have happened."

On April 15, Trump confirmed there was an investigation into whether Covid-19 had leaked from a laboratory. At the daily coronavirus pandemic press conference, he was asked by Fox News reporter John Roberts about reports that multiple government sources had said a naturally occurring virus had leaked from a virology lab in Wuhan where there were lax safety protocols. "Well, I don't want to say that, John, but I will tell you, more and more, we're hearing the story and we'll say, multiple sources, that's a case where you can use the word sources, we're doing a very thorough examination of this horrible situation that happened," he said. For Trump, this was fairly benign and calm language.

That same day, Pompeo told Fox News, "What we do know is we know that this virus originated in Wuhan, China. We know there is the Wuhan Institute of Virology just a handful of miles away from where the wet market was. There is still lots to learn. You should know that the United States government is working diligently to figure it out."

On April 30, Trump was asked by a reporter if he had seen anything that gave him "a high degree of confidence that the Wuhan Institute of Virology was the origin of this virus?"

Trump responded, "Yes I have, and I think that the World Heath Organization should be ashamed of themselves, because they're like the public relations agency for China. This country pays them almost $500 million a year and China pays them $38 million a year, and whether it's a lot, or more, doesn't matter, but still, they shouldn't be making excuses when people make horrible mistakes."

He was then asked, "Maybe you have evidence this was not a naturally occurring virus?"

The President responded, "We're going to see where it is, we're going to see where it comes from and you know every theory, the theory from the lab, you had the theory from the bats, and the type of bat and the bat is 40 miles away so it couldn't have been here and it couldn't have been there. There's a lot of theories but yeah we have people looking at it very, very strongly, scientific people. Intelligence."

Asked what gives him a high degree of confidence that this originated from the Wuhan Institute of Virology, the President said, "I can't tell you that."

Pompeo, not mentioning the Wuhan Institute of Virology by name, said on May 3 that there was "enormous evidence" that the virus began in a laboratory. When pressed, he could not divulge the specifics. "I can tell you that there is a significant amount of evidence that this came from that laboratory in Wuhan," he said.

Then on May 6, Pompeo continued to alert the public to the possibility the virus had escaped from a laboratory. "You should know that the US government is working diligently to figure this out. We really need the Chinese government to open up. They say they want to cooperate. One of the best ways they could find to cooperate would be to let the world in, to let the world's scientists know exactly how this came to be, exactly how this virus began to spread."

The backlash to these comments from Pompeo and Trump was fierce. The laboratory origin was called a debunked conspiracy theory and the administration was soundly criticised for making the claim that there was enormous evidence the virus had come from the laboratory. Hostile media commentators and political opponents ridiculed them and demanded they produce evidence to support their claims. The attitude from the mainstream media outlets was that they were making it all up.

CHAPTER ELEVEN

The Cables

MARCH 2018, BEIJING, CHINA

It's late March 2018 and US career diplomat Rick Switzer has just flown home to Beijing after a trip to Wuhan. Along with his colleague, US Consul-General to Wuhan Jamie Fouss, he'd led a delegation of American environmental, science, technology and health consular staff to inspect the Wuhan Institute of Virology, where he'd met with 'batwoman' Shi Zhengli.

It was two years before a pandemic would arise from that very city – perhaps even that very laboratory – and he was deeply concerned about what he saw during his visit. The consular official at the US Embassy in Beijing tapped out a "Sensitive but Unclassified" cable to send back to the State Department. He needed to let Washington know just what was going on inside China's new level-4 biocontainment facility dealing with the world's deadliest and most contagious pathogens. The cable warned of poor safety practices at the laboratory.

Switzer pressed send on the cable two weeks later, on April 19, 2018, with the subject line: "China Virus Institute Welcomes More US Co-operation on Global Health Security". It was an unusual choice of email subject, because the contents of his cable outlined how the opposite was true. The laboratory, built on the condition

127

of international collaboration, was severely limiting the number of international researchers who could work inside its walls.

The Wuhan Institute of Virology level-4 lab had originally been built in conjunction with the Jean Mérieux BSL-4 Laboratory in Lyon, France. It was to be China's first high-containment laboratory under the direction of the Chinese Academy of Sciences, which is under People's Liberation Army control. Construction of the laboratory began in 2004 and took 11 years to complete, finally finishing on January 31, 2015. The project cost US$44 million. It is a vast building, with four floors stretching over 300 square metres (32,000 square feet). It was accredited in February 2017 by the China National Accreditation Service for Conformity Assessment, and began working on live viruses by 2018.

There were "intense clashes" between the French and Chinese parties during the construction phase, according to a Chinese Academy of Sciences video. It was far from a smooth process. Even before the deal was signed, there was strong objection in France to cooperating on such a laboratory in Wuhan, but the scientists advocating for the collaboration won.

Once the laboratory was up and running, the French were soon kicked out. While the initial funding, training and construction was in conjunction with the French, according to Switzer and Fouss's cable, "it is entirely China-funded and has been completely China-run since a 'handover' ceremony in 2016". And despite being built in the name of international scientific collaboration, few international researchers were welcome to work inside the facility. "Institute officials said there would be 'limited availability' for international and domestic scientists who had gone through the necessary approval process to do research at the lab," the cable states.

The cable indicated the French were unhappy with this. "A Wuhan-based French Consulate official who works on science and technology cooperation with China also emphasised that the lab, which was initiated in 2004 as a France–China joint project, was meant to be 'open and transparent' to the global scientific community. The intent was to set up a lab to international standards, and open to international research," it said.

So a laboratory working with the most lethal pathogens known to humankind had effectively cut off collaboration with the international community. Multiple US and UK government sources tell me the French government was furious. Former head of British intelligence service MI6 Sir Richard Dearlove, who spent a good deal of his career in France, speaks fluent French and maintains intelligence contacts there, says, "They were really fed up with the Chinese reneging on the deal over that laboratory. It was meant to be based on the international cooperation between the two countries."

A former member of a French presidential commission on defence and security, Francois Heisbourg, also confirms this, saying former President of France Jacques Chirac signed off on the collaboration with China "and it should have been collaborative but at the conclusion of building the lab the French were thrown out".

What made this particularly alarming was the work the laboratory was conducting. Disturbingly, Switzer and Fouss discovered the laboratory was setting up its very own database identifying all deadly viruses with pandemic potential. It would be its own version of a concept called the Global Virome Project (GVP), the cable stated. "The GVP aims to launch this year as an international collaborative effort to identify within 10 years virtually all of the planet's viruses that have pandemic or epidemic potential and the ability to jump to humans," the cable read.

The cable quoted a Wuhan Institute of Virology official saying, "We hope China will be one of the leading countries to initiate the Global Virome Project." But in the meantime, the WIV official told Switzer and Fouss that they were already running a similar project of their own. "The officials said that the Chinese government funds projects similar to GVP to investigate the background of viruses and bacteria," the cable stated. "This essentially constituted China's own Virome Project, officials said, but they noted the program currently has no official name."

The US State Department has redacted part of the next sentence of the cable, but the words that remain are as follows: "The Wuhan Institute of Virology ... is the ... which is designed to show 'proof of concept' and be a forerunner to the Global Virome Project ... with the EcoHealth Alliance". The cable noted that other countries "are skeptical on whether China could remain transparent as a 'gatekeeper' for keeping this information." In other words, the EcoHealth Alliance, an animal-sampling group based in New York, was working with the Wuhan Institute of Virology on developing an extensive database of deadly viruses.

This revelation – of such a database being developed by a laboratory where the US had no oversight – should have been highly alarming at the time. Except it's unclear whether anybody with any level of seniority ever read this cable after it was sent to the State Department and intelligence apparatus in Washington.

The cable also makes clear the extent of the United States involvement with the Wuhan Institute of Virology. "In the last year, the institute has also hosted visits from the National Institutes of Health (NIH), National Science Foundation and experts from the University of Texas Medical Branch in Galveston." It said the Galveston branch had trained the Wuhan lab technicians in lab management and maintenance while the US National Science Foundation had just concluded a workshop with the Wuhan Institute in Shenzhen involving 40 scientists from the United States and China.

It also made clear – at this early stage – how America was funding the coronavirus research at the Wuhan lab. "NIH was a major funder, along with the National Science Foundation of China, of SARS research by the Wuhan Institute of Virology," the cable states. The paragraphs that follow it are redacted.

It wasn't the first cable the US Embassy in Beijing had fired off to Washington about the Wuhan Institute of Virology. The subject of an earlier cable, dated January 19, 2018, stated that the institute had "a serious shortage of appropriately trained technicians and investigators needed to safely operate this high-containment laboratory".

This cable detailed the work the laboratory was doing on coronaviruses, into SARS and bats. It also made clear that US government funding was supporting this risky research through the EcoHealth Alliance, the NIH, the United States Agency for International Development (USAID) and the National Science Foundation. It says that over a five-year study, the Wuhan Institute of Virology "widely sampled bats in Yunnan province with funding support from NIAID [National Institute of Allergy and Infectious Diseases]/NIH, USAID, and several Chinese funding agencies."

This cable warned that the "WIV leadership now considers the lab operational and ready for research on class-four pathogens, among which are the most virulent viruses that pose a high risk of aerosolised person-to-person transmission."

In another revelation, the cables spell out that the Wuhan Institute of Virology was doing research on coronaviruses, including how the deadly virus transmits from bats to humans. "Most importantly, the researchers also showed that various SARS-like coronaviruses can interact with ACE2, the human receptor identified for SARS coronavirus. This finding strongly suggests that SARS-like coronaviruses from bats can be transmitted to humans to cause SARS-like disease."

A report about Switzer and Fouss's visit featured on the Wuhan Institute of Virology's website, along with a photograph of them standing with Shi Zhengli and other scientists. The report stated that American organisations, including the National Science Foundation, EcoHealth Alliance, the University of Texas Medical Branch and the Galveston National Laboratory, are "major strategic partners" with the Wuhan laboratories.

Switzer and Fouss had tried to visit the Wuhan Institute of Virology twice in three years, before they eventually gained access.

"The Consulate had twice in the past three years made official requests by DipNote to visit the lab, both of which were rejected," states documents obtained by the US Right to Know group under the *Freedom of Information Act*. The Wuhan Institute of Virology also cancelled a coffee meeting to discuss the visit with the US

Consulate in December 2017. This followed the Institute cancelling an invitation for Consular Chief Terry Mobley to attend a tourism conference on Sunday, December 10 at 11pm the night before. Earlier in the year, in January, Fouss had planned to speak at a joint "Sino–US Energy and Environment Forum" but "the organisers postponed the event from October until December 4–5, when the CG was on leave." When the US Consulate told them another official would attend in his place, the reply came back just one day before the forum that the two diplomats were uninvited, claiming they needed one month's notice to get permission to invite diplomats to the event and it was too late.

"When the Wuhan CG attempted to directly complain to the Huanan FAO director, who had just a few weeks earlier hosted him for lunch, the Huanan FAO's Yang Qi told Consulate staff the director was 'busy these days'. Calls to the cell and office numbers on the FAO director's business card went unanswered."

These cancellations should have raised concerns about the secretive nature of the Wuhan Institute of Virology, along with questions about why United States agencies like the NIH were funding research at a laboratory that officials had no oversight or access to.

When the cables were sent back to Washington, they went to the State Department and the NSC. The NSC, the President's forum for national security and foreign policy matters, has been around since President Truman. The officials say if they could turn back time, and dig those cables out and demand action, they would. But they slipped unnoticed amid the thousands of other cables coming in.

If the cables didn't make their way to the desk of NSC officials, they certainly didn't come to the attention of then NSA director Mike Rogers. The NSA is the top-secret intelligence agency responsible for global monitoring and data collection for foreign and domestic intelligence, specialising in signals intelligence. Rogers never saw the cables. He didn't even know of their existence until they emerged in the wake of the pandemic. "While there were certainly concerns expressed in some areas, I don't remember this getting to a red-flag level where the senior-most leadership was focusing on this," he tells me. "It's the country team reporting on activities within their area which they think the broader community should be aware of, but you can tell from the tone they're not written to elicit a red flag to say, 'Hey look we've really got a fundamental problem here.'"

It seems Switzer and Fouss's warning was a waste of time. Nothing was done. Instead, unbeknown to most in the Trump administration, funding continued to flow from American taxpayers through to the Wuhan Institute of Virology for its risky research genetically manipulating bat coronaviruses.

Two years later, in the months after the pandemic, the cables were finally dredged out during the US State Department investigation into the origins of the pandemic and the Wuhan Institute of Virology. They landed on Pompeo's desk. "I learned of the cables sometime in early 2020. I was unhappy that I had not seen the cables previously," Pompeo tells me. "I immediately asked the team to go validate the cables, talk to the person who wrote the cables, make sure we understood what they said, what they didn't say, what the basis of knowledge was. Cables are what they are, they are communications."

During this period of validation, Pompeo did not want the cables released. He was concerned they may be misleading to the American public if they claimed to show there were safety concerns at the Wuhan Institute of Virology that were not, in fact, substantiated. Or, if they claimed to show that the Institute was doing risky research on bat coronaviruses and how they infect humans via ACE2 receptors, if that wasn't unusual.

He needed to be certain exactly how much substance was behind the cables before he thrust them into the public domain in what would surely be a powerful statement.

"The person writing them was not himself a virologist so I wanted to make sure we could validate the facts that were in the cables," Pompeo says.

"The moment I was confident that we had our act together and we knew what we knew and we knew what we didn't know, I was working my tail off to get that information released to the public as fast as I possibly could. There was a pause, once I had seen the cables, there was a pause for a couple or three weeks to go do our homework, and from that moment forward I was advocating for the release of those cables as quickly as we could get them declassified."

One would imagine, as Secretary of State, it would be a matter of deciding what information should be declassified and then releasing it. But it wasn't so simple. Ultimately, the sole decision to declassify the cables did not fall to Pompeo. I asked him who would possibly say no to him releasing information. His response was careful. "Some of the information isn't just ours, it's an interagency process," he said.

News of the cables broke in Josh Rogin's weekly *Washington Post* column on April 14, 2020. He wrote in his global scoop, "The cables warned about safety and management weaknesses at the WIV lab and proposed more attention and help. The first cable, which I obtained, also warns that the lab's work on bat coronaviruses and their potential human transmission represented a risk of a new SARS-like pandemic." They were later released under a Freedom of Information lawsuit by the paper, but parts remained redacted.

Even writing about the cables, and suggesting that the Wuhan Institute of Virology may not have followed adequate safety procedures, saw Rogin suffer blowback. He was not dissuaded by the pressure, including from his own peers, and has been one of the only English-speaking journalists internationally to consistently investigate a potential laboratory leak from early 2020, when it was unfashionable to do so, along with UK journalist Ian Birrell, the *Washington Times*'s Bill Gertz, investigative reporter Alison Young, me and several others. Science writer Nicholson Baker did a thorough piece looking at the science for *New York* magazine's Intelligencer in late 2020; and Nicholas Wade's May 2021 article, originally on *Medium*, played a crucial role in changing the public narrative when Trump was no longer in office.

American journalists and others around the world were determined to debunk anything the Trump administration raised, turning genuine reporting of facts into a partisan political exercise. Other journalists were captured by compromised scientists with abundant pre-existing relationships with China, who insisted any question of a laboratory leak was "misinformation", or who were not prepared to weather the storm of being publicly labelled a conspiracy theorist.

Journalists who investigated the Wuhan Institute of Virology, even simply reporting that intelligence agencies were making inquiries about the matter, were ridiculed, humiliated and shamed by other media outlets.

Birrell, who is known for fighting battles across the political spectrum, says he was surprised so many of the journalists investigating the origins of SARS-CoV-2 were largely ignored or dismissed for more than a year into the pandemic. "It fascinates me how so many people in our profession just accepted the word of clearly conflicted scientists or presumed that Trump saying something made it wrong," he said. "This has been such a failure of journalism, as well as science and some leading medical journals, which is why the rather lonely efforts of a few select journalists stood out."

CHAPTER TWELVE

A Failure to Investigate

APRIL 2020, AUSTRALIA

It was 9am on the second-last Sunday in April when Australia's Foreign Minister Marise Payne went on Australian national television to call for an investigation into the origins of Covid-19. It was left to the most senior woman in Australia's Cabinet to calmly utter words deemed so incendiary by China they would spark rolling retaliatory trade tariffs and export bans.

"It's fundamental that we identify, we determine an independent review mechanism to examine the development of this epidemic, its development into a pandemic, the crisis that is occurring internationally," Payne said on the public broadcaster. "We need to know the sorts of details that an independent review would identify for us about the genesis of the virus, about the approaches to dealing with it, and addressing it, about the openness with which information was shared, about interaction with the World Health Organization, interaction with other international leaders. All of those sorts of things will need to be on the table."

It was an action Australian Prime Minister Scott Morrison took while other world leaders were besieged with the crippling health crisis within their own borders. Australia had recovered relatively early after shutting its borders and enforcing two-week hotel quarantine for returning citizens. Senior sources tell me that Morrison and Mike Pompeo had spoken before the Payne interview about the need for an investigation into the origins of Covid-19. Payne had also spoken to other international counterparts.

Morrison and Pompeo hold the same view of China's culpability for the outbreak of Covid-19. The two men are close, sharing many of the same values and beliefs. Their relationship extended beyond politics; they had become friends and were in regular contact. They still are.

Their senior national security and intelligence officials share close relationships, too. The head of Australia's Office of National Intelligence, Andrew Shearer, is a long-time friend of then Trump Deputy National Security Advisor Matt Pottinger, and they had numerous, lengthy conversations in an official capacity about the evidence surrounding a laboratory leak and the origins of Covid-19.

The official Australian and British analysis in 2020 was more circumspect than the view from some parts of the American intelligence community. In terms of calling for an inquiry publicly, there was no formal agreement before Payne's interview, but the US was happy to let one of the Five Eyes allies take the lead; it would be taken more seriously by the international community, whereas if Trump had made the call it would have been dismissed as racist. It also helped the US frame the crisis as a free world versus tyranny issue – rather than simply a battle between China and America, which the origins of Covid-19 were absolutely not.

Indicating this had been a discussion point with foreign leaders globally, Payne added in that interview on April 19, "The international community wants the same thing."

Asked by Australian Broadcasting Corporation (ABC) host David Speers if the leader of the investigation "could be the World Health Organization, or do you agree they're too beholden to China?" Payne dismissed the notion of the WHO conducting the inquiry. "Well, I don't think that it is so much about whether they are or are not beholden to China. And we share some of the concerns that the United States have identified in relation to the World Health

Organization. That is certainly correct," she said. Payne said the idea of the health body "responsible for disseminating much of the international communications material" also acting as the "review mechanism"… "strikes me as somewhat poacher and gamekeeper".

At that point, Morrison wanted an inquiry with more teeth, where health inspectors could automatically go into a host country to investigate, similar to the powers held by the International Atomic Energy Agency. He even made the comparison to a weapons inspector.

After Payne's comments, Morrison wrote to the G20 nations, formally pitching a review into the pandemic response. "What's really important is that we have a proper review, an independent review, which looks into the sources of these things in a transparent way so we can learn the lessons," he said.

Australia's Defence Minister Peter Dutton says that at the time "there was enough suspicion" about a potential laboratory origin, although the formal advice provided to government said zoonotic (animal-to-human) transmission was more likely. "There was a desire from Australia to know more about the origin so that we could respond appropriately and so that science could be properly understood, and that our response to it could be more effective," Dutton tells me.

For this standard, benign call for an inquiry into the origins of Covid-19, Australia was subjected to horrific economic coercion by Beijing. China's aggressive response included punishing Australia with trade sanctions. Beijing slapped high tariffs on or banned Australian barley, beef, cotton, wine, timber and lobster exports.

The situation on the ground in China became untenable for Australian journalists. Cheng Lei, an Australian television presenter at China Global Television Network, disappeared, wiped from the state broadcaster's website. Her family and friends had no contact with her and diplomats were only granted access two weeks after Australia was finally notified she had been detained under "residential surveillance". This form of detention can involve interrogation, torture and isolation. Six months later she was finally charged, and in February 2021 Lei was arrested on the suspicion of illegally supplying state secrets.

Australia's Department of Foreign Affairs and Trade quietly warned media organisations their journalists were no longer safe on the streets of China. Two of the remaining Australian journalists were subjected to an intimidating midnight visit by Chinese authorities, and their departure from China involved protracted negotiations over five days. Australian media companies now have no reporters on the ground in mainland China.

It's clear China used the pandemic to its strategic advantage in the region. "The whole thing has massively played into Chinese hands and it's very disturbing, particularly in a country like Australia, where you're on the Pacific rim and the other main occupant on the Pacific rim is China," former MI6 chief Sir Richard Dearlove said in an interview for this book. "If you look at the consequences for the Chinese state of what's happened, if they wanted to accelerate their success internationally and their domination of their main opponent countries, they couldn't have done it more effectively. Look at what's happening in India. Look at what it has done to the US economy, and it's clear that authoritarian states are better equipped to control their population in the face of a pandemic because they can immediately institute controls which the population don't question."

Despite the mounting pressure, Australian politicians held firm and continued to strongly call for an international inquiry into the origins of Covid-19 that would look specifically at the possibility of a laboratory leak. The Chair of the Parliamentary Joint Committee on Intelligence and Security, Senator James Paterson, said an independent international investigation was essential. "The only question is whether the Chinese Communist Party cooperates with it or not," he told me at the time. "There is no valid reason why they shouldn't. But if they don't, they will be harshly judged for it by the entire international community."

His predecessor, now Assistant Minister for Defence, former SAS Commander Andrew Hastie, agreed, saying, "We have to be open-minded about all possibilities. We can't rush to any sort of judgement; we should have an open mind and an open mind is for closing." Asked why he thinks large swathes of the left-wing media were intent on excluding the possibility that Covid-19 may have leaked from a laboratory, he said, "Politics it seems is everywhere, including in the media. As far as I'm concerned we should be open-minded and we shouldn't jump to conclusions, so let's hope this issue isn't weaponised any further and we get to the bottom of it."

Former Ambassador to Israel Dave Sharma, now an Australian federal politician, said both the origins and handling of the outbreak needed to be investigated, and that "there's a conceivable chance it came from a virology lab. I envisage something like a world eminent-person's panel, like the former Prime Minister of Spain and former head of the WHO. It should be not a score-settling exercise, but as part of that there would inevitably be findings of fault, and I suspect several of those will land at China's feet."

But the investigation that took place would be nothing of the sort Australia had envisioned. It would be a whitewash by the WHO, which had appointed investigators with fully formed views about the origins of the virus.

By the first week of May, while Pompeo was pointing towards a potential laboratory leak, Australian intelligence agencies were growing increasingly uneasy with these claims. The central concern emerging from the Australian government and its security agencies was that the US might be putting undue emphasis on the theory that the virus originated in a Wuhan laboratory.

In an extraordinary comparison, one senior Australian federal source told me at the time there were emerging fears in the intelligence community that the US administration could be repeating the mistakes made by George W. Bush and Tony Blair when they pressured the UN weapons inspector to declare Saddam Hussein possessed weapons of mass destruction. The story ran under my by-line on the front page of Australia's *Daily Telegraph*. A split in the Five Eyes intelligence agencies was news.

Their fears were realised. As with weapons of mass destruction, the intelligence was wrong. But it was wrong not because of the undue emphasis that it came from a lab but because of the undue emphasis that it came from a wet market. The advice the Office of National Intelligence would release publicly – in a rare statement on April 30 – would prove to be false.

Former NSA Director Mike Rogers rejects the notion that the intelligence community was politicised and also strongly dismisses the idea that Trump may have in any way instructed the intelligence agencies. "I worked with President Trump and I never once had him talk to me about what the priorities of my organisation should be, what I should or should not do from an intelligence perspective," he says. "I knew President Trump and he would tell me he was in a different place on Russia than I was, but I would always tell him, 'Sir, my job is to provide you our assessments, and what you choose to do with them and if you agree or disagree with them is your call, what you believe is your right, but we'll continue to make those assessments.'"

Despite the bureaucratic angst, Morrison, senior Cabinet ministers and national security figures privately agreed with Pompeo. They didn't publicise their personal views to avoid further inflaming tensions with China, instead allowing the official investigation to take its course. The US Ambassador to Australia, Arthur B. Culvahouse Jr, said as much publicly. He told me at the time that the origins of the outbreak needed to be investigated, adding that the phone call between Donald Trump and Scott Morrison on April 22 showed there is "no daylight" between the US and Australia's position on a probe. "I commend Foreign Minister Payne and her call for a hard, dispassionate look at the origins of the epidemic," he said. "This isn't about pointing fingers. It is about what could have been done better to prevent the disease, communicate its existence and prevent it from becoming a global pandemic."

But every word Australia utters is closely examined by China. It meant Morrison and Defence Minister Peter Dutton did not have the freedom to say precisely what they thought. A sentence as innocent as a call for an inquiry into the origins of the virus had set off rolling tariffs, hurting businesses and families. Morrison's language in public is careful.

While the end goal of holding China accountable is consistent, the schism between the US executives' position on China's culpability for the outbreak and the Australian intelligence agencies also put Morrison in an awkward position.

Disease-ridden exotic animals at unhygienic wet markets in China were blamed at first for the outbreak of Covid-19. Governments globally called for a ban on wet markets. Soon, the notion that the virus had emerged in a wet market looked less credible and came under intense scrutiny.

Scientific studies as early as January 2020 had ruled out the wet market as the source of the virus – and even Chinese officials admitted by May that this was not where the virus originated. The Huanan Seafood Wholesale Market was closed on January 1, 2020, and disinfected. Any evidence that may have gone towards proving its link to the outbreak was permanently destroyed. Wet market stalls were bleached and animals were killed.

Chinese scientists "prospectively" collected and analysed data, in a study published in *The Lancet* on January 24, 2020, on the clinical features of early patients who had been infected with Covid-19. "The symptom onset date of the first patient identified was Dec 1, 2019." This first patient had no epidemiological link to later cases. They found that only 27 of the 41 patients had direct exposure to Huanan Seafood Market.

As early as January 2020, Chinese officials knew the wet market was unlikely to be the source of the virus.

Just as significant as this *Lancet* study were comments made by the Chinese Centre for Disease Control Director Gao Fu, who said the wet market helped spread the virus but was not the original source of the outbreak. This is an important point. When asked in an email interview by *Science* in March 2020 whether he thought the seafood market was a likely place of origin or an amplifying factor but not the source, he replied, "That's a very good question. You are working like a detective. From the very beginning, everybody thought the origin was the market. Now, I think the market could be the initial place, or it could be a place where the virus was amplified. So that's a scientific question. There are two possibilities."

In a separate interview with CCP propaganda outlet the Global Times two months later, in May 2020, Gao said samples collected from animals in the market in early January did not contain traces of the coronavirus, which were only found in sewage. "At first, we assumed the seafood market might have the virus, but now the market is more like a victim," he said. "The novel coronavirus had existed long before." This was an extraordinary statement from a leading member of the Chinese health and scientific community.

Other scientific papers also distanced the original outbreak from the wet market. Former Stanford University School of Medicine professor Dr Steven Quay authored a paper in October 2020 titled: "Where Did the 2019 Coronavirus Pandemic Begin and How Did It Spread?" In it, he said the Huanan Seafood Market "has been ruled out as the source, although it became an early case cluster".

He investigated the Wuhan Metro System Line 2, which services the Wuhan Institute of Virology, the major hospitals and the wet market. "At this point, the local wet market, farmed animals in Hubei province, indigenous bats in Hubei province, and the rare, endangered pangolin have all been considered but ultimately ruled out by Chinese scientists and the Chinese CDC," he said.

Bats were not sold at Wuhan's wet market. When the virus broke out, videos went viral showing Chinese people eating bat soup. It was all nonsense and was completely unrelated to the Huanan Seafood Market. It's a point the University of Hamburg's Roland Wiesendanger makes in his February 2021 paper. "Bats were not offered for sale at the suspected fish market in the center of Wuhan city. However, the Wuhan City Virological Institute has one of the world's largest collections of bat pathogens, which originated from distant caves in southern Chinese provinces," he said. "It is extremely unlikely that bats from this distance of nearly 2,000 km would have naturally made their way to Wuhan, only to cause a global pandemic in close proximity to this virological institute."

Another scientific paper by the Broad Institute of MIT and Harvard and the University of British Columbia, still awaiting peer review, stated that there is currently no evidence to show that the coronavirus originated in the wet market – or anywhere, for that matter. "There has been considerable debate among scientists and the public on whether SARS-CoV-2 originated from the Wuhan Huanan Seafood Market," the paper states. "However, phylogenetic tracking suggests that SARS-CoV-2 had been imported into the market by humans."

The WHO report, when it was eventually released in 2021, would also find no evidence that the wet market was the source of the virus. "Environmental sampling in the Huanan market demonstrated widespread contamination of surfaces with SARS-CoV-2, compatible with the virus shedding from infected people in the market at the end of December 2019," it states. "However, through extensive testing of animal products in the market, no evidence of animal infections was found."

China's search for an animal source or intermediary has been exhaustive. "Sampling and testing of 38,515 livestock and poultry samples and 41,696 wild animal samples from 31 provinces in China during 2018 to 2020 resulted in no positive SARS-CoV-2 antibody or nucleic acid tests," the WHO report states. "No evidence was found of circulation of SARS-CoV-2 among domestic livestock, poultry and wild animals before and after the SARS-CoV-2 outbreak in China."

But one of the WHO team who went into China, EcoHealth Alliance's Peter Daszak, who has worked with Shi Zhengli for 15 years and calls a lab leak a "conspiracy theory", thinks the virus could still have emerged at the wet market. He argues that China's initial investigation was incomplete. "People don't realise how sensitive China is about this," he said in a May 2021 media interview with Kaiser Health News. "It's plausible that they recognised there were cases going out of a market and they shut it down."

Monash University Senior Lecturer in Chinese Studies Dr Kevin Carrico was living in China in 2002 and 2003 as a graduate student during the first SARS outbreak. "There was a massive cover-up of SARS in 2002 and 2003, but when that passed, the way the Chinese state handled potential animal sources really contrasts quite markedly with the way that they've responded to Covid-19," he says.

"Throughout 2003, 2004 and even into 2005 one would regularly see reports in Chinese media about the mass culling of civet cats in Guangdong province, where these cats are in certain contexts served as some type of delicacy at banquets or other settings." Dr Carrico recalls a "very, very proactive approach to eliminating potential animal sources of the SARS virus." It's an approach the CCP has not taken since Covid-19.

"What has made me very suspicious about the way the Chinese state has responded to Covid-19 is that there doesn't seem to be any of that anxiety or urgency about animal sources that we saw after SARS," he says. "We haven't seen that type of proactive approach, and instead we've seen a certain casualness about these animal sources, which would suggest the Chinese Party state knows where this virus comes from and as a result isn't all that worried about the virus leaping from animals to humans again."

Trump's National Security Advisor Robert O'Brien said both the wet markets and the virology laboratories in China are public health dangers to the world, and so whether Covid-19 came from the one or the other is "almost immaterial". "Most of the evidence suggests that the supposed carrier bats were 1000 miles away, so the lab leak looks more credible," he said.

Former NSC official in the Clinton administration Jamie Metzl, who is a current serving member of a WHO committee on genetic engineering, agrees the wet market is an unlikely source of the outbreak. "We know that the backbone virus in SARS-CoV-2 is a horseshoe bat coronavirus," he explains. "Those horseshoe bats live in southern China. Wuhan is well beyond their range. Wuhan doesn't have horseshoe bats. This pandemic began in the middle of winter. But what Wuhan does have is China's only level-4 virology institute, with the world's largest collection of bat coronaviruses, that was doing aggressive gain-of-function research, including to make those highly pathogenic viruses more transmissible to human cells. We know that when the outbreak began, the SARS-CoV-2 virus was almost perfectly adapted for transmission to humans."

In June 2020, frustrated with the WHO's failure to conduct any sort of genuine inquiry into the origins, Donald Trump announced America would withdraw funding from the organisation. There was no pre-determined plan to make this announcement at that time. It was an impulsive move. Trump had planned to give a speech in the Rose Garden on the afternoon of June 3 but, according to sources familiar with the events that unfolded, he thought it was "a bit meh" and needed to be stronger.

The shock announcement was met with international outrage, particularly from the Europeans. Australia agreed with the Trump administration's concerns about the WHO's handling of the Covid-19 outbreak but felt it was better to stay within the organisation and try to exert influence that way.

America's Ambassador to Geneva Andrew Bremberg, who was blindsided by Trump's move, held an urgent meeting with Tedros on June 4 to try to get the relationship back on track. His plan was to get Tedros to agree to a list of demands Bremberg could take to Trump to show the WHO was willing to work towards finding the origins of the virus and ensuring transparency from China. He had run the list by ambassadors from several US allies first, and felt he had their support.

At the meeting in Tedros's Geneva office, on the Saturday morning of June 4, was Bremberg, Tedros's Chief of Staff Bernhard Schwartländer and the WHO's Health Emergencies Programme Executive Director, Michael Ryan.

It would be an excruciating meeting.

They went item by item through the list Bremberg had first given him on May 29. It included the WHO asking China for live virus samples, ensuring that countries that contributed heavily to the WHO were proportionally represented on the organisation's staff and correcting the advice on travel restrictions during the pandemic.

"It was the most painful experience," Bremberg recalls. Tedros would indicate he supported an item, so Bremberg would say, "Great, can we do it?" And Tedros would reply, "Well, no, not exactly" and vacillate.

As the hours dragged on, Bremberg tried to incentivise Tedros to reach a compromise. "You need to tell me what you can agree to," Bremberg implored Tedros. "If you want to say July instead of June for starting the independent panel, just tell me."

Tedros, proud by nature and hurt by the President's criticism of his leadership, did not want to be seen to be caving into America's demands. "I can't commit to starting by June or July," he allegedly said to Bremberg.

"What about an interim report by November?" Bremberg asked.

"No, that would throw into question the independence of the WHO, because it would be at the same time as an assembly," Tedros said.

This was an unbelievable excuse.

It became apparent to Bremberg that Schwartländer in particular seemed to have little appetite to strike a deal. He felt that Schwartländer was "pulling Tedros back from getting to yes" and frustrating the process. "It was four hours of a run-around," Bremberg says. All those hours of intense negotiation later, Bremberg left the meeting without reaching an agreement on a single point. He walked away with nothing. He was disappointed.

Both Tedros and Schwartländer personally have a long-term relationship with the Chinese government. Six weeks after Tedros's appointment to the role of Director-General of the WHO on July 1, he led the WHO delegation to the Belt and Road Forum for health cooperation. The partnership between the WHO and the Belt and Road Initiative pre-dated Tedros's time at the organisation and was originally signed under former WHO Director-General Margaret Chan.

Standing in a photograph to mark the Belt and Road forum is Schwartländer. Since 2013, he had been the WHO Representative to China, and before that he worked as the United Nations Country Coordinator on AIDS in Beijing. Schwartländer also appears in a

2015 photograph to mark AIDS prevention with Chinese President Xi Jinping's wife, Peng Liyuan, who is a "goodwill ambassador" for the WHO.

Schwartländer praised China's First Lady in an interview with Guangming News in 2017, saying she had "made a remarkable effort and service for public health. It's just remarkable and so important. She is a role model for me and other people all around the world." Inexplicably, he praised China's health leadership during the pandemic, in an October 2020 interview in the Global Times. "He said in particular during this Covid-19 pandemic, China has been able to 'really help' some of the poorest nations who didn't have access to the basic tools to fight the disease," the Global Times reported.

Since 2015, Schwartländer has supported and attended many events promoting Traditional Chinese Medicine, which Xi Jinping endorsed as a cure to Covid-19 during the pandemic, including in his conversations with Trump. Journalists have criticised the WHO's support for traditional Chinese medicine. There is nothing wrong with WHO officials cooperating with China, of course; it is to be expected. But this is a problem if the WHO leadership is beholden or too close to the Chinese government to ensure transparency during a pandemic. It's telling, for example, that Australia declared a pandemic a full fortnight before the WHO did.

From the very time Tedros ran for election for the position of WHO Director-General, he was sympathetic to China, Pompeo tells me. "The upshot of the election that was held for Dr Tedros to become the leader of the WHO put Dr Tedros in a place where he was under the thumb of the Chinese Communist Party, and the capacity to influence his behaviour was very significant as a result of the way his election proceeded," he says.

Pompeo's Senior Policy Advisor Mary Kissel confirms Trump's withdrawal from the WHO "wasn't part of the script that day". "That was the President's prerogative to do that and in hindsight it looks courageous and prescient because the more we learn about China's behaviour inside other international organisations, the more worrisome it becomes," she says. "It's not enough to say we're going to hold them to account. Rhetoric is one thing, action is another. We need real cooperation so the world doesn't face another one of these killer pandemics."

Kissel says China's manipulation of the WHO started far before this current pandemic. "We confronted a very difficult problem, namely what do you do when a member of an important multilateral organisation simply refuses to follow the rules that it signed up to follow and then lies about it?" Kissel says. "If we don't have a way to eject said member from the organisation, what do you do? We really wrestled with that problem. It's not an easy problem to solve."

AUGUST 2020, THE WHITE HOUSE

Sitting in his office in the White House, with enough of a stockpile of hydroxychloroquine to last the entire Trump family a lifetime, Navarro rang Pompeo excitedly. He had an idea and wanted to pitch it to the Secretary of State. "We need to have a Presidential Commission," came his gravelly drawl down the line. "We had a Presidential Commission for Pearl Harbor, for the BP oil spill and for the Kennedy assassination. We need one into the origins of the coronavirus as well."

Pompeo loved it and backed it. As the months had rolled on, it had become apparent there was no specific agency or individual in the White House charged with overseeing an investigation into the origins of the virus. There was no central unit to which people like Pottinger or Miles Yu could send new information. There were also many academics and scientists on US soil who potentially held crucial information relating to the Wuhan Institute of Virology. Very clearly, there needed to be an inquiry. "There was actually no government agency to coordinate it," Yu says. "The only person at the White House who actually tried to put everything together was Peter Navarro."

After getting the tick of approval from Pompeo, Navarro devoted his energy to developing the concept and draft terms of reference. There would be three main areas of focus: firstly, investigating the origins of the virus; secondly, calculating how much damage the virus had caused to the United States economy – and working out how to claim the reparations; and thirdly, finding out whether China was exploiting the virus for its political and military advantage.

He then presented the plan to the President. Trump was enthusiastic. They spoke about using people both inside and outside the administration to lead the proceedings. Miles Yu, Tom Cotton or Mary Kissel would be the co-chair, vice-chair or executive director. Retired Air Force Brigadier General Robert Spalding could lead the sessions on geopolitics, and a Brigadier General and scientists from Fort Detrick would handle the virology portion. There would be public hearings. Fauci would be hauled in to give answers about funding virus research at the Wuhan Institute of Virology and EcoHealth Alliance would be invited to appear to answer questions about its own collaboration with the Institute, among many others.

The plan progressed and it was looking very promising. A White House executive order was drawn up. It stated: "By the authority vested in me as President by the Constitution and the laws of the United States of America, it is hereby ordered as follows: The National Commission on the Origins and Costs of Covid-19 is hereby established." Its Mission and purpose: "The Commission shall investigate the origins of the Covid-19 pandemic; the economic, political, social, human, and other costs of the pandemic borne by the United States; and whether the People's Republic of China or the Chinese Communist Party have used the pandemic to advance their own economic, geopolitical, military, or territorial agendas."

The draft executive order also stated that the commission shall "identify actions of governments, actors, organisations, and other entities that may have played a material role in concealing the dangers presented by Covid-19, including human-to-human transmission of the virus." Another commission item stated: "The Commission shall recommend actions that the Federal Government may take to recover any damages as well as all costs estimated … from any entities identified during the investigation."

Such a commission, determined to hold the CCP to account and ask it to pay reparations for the economic and human damage caused by the virus, would have been explosive. Miles Yu had an office set up in the White House. "We almost got to the finish line," Navarro says. But the presidential commission never materialised. It was killed off. Yu says the commission met resistance within the White House simply because it was Navarro who wanted to do it.

In the Oval Office, Trump held a meeting to discuss the concept. Navarro was overruled by the economic hardheads, he says, who didn't have any enthusiasm for a public trial. "They are all China apologists," he said. "[Larry] Kudlow is just stupid, dumb, you can quote me on that." Pompeo was not there, he was busy with "other fish to fry", says Navarro.

There was some personal animosity towards Navarro. "People treat Peter as a crank but he was more right about this than just about anybody from an early stage," one senior Trump official says.

Yu puts it more strongly: "Pete Navarro was the hero of the White House."

Privately, others who supported the notion of an investigation were not convinced that a presidential commission under Trump was the best way forward and was not a realistic proposition. "What you really need is something that's bipartisan, preferably international, and it was not likely that we were going to be able to piece that together given the politics of the Trump administration as we approached a presidential election," a former senior White House official says. "In other words, an inquiry like that is exactly the right thing but it was going to be almost impossible for President Trump to appoint a commission that was going to be viewed as bipartisan. People were too crazed on the left. I don't think the left would have participated in it."

The President's interest in the commission waned as his advisors warned him against it. The Executive Order sat unsigned. "It was actually an excellent idea, just floated way too late," another insider tells me. "It would've looked very political, and [we] had tried very, very hard to make the China issue non-partisan."

Navarro was devastated. "That was the biggest heartbreak in my four years at the White House. I worked really hard to get that commission established," he says.

CHAPTER THIRTEEN

Nikolai Petrovsky

"Bloody hell," Nikolai Petrovsky said to himself as he sat alone in his laboratory in the city of Adelaide in South Australia. He had a sense of apprehension – a feeling he sat with for a week until he felt he was able to voice it to his colleagues. He feared they wouldn't believe him or – worse – would think he had become a conspiracy theorist.

The scientist of more than 35 years had been hard at work since January developing a vaccine for the new coronavirus. It was now March 2020. He'd already led the world in developing more than 10 pandemic vaccines over the past 20 years, including for Ebola, avian influenza, Japanese encephalitis, West Nile virus, African horse fever and against the SARS and MERS coronaviruses.

Petrovsky looks like how you'd picture an academic. He often wears a similar outfit to work: a button-up shirt with a red vest over the top, whether or not he's on clinical duties. He has mettle and a strong independent streak. He's happy to stand up to the conservative Australian government on issues of the day, like its lack of funding for Australian-made vaccines, and is comfortable in the media landscape.

Highly respected, Professor Petrovsky studied at the University of Tasmania, doing medicine before he trained as a physician and moved to Melbourne to complete his PhD in type 1 diabetes at the Walter and Eliza Hall Institute. He grew up in a medical family: his father ran the Launceston Hospital and his mother was a GP.

He is very much an establishment scientist. After completing his PhD, he headed to a country hospital in Mildura, in rural Victoria, taking the place of five physicians who had all deserted the hospital over a pay dispute. He was the sole physician running the hospital wards and intensive care unit. "I went for a week-long locum and ended up staying two years; even having my daughter Isobella born there," he says. "My desire was to get back to being a clinician researcher as quickly as possible but I simply couldn't morally leave the local population of 200,000 doctorless."

Resuming his academic career after a new team of physicians arrived, he was employed as a senior endocrinologist at Canberra Hospital and worked as an academic at the Australian National University, before moving to Adelaide in 2004 to take up a position as Director of Endocrinology at Flinders Medical Centre and Professor in what is now the College of Medicine and Public Health at Flinders University. It was while in Canberra that Petrovsky started his vaccine-development company, Vaxine.

The 62-year-old lives a quiet life in Adelaide. Happily married, he has three children now in their 20s. Theirs is a tight-knit family. But when the news of a new coronavirus hit, Petrovsky was at his mountain home in Colorado in the United States, where he goes each year to escape the scorching heat of the Adelaide summer. Retreating to his home office, he immediately set to work developing a vaccine with the help of his Vaxine team in Australia. He needed to quickly understand the properties of the virus, to analyse what made it spread and what made it infectious, to help him develop a vaccine candidate.

Just before the pandemic struck, Petrovsky had set up an alliance with the global computer company Oracle Corporation, which had provided him with access to their cloud-based supercomputer to undertake joint futuristic research into the use of artificial intelligence to accelerate cancer research, another area in which he is deeply involved, having developed a promising cancer vaccine approach. With talk of a vaccine for Covid-19 at least 18 months way, Petrovsky wondered if Oracle might give him permission to temporarily set aside the cancer project and instead use the powerful supercomputer to help him develop a Covid-19 vaccine more quickly.

Oracle is the type of company that gives its executives titles like "visionary" instead of "strategic director". Pete Winn at Oracle is one such senior executive whose title is "visionary". Petrovsky picked up the phone to Winn to ask him if he could repurpose the supercomputer to understand the new coronavirus. Winn sought permission from his boss, Oracle's co-founder and executive chairman, billionaire playboy Larry Ellison.

The 76-year-old Ellison is famous for his rags-to-riches story and his lavish lifestyle. He owns the Hawaiian island of Lanai, where he now lives, and has yachts and waterfront properties around the world. He was reported to be one of the few tech leaders who was friends with Donald Trump, hosting a fundraiser at his home in Rancho Mirage, California. It's been reported that Ellison and Trump spoke on the phone about possible coronavirus treatments, and Trump backed Oracle's failed bid to buy the American arm of Chinese social media platform TikTok, describing Oracle as a "great company".

Oracle agreed to Petrovsky's request to use their supercomputer to help develop a Covid-19 vaccine and also search for drug therapies that might be used to treat infected patients. Petrovsky was keen to use it to design the vaccine and to explore the transmission path of SARS-CoV-2 from animals to humans. He innocently wanted to see if he could work out which animal host the coronavirus had infected before being transmitted to humans.

Traditional laboratory methods using actual animal or human cells could answer these questions, but it could take years to run the experiments. The supercomputer's "in silico modelling" approach could give a good indication within weeks. Petrovsky told Oracle the plan was to find the most likely animal host using the supercomputer and then publish a scientific paper based on the results.

To understand how Petrovsky used the supercomputer – and to comprehend the arguments about whether SARS-CoV-2 is man-made or has a natural origin – it's important to grasp two crucial terms: "spike protein" and "ACE2 receptor". They're bandied about often but rarely explained. At this point, it would be very helpful to have Margot Robbie in a bubble bath, à la *The Big Short*, to explain those scientific terms.

The ACE2 receptor (its full scientific name is angiotensin-converting enzyme 2 receptor) is a protein on the surface of human and animal cells. Its function is to regulate our blood pressure. But the ACE2 receptor is also how the coronavirus enters cells in order to reproduce. The coronavirus particles (called virions) attach to the ACE2 protein on human airway cells, and then do their best contortionist impression to burrow inside those cells, thereby infecting them. Cells coated with ACE2 are present in the nose, mouth and lungs, explaining why the virus is so efficient at transmitting from person to person through respiratory droplets, sprayed out when a person coughs or sneezes, which are then breathed in by those close by.

The well-known image of a coronavirus is a circle or ball (representing the rounded virus particle) covered with red spiky bits that look like coral on the Great Barrier Reef. These coral bits are called spike proteins. It's these spike proteins that latch onto the ACE2 receptor on the surface of the potential victim's airway cells. So the spike protein on the coronavirus attaches to the ACE2 receptor on human airway cells and that's how, technically speaking, SARS-CoV-2 infects humans. When scientists talk about SARS-CoV-2 being more infectious than other viruses, this is because its spike protein latches onto the human cells 10–20 times as tightly as, for example, the original SARS spike protein did.

Petrovsky and his team uploaded all the genetic sequences for ACE2 from potential animal hosts including bats, cats, dogs, pangolins, mice, civets, monkeys, hamsters, ferrets, horses, tigers, cattle and snakes, as well as humans, to the supercomputer. Petrovsky says it's best to think of the ACE2 receptor as the lock in a door, and the spike protein as the key that opens the door. "We were trying to find which species of lock the Covid-19 key was best designed to unlock," he said. Using the supercomputer, "you can try and fit the SARS-CoV-2 spike protein structure shape into all of the ACE2 structures from different animals to see which one fits best, just like solving a jigsaw," Petrovsky explains.

By March 2020, the supercomputer was operational and they were running simulations using the spike protein and ACE2 models. Very quickly, he had a result – and it was a result that caused him a great deal of angst.

"Strangely, humans came out at the very top of the list." Petrovsky pauses. "That was not what we were expecting, as the animal host from which the virus had been transmitted should have been at the top of the list. This presented a puzzle as the data suggested the SARS-CoV-2 spike protein had uniquely evolved to bind and infect cells expressing human ACE2. Normally with a new pandemic virus, whatever species that virus originally came from would be the best fit and the virus would initially only half fit the human lock but then mutate over time to try and become a better fit. A virus should not be able to evolve to be a perfect fit for a lock it has never seen, and yet this is what the data was telling us. The virus spike protein looked like it couldn't have been better designed to fit the human ACE2. Go figure."

Petrovsky's research partner at Melbourne's La Trobe University, Professor David Winkler, was equally flummoxed when he later learnt the result. "We both expressed surprise that the human ACE2 came out on top," he said.

When Petrovsky thought more closely about this, he rapidly grasped the finding's potential ramifications, as unpalatable as they might be. If the Covid-19 virus is perfectly adapted to humans, there was a possibility it had been worked on in some capacity in a laboratory to provide it with the opportunity to learn about and adapt to the human lock. Given the scientific consensus globally seemed to be that the virus had a natural origin, despite no evidence for this, sharing this contrary result that suggested the virus may be man-made could have major negative implications for his scientific career, never mind the fact that the result had been unequivocally generated from a supercomputer. A supercomputer cannot possibly have political leanings.

It would be another six weeks before Pompeo and Trump would float the possibility the virus had originated in a laboratory, on April 15.

Petrovsky did not want to be seen as a conspiracy theorist rather than the rational scientist he is, with an excellent reputation he had cultivated over the past four decades, attracting a sizeable amount of research funding from the United States National Institutes of Health, despite never having worked in the US and always being based in Australia.

Petrovsky isn't impulsive. Despite the astonishing findings, he didn't share the news with anyone for days. He sat with it, contemplating what action to take and how to proceed. As his weekly meeting with David Winkler and Oracle rolled around, he knew he needed to get their approval to make the findings public, something they might be reluctant to do given the vitriol being levelled at any scientist who challenged the natural origins story. During their Zoom meeting, Petrovsky summoned the courage to explain the unusual result.

Like many academics, he speaks carefully and calmly. He is articulate, considered and is rarely animated or expressive. It was in this steady, slow tone that he told his colleagues about his explosive findings that the virus may have originated in a laboratory. "Please don't think I'm crazy or a conspiracy theorist, I'm really truly not," he began, "but basically, I've formed a conclusion that we can't exclude the possibility that what these results might be telling us is this could be a man-made virus, or at the very least something that was generated in a lab and then got accidentally released." He paused. There was silence. He ploughed on. "I understand this might be difficult to publish. I understand there's going to be a backlash. But these are the findings and surely we have a responsibility to try and make the world aware of them." Petrovsky then, slowly, took the

Oracle "visionaries" and his fellow scientists through, in detail, the findings of the supercomputer studies.

The reaction was not what he'd expected. "Everyone was a bit incredulous and initially just tried to make light of it," he said. "But they could see that I was serious and I realised they needed more time to process this. I knew they were very smart and logical scientists and hoped they would eventually come around to seeing my side of the argument."

After a few more meetings, most of the team started to warm to the idea of having a go at publishing the results, as they agreed the point of science is to share the knowledge gained. Oracle was clearly more than a little nervous, concerned their reputable corporation would become associated with a sensationalist story. None of the authors knew just how difficult this publishing endeavour would be. It would be more than a year of battling the establishment before their research paper would finally be accepted in June 2021 in the prestigious journal, *Nature Scientific Reports*, after extensive rounds of peer-review and appeals.

"The easy answer seems to have been, rather than make the obvious decision to accept the paper and let it be published so that the scientific community could make their own assessment, they took the decision to stall any acceptance and thereby just held up the ability to get it published," Petrovsky says.

When the La Trobe and Flinders University paper was finally ready, it was intentionally subdued, calm, conservative. It simply said the possibility that the virus arose from a lab leak could not be discounted and that the most likely source was still an unknown animal species. The innocuous title was: "In silico comparison of spike protein-ACE2 binding affinities across species; significance for the possible origin of the SARS-CoV-2 virus".

The paper said: "Notably, SARS-CoV-2 spike protein had the highest overall binding energy for human ACE2, greater than all the other tested species including bat, the postulated source of the virus. This indicates that SARS-CoV-2 is a highly adapted human pathogen ... This finding is particularly surprising as, typically, a virus, would be expected to have highest affinity for the receptor in its original host species, e.g. bat, with a lower initial binding affinity for the receptor of any new host, e.g. humans."

Petrovsky's findings were that after humans, it was the ACE2 of pangolins to which the virus spike protein had the next tightest fit. The pangolin is an endangered, rare, scaly-skinned ant-eating mammal that picks up food with its sticky tongue. It's one of the world's most smuggled animals. The paper, however, argued that it was extremely unlikely the pangolin could have been the original host or the intermediary species by which the coronavirus crossed from bats to humans. "However, this does not mean that pangolin ACE2 was the receptor on which the SARS-CoV-2 spike protein RBD [receptor binding domain] was initially selected, with the strength of binding to pangolin ACE2 lower than binding to human ACE2," the paper stated. "This makes it unlikely that pangolins are the missing intermediate host."

The paper explored the possibility that SARS-CoV-2 could have come into existence if a pangolin had been infected with two different coronaviruses at precisely the same time – one of them a pangolin coronavirus and the other a bat virus. This could have allowed for a "recombination event" to occur, where the two viruses merged in the pangolin to create an entirely new virus: SARS-CoV-2.

A virus that results from a recombination event is called a chimeric virus. Viral recombination occurs regularly in nature in the right circumstances. The point here, however, is that bats and pangolins don't really mix. Pangolins are solitary animals and unlikely to act as a holding reservoir of evolving viruses. "Such events are by necessity rare as they require co-infection of the one host at exactly the same time," Petrovsky's paper stated. "Most importantly, if such a recombination event had occurred in pangolins it might have been expected to have similarly triggered an epidemic spread of the new highly permissive SARS-CoV-2-like virus among pangolin populations, such as we now see occurring across the human population. Currently there is no evidence of such a pangolin SARS-CoV-2-like outbreak, making this whole scenario less likely. Plus, what would an infected pangolin have been doing in Wuhan, thousands of kilometres away from their natural homes in South East Asia? And evidence from the Wuhan markets shows no pangolins were being sold there prior to the pandemic," Petrovsky explains.

Petrovsky and his team then presented another scenario where this virus might have come into existence – the same recombination event described above could have happened but, this time, in a laboratory.

It could have happened on purpose during deliberate experimentation to manipulate viruses, or it could have happened accidentally.

"Another possibility which still cannot be excluded is that SARS-CoV-2 was created by a recombination event that occurred inadvertently or consciously in a laboratory handling coronaviruses, with the new virus then accidentally released into the local human population," the paper stated. "Given the seriousness of the ongoing SARS-CoV-2 pandemic, it is imperative that all efforts be made to identify the original source of the SARS-CoV-2 virus. In particular, it will be important to establish whether Covid-19 is due to a completely natural chance occurrence where a presumed bat virus was transmitted to humans via an intermediate animal host or whether Covid-19 has alternative origins."

When Petrovsky and his partners at La Trobe submitted the paper for publication, they hit roadblocks immediately. They submitted the paper in April to a pre-print server – which is meant to allow publication of any research prior to peer review – but, to Petrovsky's frustration, it was flatly rejected, with the pre-print server managers effectively saying it was too hot. The researchers were stunned by this response. It was unheard of for a pre-print server to refuse to post a legitimate manuscript. The same experience occurred over and over again.

"The paper was clearly being seen as going against the prevailing scientific political orthodoxy," he says. "They said the paper should be peer-reviewed first, but this was a nonsense as the whole point of pre-press servers is to make papers available before peer review. Obviously it was seen as political dynamite and the scientific community had already decided that only research suggesting a natural origin should be allowed to see the light of day. We were trying very hard to be guarded and not say too much about the implications of our results in the discussion part of the paper, but the very fact that this could point to a non-natural origin meant that everyone treated it like we had sent them a stick of dynamite."

Petrovsky spoke to his family and his colleagues about going public with his findings. Aside from the fear of reputational damage, his main concern was the risk of retribution that could be inflicted on his Covid-19 vaccine-development program. "Our work could be in jeopardy by going public on this issue. There could be a backlash on our vaccine program and our NIH funding," he agonised to Winkler.

Winkler agreed with his concerns but suggested if they stayed within the bounds of what their data showed, they'd be on safe territory. "The origin issue is very political, there is potential for us to be discredited or labelled conspiracy theorists if we're not rigorous in providing evidence for any statements we make," Winkler said. "Even so, we may suffer criticism or attempts to discredit us that would clearly have the potential to impact on [your] vaccine project."

Petrovsky's family was supportive. "They strongly supported my view that the responsibility of a doctor and scientist is not to tell people only what they want to hear, but to get the truth out," Petrovsky says. "Whether the truth is palatable or not is irrelevant; you're either honest or you're not. My father was scrupulously honest and I guess I have followed in his footsteps. When Singapore fell to the Japanese in World War II, my father was offered an easy exit by his commanding officer in the British army as he had enlisted only weeks before in the hope the British army would ship him to the Eastern front to help the Russians, Britain's allies, fight the Germans – a crazy idea when you look back on it. Even crazier, he declined his commanding officer's offer to rip up his enrolment papers so my father, a Russian, could walk away from Japanese imprisonment in Changi. He refused the offer, saying 'I signed my allegiance to the Queen when I signed the papers – I could not go back on that.' The price for his integrity was five years being brutalised by the Japanese as a prisoner of war on the infamous Siam–Burma Railway, an experience very few survived. Yet he never regretted his decision to honour his word. With precedents like that, what hope do I have?" Petrovsky asks. "I have always believed science is about truth, not political correctness, so there really was no choice but to stand our ground and try get this information out there."

Some of his family members warned him about the repercussions from China and were concerned for his safety. "My sister was concerned the Chinese might start chasing me, but I didn't take that terribly seriously," he says. "All the Chinese officials I have met have had high integrity, and I don't believe they would target a foreign scientist just because of their research findings. If this [pandemic] did occur because of a lab leak, it was clearly an accident that was suppressed at a local level. The issue here is not about pointing fingers but just to come to an appropriate scientific conclusion about the true origin of the virus and then find ways to prevent such events in the future. I am sure my Chinese medical and scientific counterparts would completely agree with me on this."

After many weeks of agonising, Petrovsky eventually came to a decision that was true to himself and aligned with his core scientific values: important scientific findings should always be made public. Transparency was vital. It was against his nature to hide something that was, potentially, of huge importance to the global understanding of the new coronavirus.

"We tried to thread a narrow course between being silenced and in making potentially useful data and information available in the public domain that may inform discussion of this very important question," Winkler says. "I think Nik, like me, is guided by the data. I think also there has been pressure more broadly to discount the lab escape theory that has not been backed up by hard evidence."

Their paper eventually made it onto the arXiv platform in mid-May 2020. It was what is known as a "pre-print", meaning it had not yet been peer-reviewed or published. A few days later, a keen-eyed person on Twitter – who had followed my newspaper reporting on the origins of the coronavirus – spotted it and sent me a link. I read the paper and was personally surprised to find the authors were Australian. I was in the middle of working on a mini-documentary for Sky News on the topic, and I instantly tapped out an email to Professor Petrovsky, asking him if he'd speak to me on air. It was May 20 at 7.54pm.

"Yes, I can do this from my office tomorrow if you like," he replied six minutes later.

Given the hostile climate for anyone to even speculate about the origins of the virus, I was taken aback that he immediately agreed. He had shied away from approaches from major US television networks, including Fox News, which, luckily for me, meant I had the world exclusive.

I was stunned by the strength of his interview. We broadcast it four days later – I brought it forward when Ian Birrell at the *Daily Mail* in London got wind of Petrovsky's research and wrote a piece in print. We let it run for 16 minutes – a very long time for prime-time television. "It really looked like this was a virus that was optimally designed to infect humans," Petrovsky said in the interview. "It's better adapted to infect humans than any other animal."

"Covid-19 could have been created from that recombination event in an animal host or it could have occurred in a cell-culture experiment. We can't exclude the possibility this came from a laboratory experiment rather than from an animal."

Petrovsky called for an inquiry – something he would still be calling for a year later. "We need an investigation into the other possibilities of where this virus may have come from and that would require an independent, scientific panel to be put together and they would then have the opportunity to investigate where the virus may have come from in China, whether it came from an animal or whether it might have come from an accidental release," he said.

The professor was also critical of the conflicts of interest from some of his colleagues in the scientific community, and said it may have prevented them from speaking out about the nature of the virus. "If it was to turn out that this virus came about because of an accidental lab release, that would have implications for how we do viral research in laboratories all around the world, which could make doing research much harder, and so I think the inclination of virus researchers would be to presume that it came from an animal until proven otherwise, because that will have less ramifications for how we are able to do research in the future," he said.

Watching it back a year on, with a greater understanding of SARS-CoV-2, I was embarrassed to hear I confused the scientific terms in my questions. But at that point, viewers had even less understanding of the virus than I did, and no one noticed.

It was a significant break from what had become established as the scientific community's dogma on the origins of the virus, from a highly credible academic who had previously developed many world-first vaccines including against SARS and MERS coronaviruses.

At that point, authorities were only really interested in investigating whether a naturally occurring virus had been collected in a cave and then held by a laboratory from which it leaked. No one credible had as yet suggested it could be a man-made virus. Until Petrovsky. This was partly because, I would later discover, scientific journals and pre-print servers were blocking papers that did not conform to the view that Covid-19 had a natural origin. Scientists who held a different view were censored, their papers blocked from publication and criticised by their peers as conspiracy theorists and anti-China racists.

CHAPTER FOURTEEN

Scientists Speak Out

After my interview with Petrovsky was broadcast on Sky News Australia, it was picked up in Europe and shared widely online, and the Flinders University scientist unexpectedly found himself at the centre of global discussion as scientists who had come to similar conclusions about the virus contacted him in droves. Many shared their own findings about suspicious features of the SARS-CoV-2 virus they'd been apprehensive about publicising.

Studying the genome of SARS-CoV-2 itself can provide many clues about its origin. Professor Richard Ebright from Rutgers University in New Jersey had been warning about the activities of the Wuhan Institute of Virology for years before the pandemic.

Ebright said he first realised that Covid-19 may not have a natural origin as early as January 8, 2020, when he heard that sequencing data indicated the virus responsible for SARS-like pneumonias in Wuhan was a bat-SARS-related coronavirus. Ebright was part of an email discussion group with scientists and policy specialists in February 2020 where they spoke about the possibility of a laboratory accident. "The main messages from the discussions were the entry of SARS-CoV-2 into humans may have occurred through a natural accident or may have occurred through a laboratory accident," he said.

He began discussing this possible laboratory-accident origin with journalists in the science press on condition that he not be named or quoted, first agreeing to be quoted as stating that a lab accident was possible in *Science* magazine on January 31, 2020. His comments then appeared in Chinese investigative media outlet Caixin Global on February 5. "By early February 2020, it had become apparent that many US and non-US science-policy specialists in a biodefense/biosafety/biosecurity email discussion group in which I have participated over the last two decades were willing to go on record stating that a laboratory-accident origin is plausible," he tells me.

Professor Ebright says there are "noteworthy unusual aspects of the sequence" of SARS-CoV-2. One is that Covid-19 has what is called a "furin cleavage site" at a very particular location in its spike protein. This greatly expands the ability of the virus to jump between species and could also make it more transmissible within a species.

I asked Professor Ebright what it is about the furin cleavage site that makes scientists suggest Covid-19 may not have a natural origin. He says, "SARS-CoV-2 is the only member of the SARS-related betacoronavirus group that contains a furin cleavage site, the SARS-CoV-2 furin cleavage site exhibits unusual codon usage, and the SARS-CoV-2 furin cleavage site is located at a position that previously has been used to engineer coronaviruses having enhanced infectivity. This is noteworthy but it is not conclusive."

He wasn't alone to focus on the unusual nature of the furin cleavage site. It became a hot topic the world over, eventually spilling into some mainstream media outlets, such as *The Mail on Sunday* in the UK and *The Washington Post*.

Petrovsky agrees the furin cleavage site is highly unusual. "The issue is that the Covid-19 virus has a furin cleavage site whereas neither the bat virus that is its closest relative nor SARS have it. A key question then is, where did Covid-19 get its furin cleavage site from?" Petrovsky asks. "Scientists in the US and China were publicly making viruses like SARS and MERS more virulent by artificially inserting furin cleavage sites into their spike protein. This then generates the question, did someone insert the furin cleavage site into Covid-19 or did it acquire this naturally from another virus?"

Eminent US virologist David Baltimore is the co-discoverer of reverse transcriptase, an enzyme used in all PCR-based Covid tests among other things, and was awarded the 1975 Nobel Prize. He is also the co-inventor of the infectious-clone technology used to engineer genomes of viruses and to construct chimeric viruses. He is the former president of Caltech, a prestigious private research university ranked alongside MIT and Harvard. It has a focus on science and engineering; Caltech's faculty and alumni have been awarded 39 Nobel Prizes.

Baltimore told science writer Nicholas Wade, in a piece published in the *Bulletin of the Atomic Scientists*, that the furin cleavage site pointed to a laboratory origin. "When I first saw the furin cleavage site in the viral sequence, with its arginine codons, I said to my wife it was the smoking gun for the origin of the virus," he said. His wife, Alice Huang, is a celebrated virologist who taught Professor Ebright. "These features make a powerful challenge to the idea of a natural origin for SARS2." Baltimore says ultimately you can't "distinguish between the two origins from just looking at the sequence". "When I first saw the sequence of the furin cleavage site – as I've said, other betacoronaviruses don't have that site – it seemed to me a reasonable hypothesis that somebody had put it in there. Now, I don't know if that's true or not, but I do know that it's a hypothesis that must be taken seriously," he told the California Institute of Technology. "I think we very much need to find out what was happening in the Wuhan Institute of Virology."

It's an analysis with which world-renowned American physicist Richard Muller, an emeritus professor at the University of California, agrees. "This is a fingerprint of genetic manipulation," he tells me of the furin cleavage site in an interview for this book. "It's like finding a fingerprint at a crime scene. If you pick up a gun at a crime scene and find a fingerprint, this is not circumstantial evidence. This is the smoking gun. The furin cleavage site, the CGG sequences that they splice in if you're trying to really attack humans, this is the fingerprint." Professor Muller says, on the other hand, "The evidence for zoonotic [animal origin] is all circumstantial."

The furin cleavage site was also of note to another esteemed scientist, the University of Hamburg's Professor Roland Wiesendanger, who also contacted Petrovsky. The German scientist specialises in nanotechnology and is a three-time recipient of a prestigious European Research Council Advanced Grant. "I have read your arXiv paper of May 13 with great interest," he wrote in an email to Petrovsky. "I am part of a network of European scientists who no longer believe in a natural origin of the SARS-CoV-2 virus after studying hundreds of relevant papers on this matter."

Professor Wiesendanger released a 100-page research paper where he provided his view on the unusual characters of SARS-CoV-2. He drew a stronger conclusion than Professor Ebright, saying he is "99.9 per cent sure that the coronavirus came from a laboratory".

"The SARS-CoV-2 viruses possess special cell receptor binding domains combined with a special (furin) cleavage site of the coronavirus spike protein. Both properties together were previously unknown in coronaviruses and indicate a non-natural origin of the SARS-CoV-2 pathogen," he says in an English-language precis on the Swiss Policy Research site. He also concludes that there is no evidence for the zoonotic theory, saying no intermediate host animal has been identified that could have facilitated the transmission of the SARS-CoV-2 pathogen from bats to humans.

Another scientist to contact Petrovsky was an Israeli geneticist working on Covid-19 treatments, Dr Ronen Shemesh. He tells me "there are many reasons to believe that SARS-CoV-2 was generated in a lab. Most probably by methods of genetic engineering. The method is very easy, nucleic acid manipulation is a standard in many molecular biology labs. An insertion of four amino acids coded by 12 nucleotides into a DNA or RNA strand by means of PCR and cloning would be an easy task for a third-year student. The planning and generation of the sequences to be entered would need some advanced thinking and could be done by experienced scientists."

In his assessment, it is more likely that the virus was generated in a laboratory than arose naturally, but he adds there is no way to prove either origin. "I believe that the most important issue about the differences between *all* coronavirus types is the insertion of a furin protease cleavage site at the spike protein of SARS-CoV-2," he says. "This site is created by an insertion of four amino acids (proline, arginine, arginine, alanine – PRRA) directly at the usual coronavirus spike protein cleavage site in the junction separating the two parts of the spike protein. This insertion of 12 nucleotides of RNA is found only in this strain, whereas the S1–S2 region of the spike protein is highly conserved in most coronavirus strains.

"Such an insertion is very rare in evolution; the addition of such four amino acids is very unlikely. More unlikely is that this insertion happened exactly at the right place – the original cleavage site of the spike protein.

"What makes it even more suspicious," he continues, "is the fact that this insertion not only occurred in the right place and at the right time, but also turned the cleavage site from a serine protease cleavage site to a furin cleavage site. This protein cleaving protein is highly promiscuous; it's found in many human tissues and cell types and is involved in many other virus types' activation and infection mechanisms. It is involved in HIV, herpes, Ebola and dengue virus mechanisms. If I was trying to engineer a virus strain with a higher affinity and infective potential to humans, I would do exactly that: I would add a furin cleavage site directly at the original, less effective and more cell-specific cleavage site."

Norwegian virologist Birger Sørensen, who is the CEO of biotech company Bionor Pharma, co-authored a scientific paper with UK oncologist and immunologist Angus Dalgleish, which claims SARS-CoV-2 has no credible natural ancestor and was created through laboratory manipulation beyond reasonable doubt. They claim Covid-19 was created by first using a natural coronavirus backbone and splicing a new spike onto it.

"We had discovered that the spike has six inserts which are unique fingerprints with five salient features indicative of purposive manipulation," their 2021 paper states. They had questioned a natural origin for SARS-CoV-2 ever since 2020. "I think the coronavirus leaked as early as the second half of August, early September 2019. There is a lot to suggest that," Sørensen told Swedish news outlet *Fria Tider* in December 2020. "The scientific community doesn't want to discuss issues that may hinder future virus research. You have to prove that it comes from nature, otherwise, it comes from a laboratory."

This goes to the heart of the cover-up: some virologists could have feared their experiments would be barred if the Covid-19 pandemic arose from gain-of-function research.

Dr Steven Quay, the CEO of public company Atossa Therapeutics, has invented seven FDA-approved drugs and was at one time on the faculty of Stanford University School of Medicine. He has written 360 papers, which have been cited more than 10,000 times. The 70-year-old, now living in Taiwan, turned his attention to the new coronavirus in late January 2020 after seeing the sequence of the virus and the structure of the spike protein and the furin cleavage site. Drawing on his science background, and in response to governments the world over advocating that masks don't help, he wrote a book *Stay Safe: A Physician's Guide to Survive Coronavirus*. He then returned to researching the virus itself.

"The polybasic cleavage site [coding for four amino acids] really caught my attention, because for five years at Stanford I was doing research on melittin, the active toxin in bee venom," he says. "It actually has the same polybasic site and I know exactly what that would do in membranes, and I knew how it would disrupt cells."

He says the virus was highly adapted for infection of humans from the start, unlike earlier natural zoonoses, and that its infectious trigger – the furin cleavage site – isn't found anywhere in related betacoronaviruses in its class, and thus he argues couldn't have come from a natural recombination, but has been repeatedly included in viruses by laboratory scientists including at the Wuhan Institute of Virology. "Since 1992, laboratories have been putting furin cleavage sites into viruses that didn't have them – 11 different laboratories, 11 different experiments, including previous Wuhan Institute of Virology experiments, and every single time it makes it more virulent, more transmissible and more lethal," he says. The end result, Dr Quay says, has always been supercharged viruses.

Dr Quay points out just how unusual the characteristics of the coronavirus are, making it so "exquisitely matched" to humans. He concludes that SARS-CoV-2 may have been well developed to adapt to human ACE2 receptors because it had been worked on in a laboratory using humanised mice. "That's exactly what happened," he says. (I'll explain exactly what the Wuhan Institute of Virology was doing with humanised mice in the next chapter.) "It was completely pre-adapted to humans," he says. "This is the first virus from nature that has strong human-to-human transfer right from the beginning."

The fact that SARS-CoV-2 was highly, uniquely adapted to infect humans from the start is widely recognised. A Russian-Canadian longevity entrepreneur, Yuri Deigin, 41, from Youthereum Genetics in Toronto, is credited as the first scientist to outline the unusual furin cleavage site, the EcoHealth grant, the gain-of-function work at the Wuhan Institute of Virology among other things in a *Medium* article he wrote in April 2020.

He then partnered with Rossana Segreto, from the Department of Microbiology at the University of Innsbruck in Austria, on a study published in *BioEssays* in November 2020 titled: "The Genetic Structure of SARS-CoV-2 Does Not Rule Out a Laboratory Origin". Their view is that SARS-CoV-2 is a "chimera virus" – the result of genetic recombination of two different viruses. For natural recombination to occur, the two divergent viruses need to infect a host at the same time. "Genomic analyses show SARS-CoV-2 likely to be chimeric, most of its sequence closest to bat CoV RaTG13, whereas its receptor binding domain (RBD) is almost identical to that of a pangolin CoV," their study states. "Chimeric viruses can arise via natural recombination or human intervention."

Like Ebright and Petrovsky, Segreto and Deigin found the furin cleavage site unusual and noted that modern genetic-engineering methods do not leave any obvious traces of genetic manipulation. Ralph Baric, a virologist at the University of North Carolina, pioneered this seamless "no-see-um" genome-assembly method in the first SARS virus in the early 2000s. "Might genetic manipulations have been performed in order to evaluate pangolins as possible intermediate hosts for bat-derived CoVs that were originally unable to bind to human receptors? Both cleavage site and specific RBD could result from site-directed mutagenesis, a procedure that does not leave a trace," they wrote.

Many scientists dismissed the possibility of an artificial recombination event or a chimeric virus early on by saying there was no evidence of genetic manipulation within SARS-CoV-2. It was something that confounded me as I investigated the topic in early 2020. But this is an argument that Professor Ebright easily refutes. His remarks are crucial. "The observation that the genome sequence of the virus shows no signatures of human manipulation rules out the scenarios for a laboratory accident origin that involve the kinds of gain-of-function research that leave signatures," he says. "But this observation does not rule out scenarios for a laboratory accident origin that involve the kinds of gain-of-function research that do not leave signatures. The kinds that have been in use worldwide, including at WIV, in the last half-decade. And, of course, this observation has no relevance whatsoever to scenarios for a laboratory accident origin that involve a natural, genetically unmodified, bat SARS-related coronavirus, e.g. scenarios that involve infection of a WIV field-collection staffer in Yunnan, a WIV field-survey staffer in Yunnan or a WIV laboratory staffer in Wuhan with a natural, genetically unmodified, bat-SARS-related coronavirus."

Ralph Baric, who has partnered with the Wuhan Institute of Virology on coronavirus research, made the same point in an interview with Italy's national broadcaster in September 2020. "You can engineer a virus without leaving any trace," he said. "If you want, you can choose to leave a trace, a kind of signature of your intervention. A bit like saying, this virus was made in Professor Baric's laboratory. In the chimera we made in America in 2015 with the SARS virus, together with Professor Zhengli Shi of the Wuhan Institute of Virology, we had left signature mutations, so it was understood that it was the result of genetic engineering. But otherwise, there is no way to distinguish a natural virus from one made in the laboratory."

Professor David Relman, a graduate of MIT and Harvard, is a microbiologist who has advised the US government on biosecurity and emerging infectious disease issues. He has been recognised with a dozen honours and awards for his scientific research. In November 2020 he wrote an opinion piece for the *Proceedings of the National Academy of Sciences*, saying the genome of SARS-CoV-2 "shows evidence of recombination between different parental viruses". "In nature, recombination is common among coronaviruses. But it's also common in some research laboratories where recombinant engineering is used to study those viruses," he wrote.

He said SARS-CoV-2 may have evolved naturally through bats, known reservoirs of coronavirus diversity. "Second, SARS-CoV-2 or a recent ancestor virus may have been collected by humans from a bat or other animal and then brought to a laboratory where it was stored knowingly or unknowingly, propagated and perhaps manipulated genetically to understand its biological properties, and then released accidentally," he said.

"Some have argued that a deliberate engineering scenario is unlikely because one would not have had the insight *a priori* to design the current pandemic virus. This argument fails to acknowledge the possibility that two or more as yet undisclosed ancestors ... had already been discovered and were being studied in a laboratory – for example, one with the SARS-CoV-2 backbone and spike protein receptor-binding domain, and the other with the SARS-CoV-2 polybasic furin cleavage site. It would have been a logical next step to wonder about the properties of a recombinant virus and then create it in the laboratory. Alternatively, the complete SARS-CoV-2 sequence could have been recovered from a bat sample and viable virus resurrected from a synthetic genome to study it, before that virus accidentally escaped from the laboratory. The third scenario, seemingly much less likely, involves laboratory manipulation or release, with the clear intention of causing harm."

Even those who insist the virus has a natural origin can't explain the unusual furin cleavage site. One such scientist is the director of the University of Pennsylvania's Penn Center for Research on Coronavirus and Other Emerging Pathogens, Susan Weiss, a microbiologist who has been studying coronaviruses for decades. She says the "furin cleavage site" is "a mystery". "We don't know where the furin site came from," she told award-winning science writer Charlie Schmidt in a piece published on the Undark website. Her position was that the virus is unlikely to have been engineered but the possibility it escaped from a lab can't be ruled out.

Professor Ebright says there are more "arguably unusual aspects" of coronavirus, including its "nucleotide and substitution frequency". But he makes the point that while these are all noteworthy and suspicious, none ultimately proves definitively that it came from a laboratory. He says that all scientific data related to the genome sequence of SARS-CoV-2 and the epidemiology of Covid-19 are equally consistent with a laboratory-accident origin and a natural-accident origin. "There are no – absolutely no – scientific data that permit a choice between a natural-accident origin and a laboratory-accident origin," he says.

But he says there is circumstantial evidence linking the virus to a laboratory. "The outbreak occurred in Wuhan, a city of 11 million persons that does not contain horseshoe-bat colonies, and that is tens of kilometres from, and outside the flight range of, the nearest known horseshoe-bat colonies," he tells me. "Furthermore, the outbreak occurred at a time of year when horseshoe bats are in hibernation and do not leave colonies. The outbreak occurred in Wuhan, on the doorstep of the laboratory that conducts the world's largest research project on horseshoe-bat viruses, that has the world's largest collection of horseshoe-bat viruses, and that possessed and worked with the world's closest sequenced relative of the outbreak virus. The laboratory actively searched for new horseshoe-bat viruses in horseshoe-bat colonies in caves in remote rural areas in Yunnan province, brought those new horseshoe-bat viruses to Wuhan, and then mass-produced, manipulated, and studied those new horseshoe-bat viruses, year-round, inside Wuhan."

This is the question: If it did come from a laboratory, how did it get out? "Documentary evidence establishes that the bat-SARS-related-coronavirus projects at WIV used personal protective equipment (usually just gloves; sometimes not even gloves) and biosafety standards, usually just Biosafety Level 2, that would pose high risk of infection of field-collection, field-survey or laboratory staff upon contact with a virus having the transmission properties of SARS-CoV-2," Professor Ebright said.

Privately, many other scientists had come to the same or similar conclusions as Professor Petrovsky and Professor Ebright, and had felt compelled to speak to the United States government – but had steadfastly refused to speak publicly. It was something that caused immense frustration for both Miles Yu and the lead investigator at the US State Department David Asher, who were tasked with examining the origins of Covid-19. "We interviewed some top scientists. We interviewed the world's first-class scientists and they all agree there's a possibility that this thing could be lab-related," Yu says. "But we just cannot release that information because the condition for them to talk was that they must remain anonymous."

Former CDC director Robert Redfield told CNN in late March 2021 that it is highly unusual the virus so readily infects humans – and humans alone. "Normally, when a pathogen goes from a zoonotic to a human, it takes a while for it to figure out how to become more efficient in human-to-human transmission. I don't think this makes biological sense," he told Dr Sanjay Gupta, CNN Chief Medical Correspondent.

It was clearly a position Redfield had held for quite some time, but even he had not expressed it. "You know, it's my opinion. All right? But I'm a virologist. I've spent my life in virology. I do not believe this came from a bat to a human," he said. Redfield also says he believes the virus could have started "transmitting" in September or October in Wuhan. "I'm of the point of view that I still think the most likely etiology [is that] the pathogen in Wuhan from a laboratory, escaped. Now, the other people don't believe that. That's fine. Science will eventually figure it out. It's not unusual for respiratory pathogens worked [on] in a laboratory to infect the laboratory worker," he said.

Ebright understands why it has been difficult for scientists to speak out. "There are strong disincentives for scientists to speak publicly on the subject," he concedes.

National Security Advisor Robert O'Brien says that, overwhelmingly, the scientific community did not want to believe that the virus may have come from a laboratory leak. "There were a lot of people who didn't even want to talk about that possibility," he tells me. "Almost from day one, there were two competing theories. It came from a wet market or it came from a Wuhan lab. Given the totality of the circumstances, it always made more sense that it came from the lab than from the wet market, just commonsense-wise."

Reflecting on that time, Professor Petrovsky believes that bias in the media played a significant role in shaping the public narrative. "It was very clear the left-wing media were only willing to tell one side of the story, and that included Australia's public broadcaster, the ABC, who were only repeating whatever propaganda China was putting out on this issue," he says. "It was maddening to hear the ABC report time and time again that scientists agreed that this virus could only come from a natural animal source. It was very clear that this issue was heavily politicised and the left-leaning media saw this as a great opportunity to beat up Trump and label him as an idiot for suggesting the virus might have resulted from a lab leak. People think of publicly funded media organisations like the ABC as the ultimate truth-tellers, but my experience during that time is that this couldn't be further from the truth, whether they were reporting on the origins of the virus or discussing vaccine policy and what were the most promising vaccines out there. The ABC was clearly out to politicise the origins issue and chose to present a very one-sided story. It was refreshing and even a little surprising to see Sky News and *The Australian* newspaper much more open-minded and prepared to explore all sides of these stories."

Professor Muller says there was a strong anti-Trump sentiment among the scientific community, which meant they were reluctant to speak out about the unusual aspects of the virus that pointed to a laboratory origin. "I learnt very quickly when speaking to well-known scientists that there was a sense that any validation that Covid-19 came from the Chinese laboratory would validate Donald Trump's position on China, and that this could throw the election," he says. "Any suggestion it was from a laboratory engaging in biological warfare was seen as supporting Trump in the election, and this was sufficient to call it a fringe theory or a conspiracy theory."

But there was another reason scientists struggled to find a voice. Scientific journals blocked their research from publication.

Petrovsky wasn't the only scientist who faced difficulty having his scientific research published in esteemed medical journals – or even on pre-print servers. The whole idea of a pre-print server is to get the science out there to help with the development of other scientific research and vaccines while it's going through the long, arduous process of peer review. But, scandalously, pre-print servers would not accept any scientific paper that questioned the natural origins of Covid-19.

This played a key role in shaping the public narrative around the origins of Covid-19. It meant that the media and government officials thought the "scientific consensus" was that the virus had a natural, zoonotic origin. In fact, this wasn't the case. It's just that the brave scientists who did decide to publish their scientific findings that questioned a natural origin were blocked from doing so by scientific and medical journals and even pre-print servers.

I asked the major pre-print server, bioRxiv – which says pre-prints are made for sharing information in times of urgency – the following: "Why did bioRxiv stop publishing papers that questioned a natural origin of Covid-19? How many papers did bioRxiv refuse to publish? Do you admit this amounts to obstructing the publication of science and distorted the narrative about the origins of the virus in the crucial early days? On what basis did you make one rule for some scientists like Nikolai Petrovsky, however, you did not ask the papers that said Covid-19 had a natural origin to await peer review?"

In his reply, co-founder of bioRxiv and medRxiv John Inglis admitted they had declined to publish some scientific papers. "A small proportion of manuscripts may have harmful consequences if posted in the open on a pre-print server before peer review," he wrote. "For example: challenges to the safety of standard medical procedures, assertions about substances' carcinogenicity, or encouragements to self-medicate. Because of the frantic pace of new information about the novel virus and overwhelming public interest, we applied this 'do no harm' policy carefully to studies of the virus (for example, claims for the therapeutic value of materials based simply and solely on the basis of molecular modeling).

"This is not a judgment of the investigations concerned or their interpretation, simply a recognition that pre print screening must be limited and fast, and certain manuscripts – a very small proportion – in our view should have the more concentrated, expert, and detailed assessment before being distributed that only journals can do. These are therefore declined with that explanation to the authors." Inglis said they implemented the policy after publishing a wildly inaccurate paper on Covid-19 claiming the virus had HIV inserts, which they had to withdraw when they were inundated with criticisms.

In my view, however, this meant the system was working, because that paper was withdrawn when it did not stack up to scrutiny. This shouldn't have meant that credible papers could not see the light of day. The effect of what he was doing, in my view, was to decide which version of science should be published. As it happens, the scientific papers he chose to publish were the ones that supported China's narrative.

Not only were medical journals banning articles that questioned a zoonotic origin from being published, but they were returning to old papers that delved into gain-of-function research and adding a note on top that read: "Editors' note, March 2020: We are aware that this story is being used as the basis for unverified theories that the novel coronavirus causing Covid-19 was engineered. There is no evidence that this is true; scientists believe that an animal is the most likely source of the coronavirus." It was a circular argument. They were blocking scientists who did not think it had a natural origin, by using the argument that scientists believe an animal was the most likely source of the virus.

The supposedly esteemed medical journals played a role in suppressing scientific research and shaping the public narrative, stopping the truth from emerging and proper discussion from taking place publicly in the scientific community.

Many scientists encountered the same problem Petrovsky faced when trying to get their papers published. Birger Sørensen and Angus Dalgleish struggled to publish their paper pointing to a possible laboratory origin. Sørensen reached out to his long-time friend Sir Richard Dearlove, a former head of MI6, for help. But Sir Richard came up against roadblock after roadblock trying to get the paper into the public domain. "It's an absolute scandal because there is a total lack of debate," he told me in an interview for this book. "We tried the *American Journal of Virology*, the *New England Journal of Medicine*, *Nature* and the list goes on. We tried bioRxiv, too." Sir Richard says that the moment the journals realised the paper presented an opposing view from the natural origin thesis, they "behaved in a totally outrageous fashion to stop it from being published".

To get the paper into the public domain, the scientists had to rewrite it entirely, presenting it as a vaccine paper. Sir Richard then reached out to Bengt Nordén, the Swedish chemist who chairs the editorial board of Cambridge University's distinguished *Quarterly Review of Biophysics*, and succeeded in having the watered-down version published. "We had to take out a whole load of stuff in order to get it published," he says.

Sir Richard adds there was blowback from Cambridge University for publishing the article in the *Quarterly Review of Biophysics*. He blames the reliance on Chinese funding for the failure to publish legitimate science. "So many of these institutions are dependent on Chinese Academy of Science funding and Chinese money that they don't want to offend the Chinese, so what happened internationally is the Chinese narrative became the truth," he said.

There were also perceived conflicts of interest at the medical journals themselves, where senior figures may have been unwilling to criticise Chinese scientists or science institutions with which they had business relationships. The Editor-in-Chief of the prestigious *Nature* journal, based in London, Magdalena Skipper, a geneticist with a long history in editorial and publishing, says in her profile she is passionate about "transparent science and clarity in science communication".

She attended the 21st annual meeting of the China Association for Science and Technology in June 2019 – a non-governmental organisation. The association's website states: "The China Association for Science and Technology (CAST) serves as a bridge that links the Communist Party of China and the Chinese government to the country's science and technology community." CAST is also a constituent member of China's peak united front forum, the Chinese People's Political Consultative Conference. Skipper sent a personalised video message to the Chinese Academy of Sciences to congratulate it on its 70th anniversary, and in November 2019, Skipper was in Beijing for the Tencent Science WE Summit, a joint initiative between Tencent, the owner of WeChat, and *Nature*.

There is nothing at all wrong with these business and scientific collaborations, of course. Unless financial relationships influenced decisions around which scientific papers to publish. Skipper says, "All editorial decisions are made independently of any business implications for the company or relationships with any part of the research community – the fundamental principle of such editorial independence is an absolute requirement for us to be trusted and read by the research community. Our editors consider all submissions on their scientific merits alone."

This follows an earlier revelation in 2017, by the *Financial Times*, that Springer Nature, which publishes *Nature*, had blocked access in China to more than 1000 articles in two political science journals that raised Taiwan, Tibet and the Cultural Revolution. They admitted the censorship of "a small percentage of our content", justifying it by saying they had to comply with local regulations to avoid the risk of Chinese readers not being able to access any of their content.

Asked why *Nature* rejected scientific papers that questioned a natural origin of Covid-19, Dr Skipper said editors make decisions "based solely on whether research meets our criteria for publication – robust original scientific research (where conclusions are sufficiently supported by the available evidence), of outstanding scientific importance, which reaches a conclusion of interest to a multidisciplinary readership – and remain completely independent. This applies to Covid-19-related submissions, as it does for all other submissions. Our editors consider all submissions on their scientific merits alone and no subject is excluded from publication because the conclusions may be controversial or go against the established wisdom."

Dr Skipper's argument is undermined by a letter published in *Nature Medicine*, part of the *Nature* portfolio, on Covid-19 on March 17, 2020, which insisted the virus had a natural origin with, as far as I can see, absolutely no conclusive evidence for making this claim. Titled "The proximal origin of SARS-CoV 2", it was written by US, British and Australian researchers Kristian Andersen, Andrew Rambaut, Ian Lipkin, Edward Holmes and Robert Garry. "Our analyses clearly show that SARS-CoV-2 is not a laboratory construct or a purposefully manipulated virus," they wrote. Yet their paper "clearly" showed no such thing. It was effectively a biased comment piece. Deigin said when he carefully read the *Nature Medicine* letter he was "flabbergasted by just how weak it was and how juvenile the logic in that paper is". Yet this piece, by "experts", was critical in allowing the natural origin narrative to take hold, and led people to believe a laboratory leak was impossible.

I asked Dr Skipper why *Nature Medicine* would publish such an unscientific piece if it was only committed to publishing "robust original scientific research". She replied, "The Correspondence section provides a forum for discussion or to present a point of view on issues that are of interest to the readership of *Nature Medicine*.

In this correspondence the authors offer a perspective on the notable features of the SARS-CoV-2 genome and discuss scenarios by which they could have arisen based on their consideration of the evidence available at the time. I hope it may be helpful to highlight that the authors state in their conclusions 'the evidence shows that SARS-CoV-2 is not a purposefully manipulated virus, it is currently impossible to prove or disprove the other theories of its origin described here'. They also state 'More scientific data could swing the balance of evidence to favor one hypothesis over another.' I hope you may find this helpful in clarifying the position that the authors have taken."

Andersen rejects the characterisation of his paper as commentary. "All our studies on SARS-CoV-2 are scientific and based on evidence, with peer-reviewed publications presenting the data and conclusions – none of them are 'commentary' as you are suggesting," he says.

Yu, in his report for Pompeo in April 2020, already understood how the scientific journals had played into China's narrative. "*Nature* seems to have prioritized political correctness over facts," he wrote. "In January 2020, the British science journal bought the Chinese government narrative by stating that 'Scientists believe the most likely source of the coronavirus to be an animal market,' while this CCP theory was being challenged by other medical journals and it soon collapsed."

A *Nature* reporter Amy Maxmen found herself in a spot of controversy when she wrote an article on May 27, 2021 saying scientists found the lab-leak hypothesis "unsettling", that the discussion had grown toxic and had fuelled bullying of scientists along with anti-Asian harassment. She also claimed the discussion offended scientists in China. Days later, conservative news outlet *The National Pulse* published an exclusive article headlined: "Explosive Unearthed Video shows Peter Daszak describing 'Chinese Colleagues' Developing Killer Coronaviruses". The article referred to Daszak, the long-term collaborator of the Wuhan Institute of Virology, speaking at a 2016 conference about the work undertaken in Wuhan. "My colleagues in China did the work. You create pseudoparticles, you insert the spike proteins from those viruses, see if they bind to human cells. At each step of this you move closer and closer to this virus that could really become pathogenic in people."

The article didn't refer to Maxmen but observers pointed out on Twitter that she was seated beside Daszak at the 2016 conference. She claimed that the photograph had been doctored and pointed the finger at the *National Pulse* editor, Raheem Kassam, saying he formerly ran *Breitbart News*, implying that editing a right-wing outlet meant he was guilty of faking a photograph. "I've never met Daszak," she insisted. But extensive evidence emerged to show that Maxmen was indeed at the conference beside Daszak and it was not a fake as she claimed. This included one of her own tweets, dated February 27, 2016, where she wrote: "Thanks for pic! Honored to sit beside such experts in cholera, Zika, HIV and more @soniashah @PeterDaszak Ian Lipkin". The Pulitzer Centre at the New York Academy of Medicine who organised the event also recorded a photograph and account of her participation but Daszak's name had been mysteriously deleted before being added on June 14, 2021. Maxmen ultimately claimed to have forgotten about the event. The entire saga raised the question of why *Nature* would be trying to hide its links to the likes of Daszak. Maxmen was also publicly critical of a podcast that interviewed journalists who raised the possibility of a lab leak, tweeting "maybe talk to actual science reporters who bother with actual science". The attitude was indicative of how scientific publications treated the entire issue.

Professor Richard Muller speaks regularly to his scientist friends who specialise in virology and are Nobel prize winners. Muller found his biologist friends were unwilling to speak out about the unusual aspects of the virus because they didn't want to offend the Chinese scientific community they collaborate with. "We know if a member of our laboratory is working on something where they are potentially accusing the Chinese of doing something wrong, they will be ostracised and their joint research will be cut off," Muller says. "I was horrified. The Chinese had taken some degree of control over our own intellectual honesty, openness and objectivity. They had manipulated us, by freely collaborating. You'd think it would mean we know more about what's going on over there, but it means they have this lever to make sure the US experts would never be involved in an investigation into Chinese wrongdoing."

There are scientists who insist it is very unlikely Covid-19 could have escaped from a laboratory. The University of Sydney's Professor Edward Holmes, the first person outside of China to obtain its genome, is one of them.

On April 16, 2020, the day after Trump and Pompeo's public remarks about a possible laboratory origin, Holmes released a press release titled: "Unfounded Speculation on the Origins of the SARS-CoV-2 Virus that Causes COVID-19". "There is no evidence that SARS-CoV-2, the virus that causes COVID-19 in humans, originated in a laboratory in Wuhan, China," he wrote. "Coronaviruses like SARS-CoV-2 are commonly found in wildlife species and frequently jump to new hosts. This is also the most likely explanation for the origin of SARS-CoV-2.

"The closest known relative of SARS-CoV-2 is a bat virus named RaTG13, which was kept at the Wuhan Institute of Virology. There is some unfounded speculation that this virus was the origin of SARS-CoV-2. However: (i) RaTG13 was sampled from a different province of China (Yunnan) to where COVID-19 first appeared; and (ii) the level of genome sequence divergence between SARS-CoV-2 and RaTG13 is equivalent to an average of 50 years (and at least 20 years) of evolutionary change. Hence, SARS-CoV-2 was not derived from RaTG13."

He also wrote that viruses related to coronavirus are found in pangolins, which he said suggests "other wildlife species are likely to carry relatives of SARS-CoV-2".

Holmes argues that a virus, RaTG13, was sampled from a different province of China from where Covid-19 emerged so it could not have come from that virus. The argument doesn't hold up, because the RaTG13 was held in the Wuhan Institute of Virology's freezers – the same city where Covid-19 broke out.

Second, he says there is an equivalent of 20–50 years of evolutionary change. This point doesn't acknowledge the possibility the virus may have been spliced, genetically altered or the subject of other risky gain-of-function experiments in the Wuhan laboratory.

In their letter to *Nature Medicine*, Holmes and his four co-authors recognise that SARS-CoV-2 is "optimised for binding to the human receptor ACE2" and that the "spike protein of SARS-CoV-2 has a functional polybasic (furin) cleavage site". But they say this likely arose from recombination of a virus found in bats with another virus potentially from pangolins.

The team propose two ways by which SARS-CoV-2 could have mutated naturally to be so infectious to humans. The first scenario suggests that the virus evolved naturally in hosts, such as bats or pangolins, and its spike proteins mutated to bind to molecules similar in structure to the human ACE2 protein. The second scenario is that a less severe version of Covid-19 had been circulating in humans for years, or even decades, and had gradually mutated to become highly infectious. The scientists were not able to provide any evidence for this.

In their conclusion they admit, as Dr Skipper noted, that it's impossible to rule out a laboratory origin. "Although the evidence shows that SARS-CoV-2 is not a purposefully manipulated virus, it is currently impossible to prove or disprove the other theories of its origin described here," it states. "However, since we observed all notable SARS-CoV-2 features, including the optimized RBD and polybasic cleavage site, in related coronaviruses in nature, we do not believe that any type of laboratory-based scenario is plausible."

The Director of the US NIH, Francis S. Collins, commented on the letter shortly after publication, arguing "this study leaves little room to refute a natural origin for Covid-19".

One of the authors of the *Nature Medicine* letter, Kristian Andersen, rejected Baltimore's assertion that the spike protein was a "smoking gun" and said it is "simply incorrect".

"The site is not a 'smoking gun', nor does it 'make a powerful challenge to the idea of a natural origin," he tweeted. "Quite the opposite … FCSs [furin cleavage sites] are abundant, including being highly prevalent in coronaviruses. While SARS-CoV-2 is the first example of a SARSr virus with an FCS, other betacoronaviruses (the genus for SARS-CoV-2) have FCSs, including MERS and HKU1. There is nothing mysterious about having a 'first example' of a virus with a FCS. Viruses sampled to date only give us a teeny-tiny fraction of all the viruses circulating in the wild. Fragments … come and go all the time. How did SARS-CoV-2 acquire the FCS? We don't know, however, we know four main mechanisms often lead to insertions: (1) mutation (2) polymerase slippage (3) template switching (4) recombination."

Israeli geneticist Ronen Shemesh rejects these arguments. "If someone would have shown me a virus strain which has the inserted furin cleavage site or even another insertion of four amino acids at the same cleavage site, I would be likely to believe it is an evolutionary process or a recombination between two species … however, this strain was never found yet," he says. "Some conservative scientists would need a 'smoking gun' in order to determine that something like this virus is 'hand made', and so they prefer to make the assumption that this was created by chance … not that anyone can say how. There is no way to prove either way really, but proving it is a lab-generated strain by methods of likelihood and circumstantial evidence is easier than proving that it was not."

Another co-author of the *Nature Medicine* letter that set the tone for a natural origin of Covid-19, the director of Columbia University's Center of Infection and Immunity, epidemiology professor Ian Lipkin, has since withdrawn his support for it. He told former *New York Times* science writer Donald McNeil Jr that he had favoured a natural origin theory in part because he assumed that all of the Wuhan Institute of Virology's 2019 work with SARS-like viruses had taken place in its top-level BSL-4 laboratory. "But later he learned of studies with Dr Shi's name on them showing that work he considers dangerous had been done in level BSL-2 labs, which he considers highly porous to leaks, not just in 2016, but in 2020," McNeil wrote. Lipkin reportedly said: "That's screwed up.

It shouldn't have happened. People should not be looking at bat viruses in BSL-2 labs. My view has changed."

A year on, in 2021, 43 international scientists would sign four letters calling for an investigation into a possible laboratory leak. The first group of 25 scientists went public with their letter on March 4, 2021 in response to the WHO's flawed inquiry, which failed to investigate the Wuhan laboratories. The scientists published a series of letters outlining the steps the WHO needed to take for a rigorous scientific inquiry into the origins of the virus. One of the essential questions they identified that needs examining is this: "Did the WIV or any other laboratory ever attempt to recreate RaTG13 or any other coronaviruses by assembling them from synthetic gene sequences?" They want to obtain the records of laboratories involved in coronavirus research in Wuhan, such as laboratory notebooks, electronic records and details of gain-of-function research, including related sequences and isolates.

Along with Professor Ebright, Dr Quay and Professor Petrovsky, the signatories included the Australian National University's Professor of Public Health Colin Butler, French zoologist Henri Cap, Emeritus Professor of Medicine Jean-Michel Claverie, evolutionary geneticist Virginie Courtier, molecular virologist Etienne Decroly, neurobiology professor André Goffinet, Japanese associate professor Hideki Kakeya, the University of Maryland's Milton Leitenberg, molecular biologist Dominique Morello and Professor of Genetics at Jena University Günter Theißen.

The co-organiser of the letter, Jamie Metzl, said any examination of the origins needs to include all hypotheses. "It cannot be credible to say we're only going to look at zoonotic jump, and we won't even lift a finger to examine the lab-leak hypothesis," he said. "It's just outrageous to try to rank which possibility is more likely than others when some of them have been examined and other lab-leak hypotheses simply have not."

Then a second powerful letter was published in *Science* magazine on May 14, 2021, signed by 18 prominent virologists, biologists and immunologists from the US, Canada, the UK and Switzerland. They were major names in the world of virology, including Harvard's Professor David Relman and Nick Patterson, Pamela Bjorkman from Caltech and Stanford University's Tim Stearns. One signatory to the letter was more fascinating than any other. The University of North Carolina's Ralph Baric had closely collaborated with Shi Zhengli at the Wuhan Institute of Virology on coronavirus research. If he thought it was possible the virus had leaked from a laboratory, it was extremely telling.

The Fred Hutch Cancer Research Center's Associate Professor Jesse Bloom, who is also an Affiliate Associate Professor in the Genome Sciences and Microbiology Department at the University of Washington, signed the letter. "Central to being a good scientist is keeping an open mind when evidence is sparse, and as a 'virus expert' who has followed this topic closely: it's clear in any objective assessment that both natural origins and accidental lab leak are plausible," he said in March 2021. "We should all be able to agree as scientists that there is a need for greater transparency about the SARS-related coronaviruses being studied in Wuhan prior to the pandemic."

Many people felt a certain level of frustration that these scientists had taken 15 months to speak publicly, allowing the Chinese disinformation that a natural origin was the only possibility to take hold. I asked one of the signatories, Director of the Harvard University Center for Communicable Disease Dynamics and Professor of Epidemiology Marc Lipsitch, why he had not spoken out earlier. He replied that he had avoided reopening the gain-of-function (GOF) issue because he was focused on pressing research related to dealing with the pandemic, and he knew he could not simultaneously do both pandemic response and the origins issue. "Second, I believe it is critical for scientists to work together right now for the good of solving the pandemic in front of us, and reopening a controversial debate that some take very personally did not seem conducive to that project," he said.

Professor Lipsitch said he had followed the origins discussion closely enough to "conclude that the group of hypotheses involving a lab accident – which include not only GOF but also more ordinary infections with a strain that had been isolated from an animal host in the lab – have some plausibility, and that they need to be investigated alongside the other hypotheses that many consider more likely."

Professor Lipsitch said the politicisation of the origins question makes it harder to investigate. "Once it is politicized, and sides are drawn, then the interest of each 'side' in winning becomes greater (to avoid embarrassment) and incentives to selectively pursue evidence grow," he said. "Having said that, it is hard to imagine that a subject of this importance and consequence would not become political."

Without knowing the origins of the virus, Professor Lipsitch said, we can't take evidence-based measures to prevent future catastrophes. "Regardless of whether this pandemic came from zoonosis or a lab, strengthening surveillance for spillover events and strengthening lab safety for potential pandemic pathogens are key efforts," he said. "But surely knowing which of these two pathways caused this catastrophe would help us prioritize and perhaps reveal countermeasures that we haven't thought of."

It is clearly incorrect for anyone to claim there is a scientific consensus that Covid-19 has a natural, zoonotic origin. World-leading virologists – the most eminent people in their fields – have stated that it could have inadvertently leaked from a laboratory, where it may have been the result of gain-of-function research.

Back on April 30, 2020, US intelligence agencies confirmed in a statement that a laboratory leak was being examined. "The Intelligence Community will continue to rigorously examine emerging information and intelligence to determine whether the outbreak began through contact with infected animals or if it was the result of an accident at a laboratory in Wuhan," it said. But the statement categorically ruled out that Covid-19 may be the result of laboratory experimentation. "The Intelligence Community also concurs with the wide scientific consensus that the COVID-19 virus was not manmade or genetically modified," the Office of the Director of National Intelligence said in the rare statement.

The Office of the Director of National Intelligence comprises US Defence, Justice, Homeland Security and other government agencies. The statement was far too hasty, and its claim of a "wide scientific consensus" is now demonstrably false. It was an inaccurate statement and has since been contradicted by prominent, world-leading scientists.

"That statement to me was despicable," says Former Assistant Secretary of State for East Asia and Pacific Affairs David Stilwell, who was at that time America's top diplomat for East Asia. "As soon as they issued that statement we were all shaking our heads saying, 'Why would they say that?' The intelligence community needs to be subject to an Inspector General review for putting that statement out. It was wrong and it was really unhelpful."

The intelligence community had released inaccurate, misleading information into the world that supported the Chinese narrative that the virus had a natural origin. What the Australian intelligence agencies feared had come to pass – but in precisely the reverse. Australian and British agencies worried about lending support to Trump's unverified theories, but in actual fact they were lending support to the CCP's disinformation that the virus couldn't possibly have been manipulated in a laboratory. The US statement was incredibly damaging, and there has been no retraction or apology from the Office of the Director of National Intelligence. At the time of writing, no one has held the intelligence agencies to account for their role in suppressing scientific facts about the origin of the virus.

CHAPTER FIFTEEN

The Scientists Who Knew

Shi Zhengli was well known in the close-knit scientific community that studied bat coronaviruses. She had become a scientific celebrity after discovering the closest virus to SARS in bats. As the Director for the Centre for Emerging Infectious Diseases at the Wuhan Institute of Virology, she became known as the "Batwoman" for her sampling of thousands of bats in remote caves.

It was nothing compared to the global fame she'd attract after the pandemic outbreak. Her institute's research, with all its risks, would be exposed for the world to judge. When questions arose in China about whether her laboratory was the source of the outbreak at the start of February 2020 – three months before Trump raised the prospect – Shi Zhengli snapped. "Those who believe and spread rumours, shut your dirty mouth," she posted on WeChat on February 6, 2020. Instead, she said, Covid-19 "is nature's punishment for uncivilized living habits of human beings. I, Shi Zhengli, use my life to guarantee that it has nothing to do with our lab."

Just how dangerous was the research she was conducting, often without the watchful eyes of international partners, at the Wuhan Institute of Virology? What were Shi and her colleagues up to, and who was funding it?

Of particular focus would be her "gain-of-function" experiments. Gain-of-function research aims to make viruses more infectious and deadlier or more virulent, often to humans. The technical definition is research that "involves experimentation that is expected to increase the transmissibility and/or virulence of pathogens". It can result in a pathogen acquiring new abilities; for example, a bat virus becoming able to infect humans or a virus that wasn't airborne having the ability to become so.

It takes separate natural viruses and, as science writer Nicholson Baker aptly put it, "hot-wires" their genomes, genetically manipulating, splicing and artificially recombining genetic sequences, then passaging them – subculturing them in a series of cell cultures and/or animals – to encourage them to mutate into brand-new viruses that never existed before in nature, which could turn out to be highly infectious and lethal to humans. This research, which has been carried out in the US and other Western countries as well as China, has been justified by scientists who claim it could help predict pandemics by discovering which viruses are capable of becoming infectious to humans. They say this allows them to pre-emptively develop vaccines and therapeutics. But only two laboratories globally were doing gain-of-function research on coronaviruses prior to the pandemic, according to Dr Ebright.

Other research projects may not strictly fall into the gain-of-function category but are equally dangerous. They include bringing back to life very old viruses and manipulating them in a laboratory. This type of research deals with what are referred to as "potential pandemic pathogens".

To many outside of the scientific community, this type of experimentation sounds absurd. How is it even legal, given the astronomical risks? Debate has raged about the grave dangers of allowing gain-of-function research to take place. There are two main concerns. Firstly, it is a subset of dual-use research. In other words, it can be misused for malevolent military purposes such as bioweapons. Secondly, it can accidentally cause a pandemic.

In a 2016 paper on the ethics of creating new, potentially deadly viruses, Michael Selgelid, Director of the World Health Organization's Collaborating Centre for Bioethics at Monash University's Bioethics Centre in Melbourne, wrote that this has been "one of the most hotly debated science policy issues during the 21st century, with controversy surrounding a series of published experiments with potential implications for biological weapons-making".

"Such research (when conducted by responsible scientists) usually aims to improve understanding of disease-causing agents, their interaction with human hosts, and/or their potential to cause pandemics," he continued. "Despite these important potential benefits, GOF research can pose risks regarding biosecurity and biosafety."

Selgelid wrote that even if the scientists who were creating these new infectious viruses were responsible, there was concern that publishing the research would provide "'recipes' for especially dangerous potential biological weapons agents to would-be bioterrorists ... Of particular concern in the context of life science research is that advances in biotechnology may enable development and use of a new generation of biological weapons of mass destruction." Gain-of-function research allows scientists to create new lethal viruses that didn't exist in nature before. There was the "genetic engineering of a superstrain of the mousepox virus in 2001, the artificial synthesis of a 'live' polio virus from chemical components in 2002, and the reconstruction of the 1918 'Spanish Flu' virus in 2005," Selgelid wrote.

Global controversy around this type of research ignited in 2012, when scientists wanted to see if it would be possible for bird flu (H5N1) to evolve naturally into a virus that was capable of human-to-human transmission, and thus cause a pandemic. Their stated intention was to be able to predict which viruses could turn into a pandemic.

The scientists, Professor Ron Fouchier from the Erasmus Medical Centre in Rotterdam, the Netherlands, and Yoshihiro Kawaoka, who holds a professorship in virology in the Department of Pathobiological Sciences at the University of Wisconsin-Madison, USA, and at the University of Tokyo, Japan, created a deadly new flu virus. It was a highly pathogenic influenza virus strain of H5N1 that was transmissible by air between ferrets, indicating it could infect humans in a similar way. Fouchier said the ferret-transmissible strain he created was "probably one of the most dangerous viruses you can make". But "critics questioned the validity of claims about such benefits – and argued that the studies might facilitate creation of biological weapons agents that could kill millions, or possibly even billions, of people," Selgelid wrote in his 2016 paper.

He was ahead of his time.

When the debate was raging, Harvard University Professor of Epidemiology Marc Lipsitch campaigned against the type of research that creates new "potential pandemic pathogens" that would be transmissible to humans. He specifically warned against the risk of creating a pandemic. "Experiments that create the possibility of initiating a pandemic should be subject to a rigorous quantitative risk assessment and a search for safer alternatives before they are approved or performed," he and co-author Thomas Inglesby wrote in the American Society for Microbiology's *mBio* journal in 2014. They raised concerns about BSL-2 and BSL-3 laboratories operating in countries with "less stringent standards than those in the United States", warning that "the rate of accidents" may be higher.

Three years later, in 2018, Professor Lipsitch's warnings became more grave when he wrote about the possibility of an accidental laboratory leak leading to a pandemic on a scale we've never seen before. "Experiments to create potential pandemic pathogens (PPPs) are nearly unique in that they present biosafety risks that extend well beyond the experimenter or laboratory performing them," he wrote. "An accidental release could, as the name suggests, lead to global spread of a virulent virus, a biosafety incident on a scale never before seen."

In potentially prophetic comments, Senior Science Fellow at the Centre for Arms Control and Non-Proliferation Lynn Klotz had also warned this type of research could cause a pandemic. In a *Bulletin of the Atomic Scientists* piece co-authored with science writer Edward Sylvester, Klotz said there are three "potential pandemic pathogens" – smallpox, the 1918 flu virus and SARS – that "are all extremely deadly, highly contagious in humans and not currently present in human populations, meaning it would be a disaster to reintroduce them into the population."

Writing in 2012, they said smallpox posed the least threat as it was, at the time, researched in only two facilities in the world by international agreement, where lab workers have been vaccinated to prevent infections to themselves. "In stark contrast to the strict controls on smallpox research, however, SARS, the 1918 flu virus, and potentially human-contagious H5N1 bird flu are studied in laboratories throughout the world, using less than the highest biocontainment, known as Biosafety Level 4, or BSL-4, and there is *no* approved and stockpiled vaccine for any of them," they wrote.

"It is SARS that now presents the greatest risk," they went on. "The worry is less about recurrence of a natural SARS outbreak than of *yet another escape* from a laboratory researching it to help protect against a natural outbreak. SARS already has escaped from laboratories three times since 2003, and one escape resulted in several secondary infections and one death. What is the likelihood that the virus's escape could lead to a pandemic? Too high," they warned, predicting that 15 per cent of the world's population could be infected by a pandemic flu virus.

They specifically called for research on live SARS coronaviruses to stop. "As noted, about 30 labs now are working with live SARS virus worldwide. The probability of escape from at least one laboratory is high; the probability of an escape that leads to a major outbreak or pandemic is, on the other hand, likely low. Would one in 10 escapes lead to a major outbreak or pandemic? One in a hundred? One in a thousand? No one knows. But for any of these probabilities, the likelihood-weighted number of victims and deaths would be intolerably high. Research on live SARS should be curtailed – perhaps even discontinued – until biological containment measures beyond BSL-3 and even BSL-4 can be put in place."

Klotz and Sylvester also called for the WHO to convene a meeting about research on pathogens with pandemic potential. "The goal should be nothing less than the elimination of the possibility that scientific research might cause a pandemic," they wrote.

Quite extraordinary comments. If only world health authorities and political leaders had listened to Klotz and his ilk.

Scientists fiercely opposed to gain-of-function research formed a body called the Cambridge Working Group in 2014. There were 200 esteemed signatories. They released a letter specifically warning that accidents while scientists were experimenting with these dangerous viruses could cause "an accidental pandemic" that could infect a quarter of the world's population. "Accident risks with newly created 'potential pandemic pathogens' raise grave new concerns," their letter said. "Laboratory creation of highly transmissible, novel strains of dangerous viruses, especially but not limited to influenza, poses substantially increased risks. An accidental infection in such a setting could trigger outbreaks that would be difficult or impossible to control. Historically, new strains of influenza, once they establish transmission in the human population, have infected a quarter or more of the world's population within two years."

Steven Salzberg, of the Johns Hopkins School of Medicine's Center for Computational Biology, said in a 2015 letter that the benefits of gain-of-function research were "minimal at best" and they could "far more safely be obtained through other avenues of research". "I am very concerned that the continuing gain-of-function research on influenza viruses, and more recently on other viruses, presents extremely serious risks to the public health," he wrote. "It seems clear that some of the scientists leading the GOF research on influenza are doing it primarily for the publicity and acclaim while downplaying the risks." He added that there was no evidence to support their claim that lab-created viruses would teach us how to avoid or pre-empt future pandemics.

Associate Professor Carlos Moreno, from the Department of Pathology and Laboratory Medicine in Emory University's School of Medicine, said he was "deeply concerned" by the "potential fatalities that could result from accidental laboratory infections that might occur in a laboratory conducting gain-of-function research on influenza and other infectious diseases". "The number of accidental releases of potentially fatal pathogens in recent years has demonstrated unequivocally that human error is inevitable and impossible to completely eliminate from experiments with deadly pathogens," he said.

This type of research carries such a grave risk of causing a pandemic that President Barack Obama paused funding for gain-of-function experiments in 22 fields in 2014, including research involving SARS, influenza and MERS viruses. This happened after an outcry in the scientific community about the dangerous experiments some virologists were conducting. "Specifically, the funding pause will apply to gain-of-function research projects that may be reasonably anticipated to confer attributes to influenza, MERS, or SARS viruses such that the virus would have enhanced pathogenicity and/or transmissibility in mammals via the respiratory route," the White House statement, dated October 17, 2014, said. "During this pause, the US Government will not fund any new projects involving these experiments and encourages those currently conducting this type of work – whether federally funded or not – to voluntarily pause their research while risks and benefits are being reassessed."

Coronavirus virologist Ralph Baric from the University of Carolina sent a letter to the National Science Advisory Board for Biosecurity objecting to the pause. He was working at the time with Shi Zhengli. He argued it focused too much on the risks rather than the benefits of GOF research, and said the research could be used to develop vaccines. "GOF experiments are a documented, powerful tool to understand viral pathogenic mechanisms, to attenuate virus pathogenesis, to identify new paradigms of disease causation," he wrote. "We are willing to participate at any level in discussions regarding this important new pathogenic human coronavirus."

Before the ban took effect, NIH Director Dr Anthony Fauci had welcomed a voluntary pause on GOF research but argued the opposite position from all the scientists I've quoted here. He specifically said the benefits did outweigh the risk of a pandemic –

a mind-boggling and incomprehensible position for an official charged with protecting the health of Americans. Writing in *mBio* about the voluntary moratorium on gain-of-function research in 2012, Fauci considered the scenario if experiments were conducted in a laboratory not subject to adequate safety regulations. "Putting aside the specter of bioterrorism for the moment, consider this hypothetical scenario: an important gain-of-function experiment involving a virus with serious pandemic potential is performed in a well-regulated, world-class laboratory by experienced investigators, but the information from the experiment is then used by another scientist who does not have the same training and facilities and is not subject to the same regulations. In an unlikely but conceivable turn of events, what if that scientist becomes infected with the virus, which leads to an outbreak and ultimately triggers a pandemic? Many ask reasonable questions: given the possibility of such a scenario – however remote – should the initial experiments have been performed and/or published in the first place, and what were the processes involved in this decision? Scientists working in this field might say – as indeed I have said – that the benefits of such experiments and the resulting knowledge outweigh the risks. It is more likely that a pandemic would occur in nature, and the need to stay ahead of such a threat is a primary reason for performing an experiment that might appear to be risky."

Fauci also defended the scientists who had undertaken the highly controversial gain-of-function research that had prompted the global debate, saying they had "conducted their research properly and under the safest and most secure conditions". He then suggested that the pause on gain-of-function research could slow down scientists performing these experiments. "Those of us in the scientific community who believe in the merits of this work have the responsibility to address these concerns thoughtfully and respectfully. Granted, the time it takes to engage in such a dialog could potentially delay or even immobilize the conduct of certain important experiments and the publication of valuable information that could move the field forward for the good of public health."

The same research that international scientists said should be banned, Fauci described as "important". "Within the research community, many have expressed concern that important research progress could come to a halt just because of the fear that someone, somewhere, might attempt to replicate these experiments sloppily," he wrote in his 2012 paper.

I discovered this paper while investigating Fauci's support for gain-of-function research for this book and was surprised to find it had never been mentioned in media reports. Fauci and his media advisors declined or did not respond to my numerous requests for comment or an interview. He only seems to agree to gentle interviews.

This mandatory "pause" or ban on gain-of-function research, introduced in 2014, was inexplicably lifted under the Trump administration in 2017. No adequate explanation has been given for why this decision was made. There was no public debate. On December 19, 2017, the NIH announced it would resume funding gain-of-function research involving MERS, SARS, coronaviruses and influenza after a new "framework" had been developed by the Department of Health and Human Services.

Multiple senior administration officials told me Fauci did not raise the issue of kickstarting gain-of-function research with any senior figures in the White House. There was one White House meeting, which Fauci requested with the Office of Science and Technology Policy, where he raised the issue of gain-of-function research. "It kind of just got rammed through," a senior source told me. "I think there's truth in the narrative that the NSC staff, the President, the White House Chief of Staff, those people were in the dark that he was switching back on GOF research."

I asked National Security Advisor Robert O'Brien about this. "I was in meeting after meeting with Dr Fauci, and that never came up," he says. "I don't know if he alerted anyone. I never heard about it until I was out of office." Pompeo, similarly, was kept in the dark. He said he didn't know if Fauci got permission from anyone to re-start the dangerous research, particularly with regard to contributing funding via sub-grants to the Wuhan Institute of Virology. Fauci didn't even tell his boss, Health Secretary Alex Azar, who only found out the United States restriction on gain-of-function research had been lifted from media reports in 2021.

In hindsight we can clearly see that health authorities, the US government and international governments all ignored the warnings from eminent scientists, and allowed the dangerous scientific research to go ahead. The public was never brought into these debates. A pandemic is something that affects all of us – we have lost loved ones, battled serious illness, lost jobs, had our businesses and ways of life destroyed. While the origins of Covid-19 have not yet been established, it's clear this type of research carries grave risks.

What was even more terrifying was that not only was the NIH funding gain-of-function research in the United States – but it was funding research in China, where it had no oversight and no way of knowing how safe the laboratories were where these risky experiments were taking place.

If there are clues in the SARS-CoV-2 virus itself about its potential laboratory origin, there are also a multitude of clues in the research papers published by Shi Zhengli and her team during this time period. They show precisely what research they were undertaking at the Wuhan Institute of Virology in the lead-up to the outbreak of Covid-19, who they were working with and just how they were splicing and cloning the viruses. They also show the passage of their research over time.

In basic terms, they were going out into remote bat caves, collecting coronaviruses, sequencing their genomes and comparing them to the known SARS and MERS viruses, to see which new ones could have the highest chance of 'spillover' to humans. The first assessment of this would be made purely by trained eye – comparing how similar the new spike proteins were to the ones of SARS and MERS, then *in silico* – by computer-modelling their binding to human receptors. After splicing the newfound spike genes, or just their receptor-binding domains, into so-called "viral backbones" (known coronaviral templates) and then turning those constructs into live viruses, they would check how well the viruses could infect various cell cultures or "humanised" animals, such as mice with human lung cells.

Shi Zhengli had been engaging in genetically modifying viruses since at least 2006. A paper published in the *Journal of Virology* that year shows she was trying to determine how coronaviruses gain the ability to skip from one species to another by "inserting different segments from the human SARS-CoV spike protein into the spike protein of the bat virus". This study specifically looked at how viruses could bind to the ACE2 receptor. "To address these unanswered questions, we cloned and expressed the bat *R. pearsonii* ACE2 gene and examined the abilities of ACE2 proteins from human, palm civet, and *R. pearsonii* to support infection by HIV-based pseudoviruses containing different S protein constructs," the paper states. "The ACE2-binding activity of SL-CoVs was easily acquired by the replacement of a relatively small sequence segment of the S protein from the SARS-CoV S sequence, highlighting the potential dangers posed by this diverse group of viruses in bats. The findings presented in this study serve as the first example of host switching achievable for CoVs under laboratory conditions by the exchange of a relatively small sequence segment among these previously unknown CoVs."

University of North Carolina's Ralph Baric reportedly taught Shi Zhengli how to use humanised mice to test whether viruses will infect humans. "It's kind of an amazing concept," says Dr Steven Quay. "So basically, you take a mouse embryo, and you inject genes that you want to humanise the mouse, so that it actually has human lungs or a human vascular system. Ralph Baric developed mice that have human lungs."

Baric published research with Shi Zhengli in the British journal *Nature Medicine* in November 2015, where they took a coronavirus extracted from Chinese horseshoe bats, called SHC014-CoV. "The authors followed a familiar path," explains longevity entrepreneur Yuri Deigin. "They took the spike-like protein from RsSHC014, which Shi Zhengli isolated from Yunnan bats in 2011, and inserted it into a murine[mouse]-adapted variant of SARS-CoV for subsequent in vivo experiments. They also tested it in human cells, and almost as an aside created a recombinant clone of the same RsSHC014 strain." Shi Zhengli and Baric said they did this in order "to examine the emergence potential [that is, the potential to infect humans] of circulating bat CoVs".

When they replaced the bat coronavirus spike protein with one that infected humans, Shi Zhengli and Ralph Baric created a brand-new infectious virus. It was lethal. The humanised mice they were experimenting on had severe lung damage with no cure. It gets worse. They looked at whether existing vaccines were successful against this new virus. They vaccinated aged mice and found the vaccine failed to protect aged animals. This is an important point.

Tellingly, in their findings, Baric and Shi Zhengli acknowledge the risk of the gain-of-function work they had just done. "The potential to prepare for and mitigate future outbreaks must be weighed against the risk of creating more dangerous pathogens," they wrote in their paper. "In developing policies moving forward, it is important to consider the value of the data generated by these studies and whether these types of chimeric virus studies warrant further investigation versus the inherent risks involved. On the basis of these findings, scientific review panels may deem similar studies building chimeric viruses based on circulating strains too risky to pursue."

Ralph Baric said in an interview with *ScienceDaily* at the time: "This virus is highly pathogenic and treatments developed against the original SARS virus in 2002 and the ZMapp drugs used to fight Ebola fail to neutralise and control this particular virus," he said.

Disturbingly, the sequence of the new virus they created (SHC014-MA15) was not deposited in GenBank until May 22, 2020 – even though the original paper was published five years earlier. This shows the Wuhan Institute of Virology (and other laboratories) does not publish all the viruses it creates or samples contemporaneously.

Professor Richard Ebright says the research Baric and Shi Zhengli did alarmed many scientists. "WIV's 2015 paper attracted controversy among scientists and science policy specialists worldwide, who noted that the work offered few benefits and risked triggering a pandemic." Baric himself had acknowledged that these types of viruses can be weaponised and used in biowarfare, in a paper he wrote in 2006 called "Synthetic Viral Genomics: Risks and Benefits for Science and Society". This shows he very clearly understood how the lethal viruses could be misused in biological warfare. He specifically mentioned the humanising of zoonotic viruses.

"It is also well established that the biological revolution, coupled with advances in biotechnology, could be used to enhance the offensive biological properties of viruses simply by altering resistance to antiviral agents (e.g. herpes viruses, poxviruses, influenza), modifying antigenic properties (e.g. T cell epitopes or neutralizing epitopes), modifying tissue tropism, pathogenesis and transmissibility, 'humanizing' zoonotic viruses, and creating designer super pathogens," he wrote. "These bioweapons could be targeted to humans, domesticated animals or crops, causing a devastating impact on human civilisation."

Science writer Declan Butler, in *Nature* in November 2015, examined how virologists were concerned about this gain-of-function research. "But other virologists question whether the information gleaned from the experiment justifies the potential risk," he wrote. "Although the extent of any risk is difficult to assess, Simon Wain-Hobson, a virologist at the Pasteur Institute in Paris, points out that the researchers have created a novel virus that 'grows remarkably well' in human cells. 'If the virus escaped, nobody could predict the trajectory,' he says."

Dr Quay, in Taiwan, says that when Shi Zhengli and Baric created this virus in a laboratory in 2015, they started with a backbone that did not exist in a natural bat-derived virus. "So, the really stupid thing the zoonosis crowd said was 'Well, because SARS-CoV-2 doesn't have a published backbone for the synthetic genetic process to make SARS-CoV-2 it couldn't have come from the laboratory,'" he says.

Shi Zhengli was also involved in another research project at the same time, submitting a paper in October 2015 with EcoHealth

Alliance President Peter Daszak and Wuhan Institute of Virology's Ben Hu. This study used the same virus she and Baric were working on, SHC014, and a new bat coronavirus called WIV1. "We recently isolated a bat SL-CoV strain (WIV1) and constructed an infectious clone of another strain (SHC014); significantly these strains are closely related to SARS-CoV and capable of using the same cellular receptor ACE2."

In this new paper, they reported a new SARS-like coronavirus strain called WIV16 that had been isolated from a faecal sample of a bat collected in Kunming, Yunnan. They described it as "not the closest strain to the human SARS-CoVs". They found that this new SARS-like coronavirus would also use ACE2 as an entry point. This is where they discovered that coronaviruses can infect humans through the ACE2 receptor. To do their test, they used cultured human HeLa cells in a Petri dish. HeLa cells are used in scientific experiments the world over and were named for and originally taken from the aggressive cancer tumour of an African-American mother Henrietta Lacks who died in 1951.

Just months later, in July 2016, Daszak and Shi Zhengli submitted another paper to the *Journal of Virology* where they said that SHC014 "has been demonstrated to use human ACE2 by the construction of an infectious cDNA clone". "In this study, we have developed a fast and cost-effective method for reverse genetics of coronaviruses by combining two approaches developed by others," it states.

Seven months later, in another paper by Shi Zhengli with Daszak, Ben Hu and others, submitted in February 2017, they created chimeric viruses from SARS-related coronaviruses they had obtained in the Shitou Cave in the Yunnan province. Dr Ebright has confirmed this is gain-of-function research. The study is called: "Discovery of a rich gene pool of bat SARS-related coronaviruses provides new insights into the origin of SARS coronaviruses."

It was the fruition of five years' worth of surveillance and sampling of bats from a single cave 60 kilometres (40 miles) from Kunming, where the temperature is 22–25 degrees Celsius (72–77 degrees Fahrenheit) and the humidity is as high as 90 per cent.

They visited the cave 10 times between April 2011 and October 2015. They disclosed the full-length genomes of 11 newly discovered SARS-related CoV strains. But there were plenty of other coronavirus samples they had found in the cave over the years. Out of 64 SARS-like coronavirus positive samples, they did not "amplify the RBD sequences" from 15 of them. "Most of these samples had comparatively low viral concentration," they state.

This study was conducted "in vitro" – meaning in a test-tube or Petri dish, rather than in an animal. They found that the main difference between SARS from 2003 and most bat SARS-related coronaviruses was "located in S gene". This, of course, is the gene encoding the spike protein in the virus. They took WIV1's backbone and replaced the S gene with one from the newly identified SARS-like coronaviruses. They used reverse-genetics to clone the viruses. "We constructed a group of infectious bacterial artificial chromosome (BAC) clones with the backbone of WIV1 and variants of S genes from 8 different bat SARS-like coronaviruses." They then looked at whether these new chimeric viruses could infect humans. They reported that three newly identified SARS coronaviruses "are all able to use human ACE2 as the receptor".

These new SARS-related coronaviruses "have been demonstrated to use the same cellular receptor ACE2 as SARS-CoV does and replicate efficiently in primary human airway cells". Shi Zhengli and Daszak say their five-year study "conclusively" demonstrated that all building blocks of the pandemic SARS genome are present in bat SARS-like coronaviruses from a single location in Yunnan.

It's not only the American NIH agency that helped Shi Zhengli and Daszak with this extremely risky gain-of-function experiment. Their paper states that the CSIRO's Australian Animal Health Laboratory "kindly provided" the HeLa cells and other cells, called "Vero E6 cell line", which were originally extracted from monkeys in Japan. Australia's CSIRO also trained some of the Wuhan scientists and funded many of their projects. This particular study was funded by the Chinese government, through the Chinese Academy of Sciences' Pioneer Hundred Talents program; and the

United States government, through the NIAID and USAID. Did anyone in the United States or Australia read or even understand the gain-of-function research they were contributing to or funding with taxpayer dollars?

Shi Zhengli's colleague Ben Hu then started to work on a project looking at two new bat coronaviruses. Ben Hu received ¥250,000 (US$2275) in funding from the Youth Science Fund Project, distributed by the Natural National Science Foundation of China, to work on a project called, "Pathogenicity of 2 new bat SARS-related CoVs to transgenic mice expressing human ACE2". The project was approved in 2018 and was set to run from January 2019 to December 2021. The results of this study, including details of which two new coronaviruses he was experimenting with – to specifically see if they can infect humans – were due to appear around the time of the outbreak but have never been published.

Luke McWilliams, a researcher for this book, discovered the title for this research project on the National Natural Science Foundation of China project website on March 17, 2020, and had it translated. But when he revisited the website on January 6, 2021, all of the projects relating to the Wuhan Institute of Virology had been wiped. Cyber-security expert Robert Potter confirmed it that same day, noting on Twitter: "Checked this and it looks more than 300 items aren't there anymore and we're all sitting here wondering how are there still things to hide at this point." Luckily, McWilliams had archived and saved the relevant website pages.

Ben Hu and Shi Zhengli's team had sampled bats from 22 provinces in China, mostly in the southern provinces, detecting 200 positive samples of SARS-like coronaviruses. But they focused on the Yunnan cave. "Since we found so many SARS-like coronaviruses here, personal protective measures were necessary each time we entered the cave for sampling," Hu said in an interview in December 2017. He also spoke about the type of genetic manipulation they were doing with these viruses. "In addition to the newly isolated strain, we obtained a series of chimeric viruses with different S genes by replacing the S genes of the newly discovered strain onto the constructed full-length infectious clones of the WIV1 strain of SARS-like coronavirus by a reverse genetics approach. Our results confirm that multiple strains of SARS-like coronaviruses without deletions in the S gene can all replicate efficiently in Vero E6 cells and invade HeLa cells using the human ACE2 receptor."

Shi Zhengli has in total collected 19,000 samples and coronavirus was detected in 2481 of them, according to information she provided to the WHO in February 2021. "Her laboratory used recombinant viruses to test whether bat CoVs could use ACE2 to bind but used bat spike protein on a bat-CoV backbone, not human SARS," the WHO report states. She told the WHO the Wuhan Institute of Virology began recombinant work in 2015 with WIV1. "It received ACE2 mice in 2016 and started recombinant experiments with WIV + SHC014 in 2018 but did not finish them owing to the COVID outbreak." This is further proof that the Wuhan Institute of Virology has not made public all of the virus samples it has been working with. "All samples are stored but not all have been examined yet," the WHO report states, based on their interview with Shi Zhengli.

Before the outbreak was publicly known, a Professor of Molecular Evolution at the University of Edinburgh, Andrew Rambaut, said on Twitter that there was little point to finding new viruses. "The more we look, the more new viruses we find. The problem is that we have no way of knowing which may be important or which may emerge," he said. "There is basically nothing we can do with that information to prevent or mitigate epidemics."

Peter Daszak publicly disagreed with him and in doing so opened a window into the worrying work he and other scientists were conducting. "Not true – we've made great progress with bat SARS-related CoVs, ID'ing more than 50 novel strains, sequencing spike protein genes, ID'ing ones [that] bind to human cells, using recombinant viruses/humanized mice to see SARS-like signs, and showing some don't respond to MAbs, vaccines," he tweeted. His mention of vaccines is also interesting, implying scientists had been looking at trying to develop vaccines for coronaviruses, a possible source of a virus leak.

A thesis by a Wuhan Institute of Virology scientist, Lei-Ping Zeng, dated April 2017, was uncovered by international research group DRASTIC. In it, Lei-Ping Zeng discusses how they can alter the spike protein and create a chimeric recombinant virus "without leaving any trace". "The S genes of the successfully cloned different strains of SL-CoV were inserted into the BAC vector together with the Es and Fs fragments and the A to D and G fragments ... respectively, to construct an S gene chimeric recombinant viral infectious BAC clone with WIV1 as the backbone and without leaving any trace sequences (e.g. incorporated enzymatic sites) in the recombinant viral genome," it states.

Dr Ebright says there are two other risky scientific experiments at the Wuhan Institute of Virology that are possible gain-of-function research and are of concern. One is a project called, "Two Mutations were Critical for Bat-to-Human Transmission of Middle East Respiratory Syndrome Coronavirus", published in June 2015. It was done by Shi Zhengli, Baric and two scientists, Lanyiang Du and Shibo Jiang, from the Lindsley Kimball Research Institute's New York Blood Centre. The University of Minnesota Medical School's Fang Li, Chang Liu and Yang Yang were also co-authors.

The second is a research paper published in August 2020 titled, "A Zika Virus Envelope Mutation Preceding the 2015 Epidemic Enhances Virulence and Fitness for Transmission". This was done by the University of Texas Medical Branch, Galveston, in conjunction with the Wuhan Institute of Virology.

Because of the type of risky research underway at the Wuhan Institute of Virology, when the SARS-CoV-2 virus broke out, Dr Ebright instantly suspected it may have originated from the Institute. "To scientists and science policy specialists who have been engaged since 2015 in discussions and debates about WIV's extremely high-risk gain-of-function research on bat SARS-related coronaviruses, the news in early January 2020 that an outbreak involving bat SARS-related coronavirus was occurring in Wuhan, on WIV's doorstep, immediately suggested a possible laboratory origin for the outbreak," he tells me. This was particularly the case since only three laboratories globally were conducting gain-of-function research on coronaviruses: the University of North Carolina, the University of Texas Medical Branch Galveston and the Wuhan Institute of Virology.

As Ebright has been at pains to point out, the type of gain-of-function research that has been undertaken worldwide in the last half-decade, including at the Wuhan Institute of Virology, does not leave signatures. You cannot tell from studying the virus if it has been subjected to genetic manipulation.

CHAPTER SIXTEEN

America's Doctor

Anthony Fauci, with his calm and measured manner of speech, has cultivated an image as a wise grandfatherly figure. Called "America's Doctor" in the media, the 80-year-old has spent 50 years in the public service, joining the NIH during the Vietnam War after studying as a physician. He was appointed Director of the National Institute of Allergy and Infectious Diseases in 1984.

Like many medical officials around the world, he became a household name during the pandemic. Populations crippled with anxiety clung onto every utterance by medical experts who were suddenly thrust into the spotlight, gaining almost deified status. Fauci's newfound fame saw him appear in flattering profile pieces in major publications, like *The New Yorker*, which entrenched his image as a saviour working hard to protect Americans during this unprecedented pandemic. "Americans have come to rely on Fauci's authoritative presence. Perhaps not since the Vietnam era, when Walter Cronkite, the avuncular anchor of the CBS Evening News was routinely described as the most trusted man in America, has the country depended so completely on one person to deliver a daily dose of plain talk," the magazine fawned. That same article would also note as fact that the "novel coronavirus emerged, first from bats and then from a live-animal market" in Wuhan.

Even Brad Pitt, in an Emmy-nominated Saturday Night Live sketch in April 2020, while impersonating Fauci, broke character to praise the health official. "Thank you for your calm and your clarity in this unnerving time," Pitt said. Fauci won popularity with Trump critics during the pandemic because he would often correct the President publicly while other officials kept their disagreements private.

During his first press conference after the handover to the Biden administration, Fauci said it was a "liberating feeling" to have Biden in office. "One of the new things about this administration is that, if you don't know the answer, don't guess – just say you don't know the answer," Fauci said.

Early in the pandemic he dismissed suggestions Covid-19 could have originated in a laboratory. "If you look at the evolution of the virus in bats, and what's out there now, [the scientific evidence] is very, very strongly leaning toward [the idea that] this could not have been artificially or deliberately manipulated," he said in an interview with *National Geographic* in May 2020. "Everything about the stepwise evolution over time strongly indicates that [this virus] evolved in nature and then jumped species."

A year later, he recast these early statements by claiming he hadn't been part of any attempt to suppress discussion about a potential laboratory leak, and insisted he had always kept an open mind. His public statements do not support these claims.

Fauci's public persona as a cautious, careful medical professional is contradicted by his central role in kickstarting exceptionally fraught gain-of-function research in the United States after the ban introduced in the Obama era, along with his role in funding coronavirus research in China in unsafe laboratories. Laboratories that intelligence agencies suspect may have sparked the pandemic.

In June 2021, halfway through a television interview that began soft and friendly, like most of the sit-downs Fauci agrees to, host Leland Vittert wanted to know why the NIH had bankrolled coronavirus research in Wuhan. Fauci's answer was truly shocking. Not only did he say it was to avoid an outbreak in America, he claimed the Wuhan Institute of Virology was safe and highly qualified. But the NIH and America had no oversight at all over the activities within the facility.

"You say why do it in China? You do it in China through a very well-known, highly qualified laboratory. Now you're absolutely correct that I can't guarantee everything that's going on in the Wuhan lab, we can't do that, but it is our obligation as scientists and public health individuals to study the animal–human interface because we had a very difficult experience that we lucked out, that we didn't get hurt too badly with the original SARS in 2002 and 2003, which was clearly a jumping of species from a bat to a civet cat to a human," Fauci told Vittert. "It was incumbent upon us to study the animal–human interface and to understand what potential these viruses have of infecting humans, which then might damage the United States. You don't want to go to Hoboken, New Jersey or to Fairfax, Virginia to be studying the bat–human interface that might lead to an outbreak, so you go to China."

David Stilwell concurs that concerns about coronavirus research sparking an outbreak in America is exactly why the United States funded it in China. "My personal view is it's the same reason we do heavy metals in China, because they don't care about their environment so we outsource all these toxic things there," Stilwell tells me. "It meant we didn't have to do it [coronavirus and gain-of-function research] on US soil with the risk of a leak here. The Chinese were very interested in SARS coronaviruses because of the SARS outbreak of 2002 and 2003 so we had this unholy overlapping interest. They were willing to accept American money and cover for the research."

Fauci's organisation was very familiar with the work undertaken at the Wuhan Institute of Virology, with the NIH and the National Science Foundation visiting the facility in the year prior to April 2018.

In total, the NIH has funded at least 60 scientific projects at the Wuhan Institute of Virology over the past decade, according to an analysis of Shi Zhengli's work at the Wuhan lab we undertook for this book in conjunction with US bipartisan taxpayer watchdog, White Coat Waste Project.

USAID funded at least 16 (10 of which were jointly funded with the NIH), the Department of Health and Human Services funded three, the Department of Defense, Department of Energy, and the China–US Collaborative Program on Emerging and Re-emerging Infectious Diseases individually each funded one project in conjunction with the Wuhan Institute of Virology.

It is concerning that, at the same time Obama cut off funding for gain-of-function research in America, US money was still flowing to China for risky coronavirus research.

Peter Daszak of not-for-profit group EcoHealth Alliance (EHA) has reportedly boasted that his China bat research project was funded entirely through NIH grants. "So with the funding terminated, we won't be able to do this work. The fieldwork will not carry on," he told National Public Radio in April 2020. He also said that he would lose the ability to study the "vast collection of new coronavirus samples already collected". "They're in freezers in China. We had free and open access while we were doing this collaboration to get the genetic sequences of the virus from those samples. But without the funding, we won't be able to get that," he said.

EcoHealth Alliance has received more than US$60 million in grants and awards from the US government since 2002, and this isn't including sub-grants from other organisations that have subcontracted work to EHA. Agencies that have awarded money include the Department of Defense (US$41.91 million) and the Department of Health and Human Services (US$11.66 million).

In May of 2015, and for the following four years, EcoHealth Alliance would send a total of US$598,500 of US taxpayer funds directly to the Wuhan Institute of Virology. The description for the sub-award was "conduct[ing] high-quality testing, sequencing, and analyses of field samples; maintenance of cold-chains from field to lab; ensuring quality control of sample storage and testing; collaborating on scientific publications and programmatic reporting." In 2016 and 2017, EcoHealth Alliance also sent US$200,000 to the Wuhan University School of Public Health.

From 2014 to July 2020, NIAID – the National Institute of Allergy and Infectious Diseases, one of 27 institutes that makes up the NIH – awarded US$3,748,715 to EcoHealth Alliance under a project titled, "Understanding the risk of bat coronavirus emergence". According to the description on US government grant website USAspending.gov, the project was to "examine the risk of future coronavirus emergence from wildlife using in-depth field investigations across the human-wildlife interface in China".

Other institutions that frequently collaborate with the Wuhan Institute of Virology include the New York Blood Centre, the University of North Carolina and University of Texas Medical Branch, Galveston.

White Coat Waste Project was the first to expose the money flow between EcoHealth and the Wuhan laboratories, with a strong campaign run by its President Anthony Bellotti and Deputy Justin Goodman. Bellotti said the NIH and other agencies should never have funded these experiments in China. "Shipping millions of US tax dollars to the dangerous Wuhan animal lab and dozens of other facilities in China where there's no real transparency and accountability about how the money is spent is a recipe for disaster," he said. "Taxpayers should not be forced to bankroll this reckless spending and new polls show that a majority of Democrat and Republican voters in the US want to cut funding for animal labs in China and other foreign countries."

United States House Intelligence Committee member and former Chair Devin Nunes told *Fox News* that when gain-of-function research was banned in America it continued in Wuhan, "likely with US dollars that we still haven't accounted for". He said it was "routed through a non-profit and routed into China. The point is when something wasn't allowed in the United States, it was going on in China. This type of activity, this gain-of-function, is really weaponising a virus. The question is something like this, that can be so dangerous and so deadly and turned into a weapon, is that something we really want … taxpayer money being involved in?"

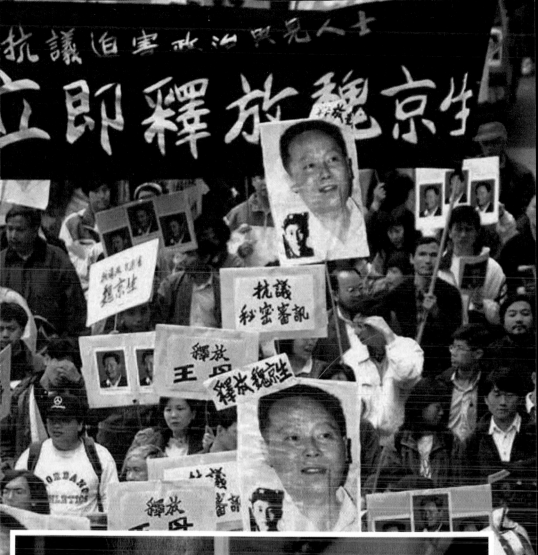

INSET: Chinese defector Wei Jingsheng first heard there was a virus in Wuhan in October 2019, alerting his well-connected friend Dimon Liu the next month. *(Jeff Pachoud / AFP via Getty Images)*

BACKGROUND: During a march on December 17, 1995, protestors in Hong Kong demand the release of Wei Jingsheng, China's most famous political prisoner. *(Thomas Cheng / AFP via Getty Images)*

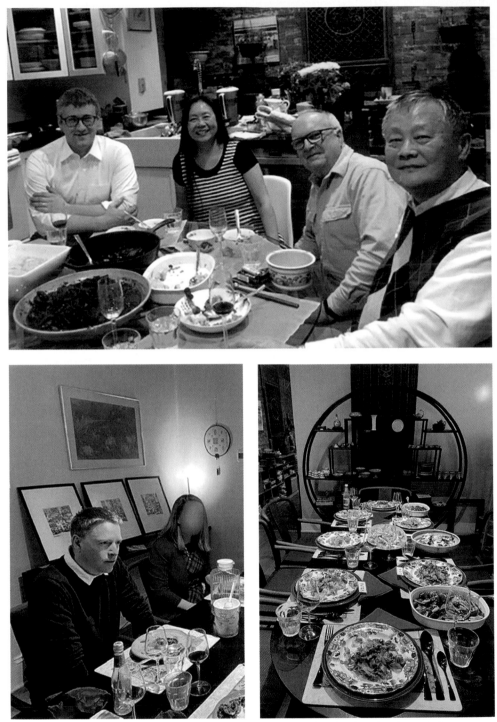

Top: Left to right: China analyst Peter Mattis, Dimon Liu, her husband Robert (Bob) Suettinger, and Wei Jingsheng. All are frequent guests at Dimon and Bob's dinner parties. March 25, 2021.
Bottom Left: Deputy National Security Advisor Matt Pottinger (left) enjoys a homemade plum and custard pie with ice cream at a dinner party thrown by Dimon and Bob in May 2021.
Bottom Right: The table laid out for a dinner party for Pottinger at Dimon and Bob's home in March 2021. *(All images on page courtesy of Dimon Liu)*

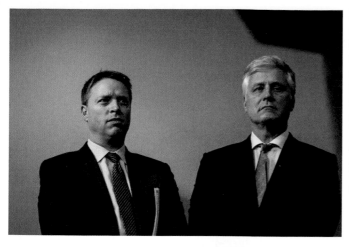

LEFT: Matt Pottinger (left) and his boss, National Security Advisor Robert O'Brien, watch on as the travel ban they'd been fighting all week to implement is finally announced at the White House on Friday January 31, 2020. *(Jabin Botsford / The Washington Post via Getty Images)*

RIGHT: Acting White House Chief of Staff Mick Mulvaney (left), stands with Robert O'Brien and the President's son-in-law Jared Kushner as the US–China "phase one" trade agreement is signed on January 15, 2020. O'Brien confirms neither side mentioned the coronavirus during the entire two-day visit: "If the Chinese knew more about the virus, they certainly weren't letting on." *(Zach Gibson / Bloomberg via Getty Images)*

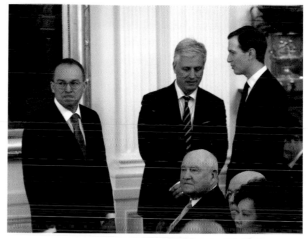

Team Pompeo (left to right: Miles Yu, David Wilezol, Mike Pompeo and Mary Kissel) in Atlanta, Georgia, December 9, 2020. The team were behind a strategy to educate Americans about the nature of the Chinese Communist Party threat. *(Photo by Ron Przysucha, US Government Archives)*

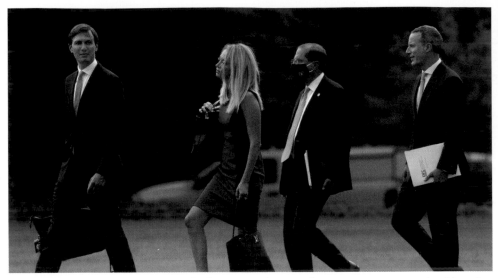

Secretary of Health Alex Azar (masked, centre-right) travels to a vaccine-supporting biotech facility with Jared Kushner, Press Secretary Kayleigh McEnany and CEO Adam Boehler on July 27, 2020. Azar was one of the first White House staffers to adopt strict mask-wearing practices, and senior Republican figures expressed their displeasure in no uncertain terms. *(Alex Wong / Getty Images)*

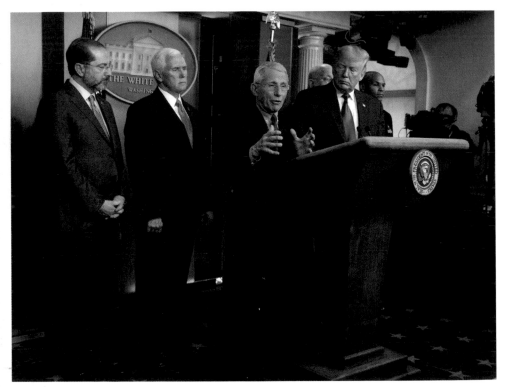

Alex Azar, Vice President Mike Pence and President Donald Trump watch on as NIAID Director Anthony Fauci speaks at a February 29, 2020 press conference to report the first United States death from Covid-19. Fauci told the American public and the White House there was no need to wear masks. Matt Pottinger didn't listen to him and was wearing a mask to work by March. *(Alex Wong / Getty Images)*

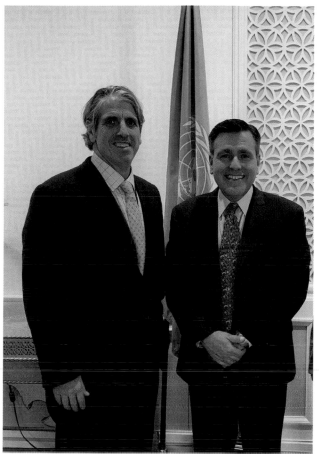

LEFT: Thomas DiNanno (left) with his colleague John Bravaco at the United Nations in 2019. Miles Yu calls DiNanno a national hero for leading an investigation into the origins of Covid-19 in the State Department, against heavy resistance.
(Courtesy of Thomas DiNanno)

BELOW: Trump's Trade Advisor Peter Navarro (right) clashed with Anthony Fauci on shutting down travel from China in a fiery January 2020 meeting. Navarro says the President trusted him and closed the borders. Here he is with Trump on the South Lawn of the White House in September 2020.
(Tasos Katopodis / Getty Images)

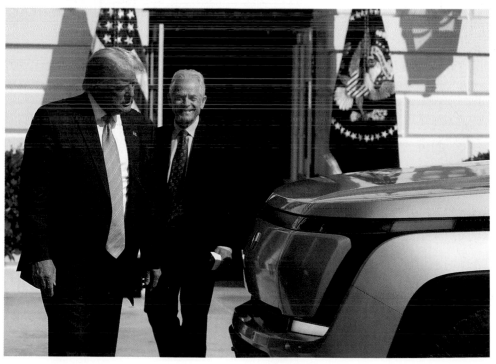

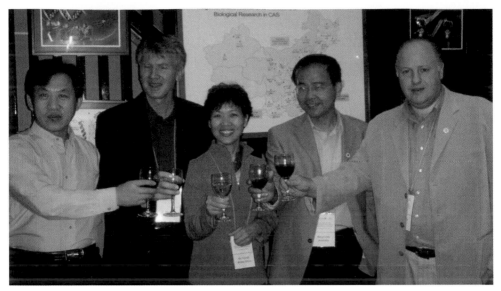

EcoHealth Alliance President Peter Daszak (far right) celebrates with the Wuhan Institute of Virology's Shi Zhengli (centre) and CSIRO's Linfa Wang (centre-right), circa 2005, around the time they co-published the article "Bats Are Natural Reservoirs of SARS-like Coronaviruses" in *Science*. Daszak would be appointed to the World Health Organization team investigating the origin of the virus and interviewing the very scientists he had worked with for over 15 years.
(Sourced from a now-deleted page on the Wuhan Institute of Virology website)

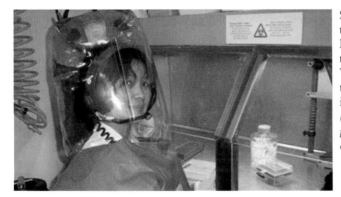

Shi Zhengli, director of the Centre for Emerging Infectious Diseases at the Wuhan Institute of Virology, pictured here at the CSIRO labs, Australia, in 2006.
(Sourced from a now-deleted page on the Wuhan Institute of Virology website)

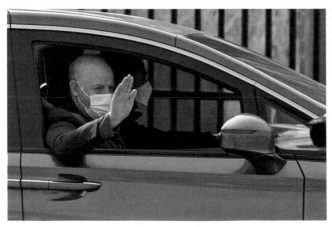

Peter Daszak waves to the media as he leaves the Wuhan Institute of Virology on February 3, 2021 as part of the World Health Organization investigation into the origins of the pandemic. Daszak, through his organisation, EcoHealth Alliance, funded research at the Institute. Pompeo describes Daszak's involvement as a "breathtaking conflict of interest".
(Hector Retamal / AFP via Getty Images)

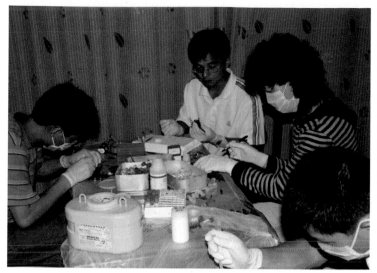

Wuhan Institute of Virology scientists show a concerning disregard for safety while processing samples, with inadequate protective equipment, such as masks, glasses or gowns.
(Sourced from a now-deleted page on the Wuhan Institute of Virology website)

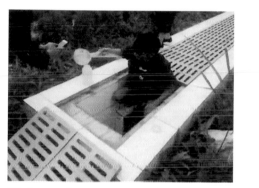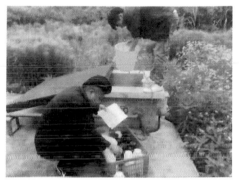

Workers collect sewage samples from the Wuhan Institute of Virology for testing, without wearing adequate protective equipment.
(Sourced from uncovered 2018 Wuhan Institute of Virology wastewater-monitoring test report documents)

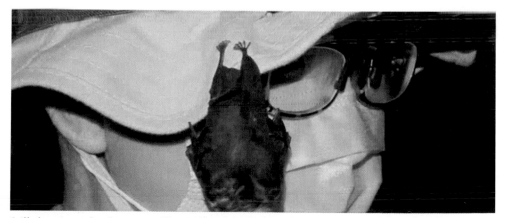

Still showing a bat hanging off a Wuhan Institute of Virology scientist's hat, taken from an official Chinese Academy of Sciences video from May 2017 titled "The Construction and Research Team of Wuhan P4 Laboratory of Wuhan Institute of Virology".

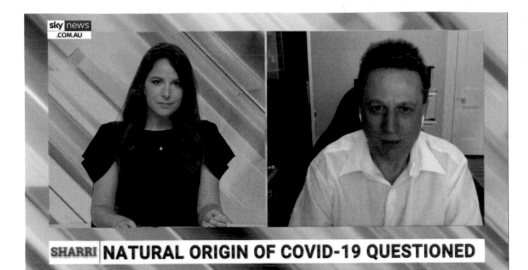

SHARRI **NATURAL ORIGIN OF COVID-19 QUESTIONED**

Top: Flinders University Professor Nikolai Petrovsky (right) in a Sky News interview with the author in November 2020. Petrovsky first raised the issue on May 24, in a world-exclusive television interview, where he told the author that Covid-19 may have been a result of a cell-culture experiment in a laboratory. At the time, this view was considered a conspiracy theory.
(Reproduced with permission of Sky News)

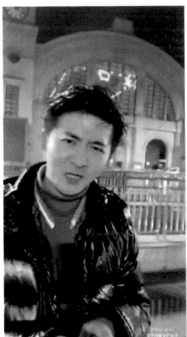

Left: Chen Qiushi, Chinese citizen journalist and activist, who caught the last train to Wuhan on Chinese New Year's Eve, January 24, 2020, to report on the plight of those in the locked-down city. "I will use my camera to document what is really happening. I promise I won't … cover up the truth," he said before signing off.

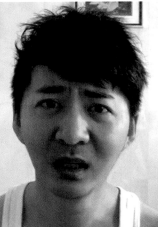

Chen Qiushi in his Wuhan hotel room in one of his last videos, less than a week before he disappeared. There is speculation he is in home detention but he remains missing and has not been seen or heard from since February 6, 2020.

The United States continued to allow funding to flow through to the Wuhan Institute of Virology until April 2020. Finally in April – four months after the coronavirus outbreak – the NIH sent a letter to EcoHealth Alliance effectively saying it was cutting off its funding unless it answered a series of questions related to the origins of Covid-19. It was sent far too late, but it was a bombshell from NIH Deputy Director for Extramural Research Michael Lauer.

"The NIH has received reports that the Wuhan Institute of Virology (WIV), a sub-recipient of EcoHealth Alliance under R01AI110964, has been conducting research at its facilities in China that pose serious biosafety concerns and, as a result, create health and welfare threats to the public in China and other countries, including the United States," it said. "We have concerns that WIV has not satisfied safety requirements under the award, and that EcoHealth Alliance has not satisfied its obligations to monitor the activities of its sub-recipient to ensure compliance."

Trump's Chief of Staff Mark Meadows made the decision to cut off funding and EcoHealth was outraged. Fauci – who knows Daszak and was thanked by him for publicly saying the virus had a natural origin – took up the case on behalf of EcoHealth Alliance. First he complained to his superior, Alex Azar, who said it was not his decision. "Tony, you have to take it up with the boss. Meadows is the one making this call," Azar told him. Fauci then had no qualms going to see Meadows to try to convince him to overturn the EcoHealth decision – even though it was now public that this not-for-profit group had been funding the Wuhan laboratories conducting gain-of-function research on coronaviruses in the same city where the pandemic started.

Fauci declined to comment but sources familiar with his complaint say he mounted a case based on the lack of process, rather than any personal relationship with Daszak. "There is a very rigorous process for establishing peer-review grants at NIH. It is meant to protect the integrity of billions of dollars of money going out and it's meant to protect the integrity of that process," the source told me. "He would be concerned about, just for geo-political reasons, pulling a grant because that didn't go through a peer-review process. There are procedures for getting rid of a grant."

NIH Director Francis Collins had formalised collaboration with the Chinese Academy of Military Sciences – the body that sits under the PLA – in 2015. He shared a photo of himself meeting with the Chinese Academy of Military Sciences President, Cao Xuetao, on June 24, 2015, tweeting: "Glad to meet with CAMS President Xuetao Cao to discuss multiple areas of health collaboration between #NIH & CAMS."

In April 2020, Collins emailed Fauci, dismissing suggestions of a laboratory leak as a conspiracy. The email was titled "conspiracy gains momentum" and it included a link to on-air comments by Fox News host Bret Baier that multiple sources had told him the virus may have originated in a Wuhan laboratory before accidentally escaping.

Perhaps the leadership at the NIH viewed this as innocent international collaboration. If so, this was naive. The United States was well aware of the inherent risks of the type of dual-use research in which Xi Jinping was engaging. It seemed the health, science and even defence community turned a blind eye to these grave national security and biosafety concerns, along with China's blatant theft of American intellectual property.

Pompeo is adamant that gain-of-function research should not be taking place in China at all – especially not with American taxpayer funding. No laboratory in China, Pompeo believes, has ever maintained the biosafety standards handling such deadly pathogens require. "We all know the complexity around gain-of-function research and that it's pretty controversial and that it creates real risk," he tells me. "We also know that there are good reasons that one wants to perform that kind of research, but having said that ... We've made clear that this can only happen in the United States under a certain set of prescriptions and rules. This kind of research should only take place in the most highly capable research laboratories with the most trained personnel and under very rigorous security and biosafety procedures, and there has not been a lab inside of China that has ever risen to that standard. And so to think that it was appropriate for that kind of research to have taken place inside of China seems to be a gross misjudgement."

Pompeo does not directly name Fauci, but he makes it abundantly clear which agency he holds responsible for American funding being funnelled into the Wuhan Institute of Virology. "What is clear to me is that the folks at NIH and the health professionals at the United States that were supervising these American researchers going to this lab also knew that this lab did not meet rigorous safety standards, the standards that we would hold an American laboratory to or a British or French or Australian or Japanese facility to," he says. "It seems like that raises an awful lot of questions about the absence of oversight and the risks that pertain to that."

If it was a shock for senior White House officials to learn through media reports that Fauci had quietly lifted the ban on gain-of-function research back in 2017, they were even more astounded to discover he knew so much about the research in Wuhan, but never said a word as the pandemic unfolded. Instead, the role of the Wuhan Institute of Virology in conducting risky coronavirus research was left to officials like Miles Yu and Matt Pottinger to uncover.

Trump's Acting Chief of Staff Mick Mulvaney, who was present for every meeting at the start of the pandemic, said Fauci did not once mention the gain-of-function research that his agency had funded at the Wuhan Institute of Virology. He didn't even mention that there was a laboratory in Wuhan doing coronavirus research. "I do not recall him saying anything of the sort, and certainly not that he may have been involved with it," he tells me. "I was surprised to recently learn of the connection. Honestly, I wish I had known about it, as it clearly would have registered as a possible source of bias in Fauci's contributions to the debate. Put another way: I knew Navarro hated the Chinese, so I knew to take his input on, say, the travel ban, with a grain of salt. I did not know of Fauci's involvement in the research in China. That certainly would have impacted the weight we gave to some of his contributions."

Fauci didn't even tell Azar that the NIH had funded research genetically modifying coronaviruses at the Wuhan Institute of

Virology. A source close to Azar says he was with Fauci all the time and yet he was never told even a penny of that grant to EcoHealth was being used for actual manipulation of the virus, only that it was for surveillance.

While Fauci did not say anything to White House senior officials while they were sitting in high-level meetings discussing the outbreak, he was privately concerned about the research his agency had funded in Wuhan and there was a flurry of activity behind the scenes. Thanks to thousands of pages of emails released under Freedom of Information Act by *BuzzFeed* we know that on February 1, 2020 Fauci emailed Deputy Director Hugh Auchincloss Jr saying, "It is essential that we speak this am. Keep your cell phone on. I have a conference call at 7.45am with Azar. It likely will be over by 8.45am. Read this paper as well as the email that I will forward you now. You have tasks today that must be done." The paper attached was the 2015 gain-of-function research where a deadly new virus was created by Shi Zhengli with the University of Carolina's Ralph Baric. It was indeed funded by the NIH. The subject of Fauci's email was: "Baric, Shi et al – Nature medicine – SARS Gain of function".

Hugh replied at 11.45am saying, "The paper you sent me says the experiments were performed before the gain-of-function pause but have since been reviewed and approved by NIH. Not sure what that means since Emily is sure that no Coronavirus work has gone through the P3 framework. She will try to determine if we have any distant ties to this work abroad."

Fauci was clearly concerned in the very earliest days of the outbreak that his agency had funded gain-of-function work at the Wuhan Institute of Virology, maybe even funding the laboratory that caused the pandemic. He had cause to be extremely worried, given scientists were telling him Covid-19 may have been genetically altered. One day earlier, on January 31, 2020, Scripps Institute scientist Kristian Andersen emailed Fauci expressing the preliminary view that the SARS-CoV-2 genome appeared to have been laboratory manipulated. "The unusual features of the virus make up a really small part of the genome (<0.1%) so one has to look really closely at all the sequences to see that some of the features (potentially) look engineered," he wrote. "I should mention that after discussions earlier today, Eddie [Holmes], Bob, Mike and myself all find the genome inconsistent with expectations from evolutionary theory. But we have to look at this much more closely and there are still further analyses to be done, so those opinions could still change."

Fauci replied the next day at 6.43pm – after he had sent his urgent email to Auchincloss – saying, "Thanks Kristian. Talk soon on the call".

Copied into the email was Jeremy Farrer, head of the world's biggest philanthropic science funding body, the Wellcome Trust. Farrer, who is also a member of the British Government's Scientific Advisory Group for Emergencies, was among those who spent the next year insisting it was a conspiracy to suggest a potential laboratory origin for the virus. Farrar, Fauci and Andersen had an initial phone call where they discussed the unusual features of the virus. Fauci later told journalist Alison Young that Andersen had spoken with Holmes and the pair both thought that "at first glance" the genome of the virus looked unusual. "I suggested we bring together a multidisciplinary team. We agreed to convene by phone the next day."

Farrar set up the larger conference call with Fauci, Francis Collins, Anderson, Holmes, British chief scientific advisor Sir Patrick Vallance and other experts on Saturday, February 1 – the same day as Fauci's email requesting urgent information on the gain-of-function SARS experiments his agency had funded. During the call, some virologists said the evidence was "heavily weighted" towards a natural origin from an animal host, but others disagreed. "It was a very productive back-and-forth conversation where some on the call felt it could possibly be an engineered virus," Fauci told Young. But just three days later, on February 3, Andersen described suggestions the virus was engineered as a crackpot theory. When I challenged him about this, he responded saying, "I know it's super mundane, but it isn't actually a 'massive cover-up'. It's just science. Boring, I know, but it's quite a helpful thing to have in times of uncertainty."

The emails shed light on how even the most prominent proponents of the zoonotic-transfer theory had acknowledged initially that Covid-19 had highly unusual features. But most importantly it exposed how Fauci was concerned in the earliest days of the pandemic that his institute had funded gain-of-function research at the Wuhan Institute of Virology. He did not mention this to any senior White House figures I spoke to. Instead, State Department officials, journalists, internet researchers and others would have to piece together the puzzle over the next year and a half, unpicking the role of the United States in funding dangerous research in Wuhan.

Fauci has repeatedly denied funding gain-of-function research that creates new deadly viruses. In July 2021, just prior to publication of this book, he was asked by Senator Rand Paul, during a US Senate hearing, "You take an animal virus and you increase its transmissibility to humans. You're saying that's not gain-of-function?"

Fauci responded, "That is correct, and Senator Paul, you do not know what you are talking about, quite frankly, and I want to say that officially." The pair became embroiled in an argument about whether the research genetically manipulating coronaviruses that the NIH was funding in Wuhan constituted the technical definition of "gain of function".

Dr Ebright has accused Fauci of not telling the truth and specifically points to research papers, already detailed in this chapter, that involve gain-of-function research funded by the NIH. I asked if Fauci could be perhaps using a different definition for gain-of-function work given his denials. "It is not a matter of definitions," Dr Ebright says. In effect, Fauci is "exploiting the deep partisan divide among policy-makers in the US, [hoping] one party will shelter him from accountability."

Dr Ebright goes further to accuse Dr Fauci of being, in effect, the father of gain-of-function research: "No person on the planet has done more than Anthony Fauci to enable, expand and excuse gain-of-function research."

Why did the world ignore the many scientists who warned that gain-of-function research could lead to a pandemic? What do Fauci and the NIH and the other agencies like the Department of Defence have to say for their role in pouring taxpayer funding into a Chinese facility that they had no way of overseeing? How could they trust the safety protocols were correct? What checks and balances were there? None.

The American connections to the Wuhan Institute of Virology run deeper, and are more concerning, than simply EcoHealth Alliance, Fauci's NIH and the University of North Carolina.

CHAPTER SEVENTEEN

USAMRIID

FORT DETRICK, MARYLAND

Inside America's highly secretive army biological research site at Fort Detrick, Maryland, are BSL-4 laboratories. Soldiers guard the premises that house America's bio-defence agency, the US Army Medical Research Institute of Infectious Diseases (USAMRIID).

It's the last place on earth you would expect to have developed ties with Wuhan Institute of Virology researchers who, in turn, are engaging in secret Chinese military activity. But its Chief Science Officer, a laboratory director, a former commander and a research contractor all have links to the Wuhan Institute of Virology, even visiting its laboratories.

USAMRIID's Chief Scientific Officer and Scientific Director Sina Bavari sits on the editorial board of the journal where Shi Zhengli is the Editor-in-Chief, *Virologica Sinica*. Sina Bavari has been at USAMRIID since 2011 and Chief Scientific Officer since September 2014, his five-year term expiring in September 2019, according to his CV.

Before he left, Bavari had agreed to attend an emerging infectious diseases conference with Shi Zhengli in September 2019, in Tofo, Mozambique. Shi Zhengli was a speaker and Bavari, who sat on the scientific committee, was planning to give a talk. Bavari had already paid for his flights and organised his Mozambique visa when he withdrew from the conference 10 days before, emailing organisers to apologise and offer to give his lectures via FaceTime or WhatsApp.

Bavari originally told me he did attend the conference, saying Shi Zhengli gave a presentation on bat coronaviruses and that he hadn't noticed anything unusual about her that week. "There was nothing that rang any bells." Five days later, Bavari said he remembered that he had attended in 2018, not 2019, although it does not appear that Shi Zhengli was at the Tofo conference in 2018.

Shi Zhengli did attend the 2019 conference, held from September 1 to 5. She gave a coronavirus presentation, according to another conference participant, who described her as friendly and sociable. A week later, on September 12, the Wuhan Institute of Virology virus database was taken offline.

Bavari had visited the Wuhan Institute of Virology in 2014 or 2015, he said, for an editorial board meeting of *Virologica Sinica*. He didn't visit the BSL-4 laboratory, which wasn't open yet, but ventured inside the lower-security BSL-3 lab, where Shi Zhengli was conducting coronavirus research.

Asked what the safety standards inside the laboratory were like, Bavari says: "Oh my God, that was like, seven years ago, so I don't remember a darn thing. I really don't. I'm not kidding you. I was jet-lagged and I got there two days after I was supposed to get there because of some screw ups with my flights and so on. So I don't really remember much about that trip, to be honest. They actually gathered a bunch of virologists together and it was the editorial board of the journal actually. They're all invited to come there and give presentation, interact with the students, things like that. I remember being in a place walking around, but I don't remember the details."

Bavari wasn't the only senior figure from USAMRIID to visit the Wuhan Institute of Virology. In October 2018, a senior USAMRIID laboratory director gave a presentation on Ebola in the facility's conference room number 1. "After the meeting, the teachers and students present and (the USAMRIID director) had a lively exchange and discussion on the operation of the P4 laboratory, related experimental techniques, and the interaction between the virus and the host," a write-up of the visit on the Wuhan Institute of Virology's website states. Researcher Xiao Gengfu presented the lab director with the "Ge Hong Forum" commemorative medal on behalf of Wuhan Institute of Virology.

There's a third connection between the Institute and Fort Detrick – and the NIH. Also sitting on Shi Zhengli's *Virologica Sinica* editorial board is Professor Jens Kuhn, the Virology Lead at Anthony Fauci's NIAID. Not only is he at the NIH, but he is listed as a contractor among Fort Detrick's "Integrated Research Facility Leadership and Scientists" under the command of Director Connie Schmaljohn. "Personnel at the Integrated Research Facility at Fort Detrick (IRF-Frederick) work in a collaborative manner within and between teams and with external partners and affiliates," the website states.

And in a fourth link, at a hotel in downtown Wuhan in May 2017, a commander at USAMRIID participated in a workshop on lab safety with the Institute's top scientists. The workshop was called the "Second China–US Workshop on the Challenges of Emerging Infections, Laboratory Safety and Global Health Security". Gain-of-function research, laboratory risks and gene editing were key topics during the conference, held from May 17 to 19.

Shi Zhengli and George Fu Gao, the Director of the Chinese Centre for Disease Control and Prevention, gave presentations at the conference hosted by China's Academy of Sciences and attended by the Director of Wuhan Institute of Virology's BSL-4 laboratory, Yuan Zhiming. A meeting report stated that the USAMRIID commander "discussed the evolution of biosecurity thinking in the US, noting only one accidental death – and not from a true select agent – is associated with the US Select Agent program (and three deaths before 1969 when the US offensive biological program was halted). He compared that to more than 700,000 hospital-acquired infections and 400,000 deaths due to medical mistakes in recent years."

The commander said there was no single solution to eliminating biosafety incidents but international collaboration would help.

Eminent Stanford University professor David Relman, who also attended this conference, said they visited the newly built BSL-4 laboratory but it "was not yet active, and there were no experiments taking place with BL3/BL4 agents".

"These discussions were cordial and useful insofar as they provided an opportunity to develop at least some superficial working relationships," Relman said. "I didn't hear about anything in particular that concerned me, but that wasn't surprising since the presentations and comments on both sides were somewhat pre-planned and a bit orchestrated."

The record of the meeting says that Yuan Zhiming and the USAMRIID commander "presented conclusions from the meeting and led a discussion on possible roles of CAS and NAS to enhance cooperation between the U.S. and China on emerging infections, laboratory safety and global health security and other topics discussed at the meeting."

Bavari denied there was any connection between USAMRIID and the Wuhan Institute of Virology, despite the back-and-forth visits. "US Army Medical Research Institute of Infectious Diseases, where I was the chief science officer there, has no connection whatsoever to Wuhan Institute of Virology or any other institute in China," he told me. "Being on an editorial board of a journal is not the same as helping a Chinese institute of this and that to do something. They're just way two different things."

He also downplayed the visits by other researchers to the Institute. "So at the institute they may have friends there, okay, they're Chinese, so absolutely, that [visits] had happened, I have no doubt," he said. "But officially, to say that USAMRIID itself was actually collaborating, for example, with Chinese Institute of Virology, or Wuhan Institute, that's just not true. We absolutely had, we absolutely had no connection to them whatsoever. Not under my watch."

The *Virologica Sinica* editorial board overseen by Shi Zhengli consists of PLA members, a virologist who was kicked out of Canada for security breaches and the director of China's Centre for Disease

Control. The journal features on the Wuhan Institute of Virology's website, in an organisational flow chart that includes the journal's "Editorial Office".

The virologist who was escorted out of Canada's only BSL-4 laboratory in July 2019 after being caught sending deadly virus samples back to the Wuhan Institute of Virology was Qiu Xiangguo. Dr Qiu Xiangguo, her husband Cheng Keding and her students from China were removed from the laboratory. Four months earlier, a shipment containing highly virulent viruses – Ebola and Nipah – was sent from her laboratory to China. It was reported that the Wuhan Institute of Virology had requested the shipment.

CBC journalist Karen Pauls, who broke the story, then wrote an article, based on travel documents, revealing Qiu Xiangguo had made at least five trips in 2017–18 alone to the Wuhan National Biosafety Laboratory at the Wuhan Institute of Virology. "IT specialists entered Qiu's office after hours to gain access to her computer, and her regular trips to China were halted," wrote Chemical and biological warfare specialist Dany Shoham, from the Begin-Sadat Center for Strategic Studies. In an unusual twist, Qiu Xiangguo had also done joint research with USAMRIID on Ebola, which was received by *Nature* in October 2018.

George Fu Gao, the Director of the Chinese Centre for Disease Control and Prevention, who rang Dr Redfield in tears on January 3, 2020, is also on the advisory board for Shi Zhengli's journal. On the editorial board is Zhang Yong-Zhen, the scientist responsible for sharing the genetic sequence of Covid-19. One of the associate editors is connected to the PLA: Tong Yigang was previously the Director of the Institute of Microbiology and Epidemiology at the Academy of Military Medical Science, which sits under the PLA. What's highly unusual is that two members of Shi Zhengli's editorial board were linked to USAMRIID, given US intelligence has tied the Wuhan Institute of Virology to the Chinese military.

But despite the regular visits, Fort Detrick scientists would become the suspected victims of intellectual property theft by scientists at the Wuhan Institute of Virology. Fort Detrick scientists, in collaboration with Gilead Sciences of Foster City, California, had success in 2015 with a treatment that blocked the Ebola virus's ability to replicate. They issued a press release heralding their achievement. The treatment was an antiviral compound called GS-5734 – more commonly known as Remdesivir.

Sina Bavari was one of the clever scientists behind this antiviral treatment and is listed as a contributor on the research, which was funded by the Defense Threat Reduction Agency and the Medical Countermeasure Systems Joint Project Management Office, under the US Department of Defense. The drug came to global prominence when it was touted as a potential treatment option for Covid-19 some five years later.

Despite the US government contributing research and funding, it didn't get credit in the Gilead Remdesivir patent. In an even bigger scandal, when it was finally patented for commercial use, it wasn't even in the United States. A patent for commercial use of Remdesivir – the drug discovered by Sina Bavari and his colleagues and patented by Gilead – was filed in China. The application was made by none other than the Wuhan Institute of Virology.

The Institute lodged the patent application on January 21, 2020 – one day after China confirmed human-to-human transmission of the virus, Ian Birrell first reported in London's *Daily Mail*. Asked about this, Bavari said he was not aware that the Wuhan Institute of Virology had lodged the patent. "For Remdesivir, the only patents that I know about are the ones that Gilead had. I don't know of any other patents," he said. "So, I mean, there all sorts of people (who) put all sorts of stuff in China, you can easily get a patent on anything you want to. It doesn't mean it's valid anyplace else." It's reminiscent of some of the concepts FBI Director Christopher Wray spoke about in his speech he designed with Pompeo (see Chapter 10) – American technology stolen and patented by China.

Bavari says he doesn't really have an opinion on whether the virus leaked from a Wuhan laboratory or arose naturally, but describes it as "almost a perfect virus". "The virus itself has a few things in it that is sort of odd, and you know it seemed like to be almost a perfect virus, the respiratory transfer cleavage site that actually matches almost any human cells. It's sort of a strange virus. But is it possible evolutionarily for something like that to pop out? Probably yes, too. So till somebody really did do real forensic studies on it and they open up their notebook so people can see through what has happened, I think it'll be a lot of guesses and a lot of finger-pointing. And, you know, that's not science also. There is another BSL-3 actually inside Wuhan [the Wuhan CDC], and I think that's the one that nobody's talking about that I can't figure out why."

As for Fort Detrick, Bavari's time at the helm was not without controversy. *The Fredrick News-Post* reported in 2016: "The Army found in a 2015 investigation that since Bavari took that position in 2014, he has created an 'environment of fear' at the prestigious lab". It added that "The Army's investigating officer urged that the leader, science director Sina Bavari, be removed from USAMRIID and re-assigned to a job without supervisory duties."

While Bavari was Director, Fort Detrick was also temporarily shut down in 2019 for two breaches of containment. USAMRIID announced in mid-November 2019 it would restart operations on a limited scale. Details obtained by *The Frederick News-Post* under Freedom of Information found the two breaches reported by USAMRIID to the CDC demonstrated a failure of the army laboratory to "implement and maintain containment procedures sufficient to contain select agents or toxins" that were made by operations in BSL-3 and BSL-4 laboratories. It was reported that while there was a breach, there was no "exposure" to scientists.

Pompeo seems surprised to learn about the connection between Fort Detrick scientists and the Wuhan Institute of Virology. "I don't believe I was aware of that," he says, pausing. "It is unusual. It's a small world, you've seen that, right. These international virologists are a very tight-knit circle. It's how you get a guy like Daszak. It's a tight circle controlling a lot of resources and money in a very closed space."

A senior administrative official working on arms compliance, who is not authorised to speak on the record, said the relationships between USAMRIID and Chinese laboratories like the Wuhan Institute are concerning given the latter's links to the Chinese military. His view is that it's likely a case of bureaucratic inertia, where the environment of encouraging international cooperation has continued for so long and no one has gone in and specifically shut the arrangement down.

Shi Zhengli's links to Ralph Baric, from the University of North Carolina, continued as well. She emailed him in February 2018, inviting him to fly to Wuhan. "It was nice meeting you in Galveston and learning your recent great work," she wrote. "As we have discussed, we would like to invite you attend our meeting 'the 8th International Symposium on Emerging Virus Diseases' to be held in Wuhan this year. Your local cost and travel between Hong Kong and Wuhan will be covered by our meeting sponsor."

Ralph Baric replied a few hours later: "Hi Zhengli, Nice talking with you in Galveston … I would enjoy the opportunity to meet with you in Wuhan for the 8th international symposium on emerging infectious diseases." That same year, Baric was also paid "an honorarium" by EcoHealth Alliance.

It wasn't just the United States that had lent support to the Wuhan Institute of Virology. International partnerships extended to Europe, to Sweden's Umeå University, Denmark's Novo Nordisk Research Centre, Germany's University of Duisburg-Essen, Spain's Campus University, and France's Institut Pasteur, Lyons P4 laboratory and Université d'Aix-Marseille.

In Africa, there are partnerships with Kenya's National Museum and Jomo Kenyatta University of Agriculture and Technology. In Asia, there's the Duke-NUS Graduate Medical School and Institution Novartis in Singapore, the Defense Science and Technology Organization in Pakistan, the National Institute of Infectious Diseases in Japan, and the National Engineering and Scientific Commission in Islamabad.

The collaboration extended to Australia, as well. Australia's CSIRO and other Australian universities engaged in at least 10 joint projects with the Wuhan Institute of Virology. Shi Zhengli had travelled to Australian laboratories, accompanied by senior members of her team, to study bats in research jointly funded by the Australian and Chinese governments. Peng Zhou – the head of the Bat Virus Infection and Immunity Project at the Wuhan Institute of Virology – spent three years at the CSIRO's Australian Animal Health Laboratory (now the Australian Centre for Disease Preparedness) in Geelong between 2011 and 2014. He was sent by China to complete his doctorate at the CSIRO from 2009 to 2010.

During this time, Zhou arranged for wild-caught bats to be transported alive by air from Queensland to Victoria, where they were euthanised for dissection and studied for deadly viruses. His work was funded jointly by Australia's CSIRO and the Chinese Academy of Sciences. It examined bat immunology and the role of interferons (signalling proteins produced in response to viruses) and how "bats are rich reservoirs for emerging viruses, including many that are highly pathogenic to humans and other mammals" and "many of which cause significant morbidity and mortality in humans and other mammals".

Dr Linfa Wang, while an Honorary Professor of the Wuhan Institute of Virology, also worked in the CSIRO Office of the Chief Executive Science Leader in Virology (2008–11). In January 2020, as the pandemic was breaking out, Linfa Wang went to Wuhan to work with Shi Zhengli.

Shi Zhengli herself spent time in Australia as a visiting scientist for three months from February 22 to May 21, 2006, where she also worked at the Australian Animal Health Laboratory. A CSIRO spokesman said it had partnered with China in "excellent research and development for over 40 years". "While there is no current research on bats at ACDP, the suggestion bat research is dangerous without context … is misleading and irresponsible," he said. "Research into bats underpins much of our understanding of zoonotic diseases. CSIRO undertakes due diligence and takes security very seriously."

The University of Queensland in Australia was involved in a study with the Wuhan Institute of Virology even after the pandemic emerged. The August 2020 paper titled "Origin and Cross-species Transmission of Bat Coronaviruses in China" lists the University of Queensland School of Veterinary Science's Dr Hume Field as a co-author, alongside Shi Zhengli and Peter Daszak. Dr Hume is also the science and policy adviser for EcoHealth Alliance.

Charles Sturt University Professor of Public Ethics Clive Hamilton says it is clear universities are not properly overseeing the collaborations undertaken by their scientists. "There are many instances of sensitive research in Australian universities being done in collaboration with Chinese scientists with links to China's military or who are likely passing valuable information on to China's companies or intelligence services," he tells me. "Universities have been very reluctant to admit there is a problem and have consistently hidden behind the Defence Trade Controls Act, which prohibits the export of sensitive technology but does not prohibit Chinese military scientists working on sensitive projects in Australian laboratories."

None of the universities that have had close collaboration with the Wuhan Institute of Virology have been forthcoming about their dealings with the laboratory. On March 14, 2021, we submitted a Freedom of Information (FOI) request to the University of Edinburgh, St George's University, London, and Southampton University, British universities listed as "international partners" on the Wuhan Institute of Virology website, to ask for details of their partnerships, research collaboration and any knowledge of the Institute's database. The link to the Institute's website where the British universities were listed as partners was provided.

One month later, on April 12, 2021, Southampton University responded with: "We have reviewed the link you have provided and cannot readily find any reference to the University of Southampton. We cannot locate any agreements or memoranda of understanding between the University of Southampton and the Wuhan Institute of Virology, Chinese Academy of Sciences."

Six days after the FOI request was sent, the Wuhan Institute of Virology's website had been edited to remove any mention of the University of Edinburgh, St George's University, London, and

Southampton University. From an initial list of 31 organisations ranging from universities to government agencies with which the Institute had international partnerships, only eight remained.

Using the internet archiving tool called the "Wayback Machine", we were able to determine that the website was altered not once but twice. Firstly, on March 22, six days after the FOI request was sent, where the references to the University of Southampton and St George's University, London, were removed. Strangely, Imperial College London and Bulgaria's Sofia University had been added in instead. The University of Alabama also remained on the website. By the next day, however, all partnerships with universities had been removed.

This was raised with the University of Southampton and an internal review requested. The University of Edinburgh is yet to comply with a March 2021 FOI request. University of Edinburgh virologist Andrew Rambaut is the founder and admin of the discussion forum virological.org, which first published the genetic sequence of SARS-CoV-2. The sequence had been given to him by Australian researcher Eddie Holmes.

CHAPTER EIGHTEEN

0.3 Per Cent

Many scientists have tried to paint a laboratory accident in a Wuhan facility as a "conspiracy theory". In fact, the scientific community knows better than the rest of us how commonplace laboratory incidents are – not just in China, but globally. The reality is, humans aren't robots and accidents happen, which can be particularly dangerous with highly infectious viruses transmissible by air whose spike protein has been passaged to increase transmissibility to humans.

At laboratories around the world there have been accidents involving smallpox, anthrax, H5N1, SARS, brucellosis and a vast range of other lethal diseases that scientists had been prodding and probing. In China in the 1980s, there were two epidemics of haemorrhagic fever in a remote region around a Chinese nuclear test site and biological weapons laboratory. Soviet defector Ken Alibek revealed in his book *Biohazard* – based on Soviet intelligence reports – that the epidemics were leaks from Chinese labs. "Our analysts concluded that they were caused by an accident in a lab where Chinese scientists were weaponising viral diseases," he said in a 1999 interview with *The New York Times*.

There was even a SARS leak from a Beijing laboratory. In 2004, the Chinese National Institute of Virology in Beijing, which operates under China's Centre for Disease Control, was studying SARS coronaviruses when an outbreak occurred.

A female laboratory researcher, aged 26, from Anhui province, fell ill on March 25, 2004, and was hospitalised in Beijing. "Her clinical symptoms were compatible with SARS, and health authorities have retrospectively diagnosed her as a suspected SARS case," a WHO press release stated. The lab researcher's mother, who nursed her at her hospital bed, then fell sick on April 8. Eleven days later, she died. A 20-year-old nurse who gave the lab researcher treatment also fell sick and was admitted to intensive care. Another lab researcher, a 31-year-old man who also worked at the Beijing Institute of Virology, fell sick and was hospitalised and isolated on April 22.

The laboratory was temporarily closed and more than 300 close contacts were placed under medical observation. About 200 laboratory staff were isolated at a hotel near another lab in Changping, 20 kilometres (12 miles) north of Beijing. At least nine people became infected during that outbreak, according to figures China reported.

At the time, WHO spokesman Bob Dietz said it hadn't been just one accident, but two. "We suspect two people, a 26-year-old female postgraduate student and a 31-year-old male postdoc, were both infected, apparently in two separate incidents," he told media. "It's a question of procedures and equipment. Frankly we are going to go in now and take a very close look. We have a team of two or three international experts that's arriving in a day or two. They are going to go into the labs with Ministry of Health people and find out what happened here." The WHO Western Pacific Regional Director at the time, Shigeru Omi, criticised the laboratory's safeguards, telling Associated Press that laboratory safety "is a serious issue that has to be addressed. We have to remain very vigilant".

China's official investigation determined "negligence" at the lab. "The cases had been linked to experiments using live and inactive SARS coronavirus in the CDC's virology institute where interdisciplinary research on the SARS virus was conducted," the *China Daily* reported. "The CDC's mistakes also include allowing researchers to experiment with biological materials infected with SARS in common laboratories, and the failure to immediately report the abnormal health conditions of its researchers."

Five health officials were disciplined. The Centre's Director, Li Liming, resigned, along with his deputy, while the Virology Institute's director and two other officials were removed from their roles. "The punishment of these officials shows our determination in strengthening the public health and our strong sense of responsibility in protecting the health of researchers and all residents," then Vice Premier Wu Yi said.

China had another horrific laboratory accident in 2011 at the College of Veterinary Medicine in Harbin. More than 110 students had gathered to dissect four goats. A few months later, 27 students began falling sick with headaches, joint pain and "debilitating weakness". They were infected with brucellosis bacteria, which goats can carry. The *Shanghai Daily* reported that one was unable to even walk, and an instructor was also infected. An investigation found safety procedures weren't followed, with instructors and students failing to wear gloves, while the goats were not properly quarantined before they were taken into the laboratory. China's Northeast Agricultural University apologised for insufficient safety practices and fired two administrators.

But it seems that Chinese laboratory supervisors did not learn from these mistakes. In December 2019, more than 100 students and staff at another two research institutes were infected with brucellosis bacteria from goats. The Lanzhou Veterinary Research Institute in central China closed its labs after the outbreak, and the Harbin Veterinary Research Institute was affected as well, *Nature* reported. *The Beijing News* disclosed that the discovery was only made when students noticed large numbers of their laboratory mice were infertile. Tests of 317 people found 96 had been infected. Lax safety standards were once again uncovered, including students failing to wear masks.

But it's not just China where lab accidents are commonplace. Science writer Nicholson Baker documents laboratory accidents dating back to the 1950s, and reveals just how common they are, in his 2019 book, *Baseless: My Search for Secrets in the Ruins of the Freedom of the Information Act*. He reports that by 1960, hundreds of American scientists and technicians had been hospitalised, "victims of the diseases they were trying to weaponise".

The laboratory accidents he details are extensive, from a microbiologist in 1951 who developed a fever and died, to a veterinary worker who fell ill with Bolivian haemorrhagic fever after being bitten by a lab animal in 1964 – his wife watching him die through a window to his quarantine room. Baker writes that a 1977 worldwide epidemic of influenza A, beginning in Russia and China, was traced to a sample of an American strain of flu that had been held in a lab freezer for 27 years. He discovered that live foot and mouth disease leaked from a faulty drain pipe at the Institute for Animal Health in Surrey, UK, in 2007. In other incidents Baker uncovered, a medical photographer at a Birmingham laboratory died after working on a hybrid strain of smallpox.

There have been accidents in Australia as well. Dennis Richardson served as the head of the Department of Defence, the Department of Foreign Affairs and Trade and spy agency ASIO before his retirement in 2017. He also was head of the Review of the Intelligence Community after the Cold War in 1992. He says there have been security breaches in Australian labs. "That is something which we need to be alert to globally. We have such facilities here in Australia, and I do know that in the past there have been one or two accidents," he told me in a May 2020 interview. "So accidents do occur. Just how good China's security is for its Level 4 laboratories I simply don't know."

Richardson said at least one breach has made it into the public domain. That was a 2016 biosecurity breach during CSIRO research experiments involving a toxic bacterial pathogen. Thirty staff were exposed. "It was not a virus, but it was a Level 4 facility in which certain research was being conducted in which protocols were not followed, which led to a breach which did not go beyond the facility and did not endanger the public," he said. "I'll say no more than that.

The point I'm making is that accidents can happen regardless of the level of security, and accidents have happened at Level 4 facilities globally, and it wouldn't surprise me if they've happened in China because they have happened elsewhere."

It's a point with which Matt Turpin, former head of the NSC China desk, agrees, saying laboratory accidents are not unusual. "It's not surprising that lab accidents happen, that researchers get sick themselves and that things they're doing get misplaced," Turpin says. "There's a long and documented history within countries that have high degrees of transparency that these things go on, and these things happen. It should not be at all surprising that similar kinds of things are being observed there, and the fact that we don't see any of that reporting out of the PRC government now and for them to respond that there were never any accidents there, this is beyond belief when there's violations of procedures everywhere. There should always be a record of the violations of procedures, the mistakes, transparency. To simply say, we didn't make any … well, did you find some way to employ people that aren't human? Because if there are humans working there, they're likely making mistakes."

The Cambridge Working Group, a US group of scientists and other experts concerned about potential pandemic pathogen research, pointed out in 2015 that even in the United States there had been incidents involving smallpox, anthrax and bird flu in some of the top laboratories. "Such incidents have been accelerating and have been occurring on average over twice a week with regulated pathogens in academic and government labs across the country," their statement said.

Lynn Klotz, Senior Fellow at the US Center for Arms Control and Non-Proliferation, has warned that gain-of-function research could cause a pandemic. He actually did some calculations about how many times laboratory accidents occur. "Consider the probability for escape from a single lab in a single year to be 0.003 (i.e. 0.3 per cent), an estimate that is conservative in light of a variety of government risk assessments for biolabs and actual experience at laboratories studying dangerous pathogens," he wrote in an article he co-authored for the *Bulletin of the Atomic Scientists* in 2012. "Calculating from this probability, it would take 536 years for there to be an 80 per cent chance of at least one escape from a single lab. But with 42 labs carrying out live PPP research, this basic 0.3 per cent probability translates to an 80 per cent likelihood of escape from at least one of the 42 labs every 12.8 years, a time interval smaller than those that have separated influenza pandemics in the 20th century. This level of risk is clearly unacceptable."

Given that scientists have been warning for years that gain-of-function research might result in a pandemic because accidents are so common, it's inexplicable and frankly baffling why any scientist would oppose an investigation into a lab leak. Or why any scientist would say it is an unlikely scenario or a "conspiracy".

This is so far removed from a conspiracy theory, yet that's what reputedly credible scientists would have had us believe.

One crucial discovery during the investigation for this book is that the most senior director at the Wuhan Institute of Virology held grave concerns about the type of research they were undertaking – and whether there could be an accident over lax safety practices. The Wuhan Institute of Virology's BSL-4 Laboratory Director, Dr Yuan Zhiming, was repeatedly sounding the alarm about China's poor laboratory safety in the year leading up to the outbreak.

"The biosafety laboratory is a double-edged sword; it can be used for the benefit of humanity but can also lead to a 'disaster'," he wrote in the *Journal of Biosafety and Security* in February 2019. "Compared with high-level biosafety laboratories that possess standardized management systems in foreign countries, 80% of the relevant specification/standard of biosafety laboratories in China belong to the specification and quality standards under the macro guidance, and only a small fraction are operational method standards, making it difficult to ensure the security of the biosafety laboratory due to lack of operational technical support."

Yuan Zhiming had held grave concerns about the standards at his own facility and others in China since at least 2016. "My country has certain problems in the construction and management of high-level biosafety laboratory systems," he wrote in an article for the *Bulletin of the Chinese Academy of Sciences*. "At present, only one Level 4 laboratory has been built in the country, and the management and maintenance of its key equipment and the personnel's mastery of the standardized operating procedures of Level 4 laboratories are not mature enough." Yuan Zhiming argued China needed to "strengthen" the "supervision of laboratory research activities", including for "sample transfer, storage and testing" and to "formulate emergency plans". He also said there was a lack of funding, and called for legislative reform, especially for high-level laboratories.

In yet another 2019 article, Yuan Zhiming acknowledged that the international regulations to govern this field might not succeed because they related only to known pathogens. In this *Journal of Biosafety and Security* editorial with James LeDuc from the University of Texas Medical Branch, Galveston, Yuan Zhiming wrote: "The rise of synthetic biology, employing novel techniques like gene editing, can create new biological pathways and even microbes not known to exist in nature … One area of research that received considerable attention recently is gain of function studies, especially those investigations attempting to identify key molecular changes that might lead to efficient person-to-person transmission of avian influenza viruses," he wrote. "Many countries are relying on regulations targeting Genetically Modified Organisms to regulate synthetic biology. As synthetic biology advances, these regulations may be insufficient to meet future oversight needs, given their focus only on known organisms."

This is a crucial document because it shows that not everyone at the BSL-4 laboratory was comfortable with the level of research that was being undertaken at the Wuhan facility. This piece was received by the *Journal of Biosafety and Biosecurity* on August 6, 2019, on the eve of the outbreak in Wuhan. These were the concerns the director of the BSL-4 laboratory had right before the pandemic.

Earlier in 2019, Yuan Zhiming had raised concerns about the laboratory safety standards in another journal article. "Currently, most laboratories lack specialized biosafety managers and engineers," he wrote in the *Journal of Biosafety and Biosecurity* in September 2019. "In such facilities, some of the skilled staff is composed by part-time researchers. This makes it difficult to identify and mitigate potential safety hazards in facility and equipment operation early enough. Nonetheless, biosafety awareness, professional knowledge, and operational skill training still need to be improved among laboratory personnel."

Wu Guizhen, a leading virologist from Beijing, also expressed concerns about China's lack of laboratory biosafety, in an article published in the journal *Biosafety and Health*. He spoke about the "pressing need to improve the regulatory standards system" and said "more biosafety laws are urgently needed" in the article received on August 20, 2019. Wu also stated that there should be a collaborative approach to revising regulatory measures for "biosafety and for providing support and guidance for the development of synthetic biology, gene editing and biological resource preservation and utilization".

Wu Guizhen raised concerns over the level of biosafety management in universities, hospitals and academic institutions, saying that they should be enhanced. He stated that regulatory and legal standards for lower level BSL-2 laboratories in China are "lacking". He also claimed that China was suffering a shortage of sufficiently trained and experienced laboratory biosafety personnel.

There are reasons Yuan Zhiming was highly concerned. The US State Department took a close look at the Wuhan laboratory that was located near the Hunan Seafood Market. The Wuhan Centre for Disease Control and Prevention has lower biosafety authorisation than the Wuhan Institute of Virology, and has a history of poor safety practices.

One senior scientist from this facility, Tian Junhua, spoke in December 2019 – a rather ill-timed interview – about how easy it is to become personally infected when taking samples from bats in the field. "We can easily get contact with the faeces of bats which contaminate everything. So it is highly risky here. I feel the fear.

The fear of infections," he said in a public video. He revealed he'd had to go into self-quarantine twice after being exposed to bat urine directly on his skin.

Miles Yu in the State Department had come across a 2017 video made by the state-owned Chinese Shanghai Media Group called "Youth in the Wild: Invisible Defenders" that features Tian Junhua. In the video, he goes into caves to collect viruses from bats and speaks about the risk of infection. The video is still online, and you can clearly see he is not wearing proper protective equipment when bat urine drips on him. Worse, bat blood is sprayed onto Tian's skin.

"In the past 10 years we have visited every corner of Hubei province. We have explored dozens of undeveloped caves and examined more than 300 types of virus vectors," he says. "However, I hope that these virus samples are kept for scientific research only and will never be used in real life. Because people not only need vaccines, but also protection from nature."

When he discovered the video on March 25, 2020, Yu sent a red alert email "all over Washington" including to the NSC and State Department, about the horrifying safety lapses in the video, along with other articles about Tian Junhua.

Two months later, former British diplomat Matthew Henderson told me that he understood intelligence agencies were taking a closer look at the Wuhan Centre for Disease Control. "It is extremely important. [Shi Zhengli] was called back from Shanghai on the night of December 30 to receive that evening samples that were passed on from work that had been done by the Wuhan Centre for Disease Control," he said. "[The Centre] had been looking for some time at samples from patients taken from hospitals who had this novel coronavirus disease."

The Wuhan Institute of Virology had similar issues, where high-level researchers did not wear proper safety equipment. This is confirmed by damning photographs of the Institute team that were deleted from their website after the pandemic broke. The photographs show researchers sitting around a table working on samples – some are wearing masks but others are not. Another photograph shows

Institute scientists in a cave with no masks, one not even wearing gloves, while collecting bat faecal samples.

And back in 2017, biosafety and biosecurity expert Tim Trevan told *Nature*, for an article on the Wuhan Institute of Virology's launch, that he was concerned an open culture would not be possible in China and that this was essential for keeping BSL-4 laboratories safe. "Diversity of viewpoint, flat structures where everyone feels free to speak up and openness of information are important," he says.

In that same article, Professor Richard Ebright also expressed concern about the Wuhan Institute of Virology, and specifically mentioned that the SARS virus had escaped from high-level containment facilities in Beijing multiple times. "These facilities are inherently dual use," he said. The article continued, "The prospect of ramping up opportunities to inject monkeys with pathogens also worries, rather than excites, him: 'They can run, they can scratch, they can bite.'"

Worryingly, even before the BSL-4 laboratory opened, the Wuhan Institute of Virology was conducting its risky experiments on coronaviruses in its BSL-2 and BSL-3 laboratories. (A level-2 lab has been compared to the biosafety level of a dentist's clinic.) This is not conjecture, it's according to the Chinese Academy of Sciences website, which states that the Wuhan Institute of Virology's P3 laboratory has been allowed to conduct small-sized animal-infection experiments for coronaviruses. It has one medium-sized animal laboratory, one small-sized animal laboratory and one dissecting room. It's where Shi Zhengli conducted many of her experiments with coronaviruses.

As Yu uncovered in his report for Pompeo, a safety and management review by the Chinese Ministry of Science and Technology found that out of China's 75 bio-research laboratories, the Wuhan Institute of Virology did not make the top 20 with an "excellent" ranking in terms of quality. Instead, it was given a B grade. "At the time the survey was conducted, in 2016, the WIV lab had completed its physical construction and was operational on a trial basis as a BSL-4 lab," Yu's report states. "By the time the survey ratings were published in

December 2017, China's in-house accreditation agency, the China National Accreditation Service for Conformity Assessment (CNAS), had already accredited WIV as a BSL-4 lab for nearly a year, and the PRC National Health Commission had already licensed the WIV to store and handle microorganisms of risk group 4, the most dangerous viruses in the world."

Yu's report stated that before its transition to a BSL-4 lab, the Wuhan Institute of Virology had housed more than 15,000 bat virus samples, the largest such collection in the world. "For a lab that only received a 'B' grade by its own national authorities, such an upgrade to handling the world's most lethal viruses is irresponsible at best, and dangerous at worst."

Yu concluded that the Wuhan Institute of Virology's transition from BSL-2 to BSL-4 "was hasty and reckless, causing great safety concern".

CHAPTER NINETEEN

The Cave of Death

APRIL 2016, MOUNT KINABALU, BORNEO

If you haven't been in a bat cave – and most people who aren't scientists or list 'adventure caving' as a hobby haven't – it is a completely putrid experience.

In 2016, 18 months after I met my now husband, Chaz, we travelled to Borneo. In between daily hikes and mountain climbing, we went "caving". This followed summiting 4095-metre high (almost 13,500 feet) Mount Kinabalu. In the rain. At 2am. His friends joked with me that he was trying to test my mettle. Clearly, if it was a test, I passed with flying colours.

The Gunung Mulu National Park in Sarawak has a tourism industry built around the caves, beautiful nature hikes and watching the bats fly in formation through the pink sky at dusk. Clad in a headlamp, hiking boots, long-sleeved shirt and leech socks, we went into pitch-black caves with a group of fellow cavers. There were thousands and thousands of bats. The smell was overwhelming. I felt squeamish simply standing in the cave and breathing in the air, before realising that bat poo, or guano, was falling from the roof of the cave into my hair and onto my face. It stuck to my skin each time I slipped while trying to haul myself up between the cave's crevices and through the dark tunnels with a rope. It was impossible to avoid the hundreds of oversized cockroaches and creepy crawlies, and I constantly checked under my shirt for leeches. It was a tough experience, and I can still clearly remember the relief of emerging from the cave hours later and immersing myself in the creek to wash off the disgusting guano.

Luckily, the effort was not for nothing. Chaz proposed later during that trip, when we were then thousands of miles away from the caves in stunning Corsica. Had I known then what I know now about disease-ridden bats, I would have steadfastly refused to go – ring or not.

My reaction was the polar opposite of Shi Zhengli's. She describes her first cave expedition, to collect samples from bat colonies in caves near Nanning, the capital of Guangxi, as "spellbinding". Shi Zhengli certainly romanticises the experience, telling *Scientific American* of the milky-white stalactites that hung from the ceiling like icicles, glistening with moisture.

The article stated: "Often guided by tips from local villagers, Shi and her colleagues had to hike for hours to potential sites and inch through tight rock crevasses on their stomachs. And the flying mammals can be elusive. In one frustrating week, the team explored more than 30 caves and saw only a dozen bats." This shows how the scientists are often collecting viruses from bats that are virtually impossible for humans to come across. The likelihood of a virus naturally crossing to humans from these remote bats, which you have to travel on your stomach into the crevasse of a cave to reach, rather than a laboratory leak, is certainly worth some thought.

The story of the potential lab-leak origin of Covid-19 starts in a similar bat cave in Yunnan province in south-western China, some 1500 kilometres (900 miles) from Wuhan. The cave, deep in green mountain valleys, had served as a copper mineshaft, but had long since been abandoned.

In April 2012, six miners were sent to clear out the mine. Literally to remove all the bat faeces. It was 150 metres (500 feet) deep, and they worked there at different times. By the end of April, one by one, they began to fall sick with severe pneumonia with an unknown cause. By the time four of them arrived at the hospital, they had "Type 1 respiration failure".

Miner Guo Shengfu, 45, was admitted to the First Affiliated Hospital of Kunming medical university on April 27, 2012. He had already had a cough for two weeks, along with tightness in his chest, shortness of breath, headache, sore limbs and a fever of up to 40 degrees Celsius (104 degrees Fahrenheit). He passed away 108 days later.

Another miner Lu Jinqui, aged 42, was admitted to Yuxi People's Hospital that same day, sent into the ward on a stretcher. He had a high fever and had already been coughing for two weeks. He had difficulty breathing in the three days before he was hospitalised. He spent a total of 48 days in hospital before he passed away.

A third miner, 63-year-old Zhou, would pass away, too, just 11 days after being admitted to hospital. He had fever, coughing, headache, difficulty breathing and chest pain for more than 10 days. Twenty-four days before hospitalisation on April 26 he had spent two weeks in the mine, working seven hours a day. His temperature, too, reached as high as 40 degrees Celsius.

The three other miners – Liu Zhongyun or Baoyun (his name is unclear in the documentation), aged 46; Wu Longjian, 30; and Li, 32 – were also hospitalised with serious illness but managed to eventually recover, although they were weak and had symptoms for more than a year afterwards. They had high fevers of over 39 degrees Celsius (102 degrees Fahrenheit), coughs and difficulty breathing.

The surviving miners were tested for a variety of diseases, including influenza, Japanese encephalitis, dengue fever and SARS, but nothing was found. But then a fascinating result: the miners were tested for SARS antibodies by the Wuhan Institute of Virology and all tested positive for an unknown SARS-like virus.

A year later, in May 2013, Li Xu submitted a master's thesis titled "The Analysis of Six Patients with Severe Pneumonia Caused by Unknown Viruses". Li Xu had obtained their medical records, analysis from doctors, radiological images, CT scans, lung scans and blood charts. The medical diagnosis reported that "The longer the time spent in the mining cave, the likelihood of death is higher. At the same time, the older patient died sooner. In terms of recovery, the fewer the working hours, the younger the patient, the better the recovery. They spend less time in the hospital.

"With the Kunming Institute of Zoology, we confirmed that the six patients were exposed to Chinese rufous horseshoe bat, which caused the disease," the thesis stated. "However, a paper published in *Science* magazine in 2005 by Scientist Shi Zheng Li and Zhang She Yu from Wuhan Institute of Virology under Chinese Academy of Science concluded that the SARS-like CoV carried by bats is not contagious to humans. This contradiction indicates the importance of these six cases: the severe pneumonia caused by the unknown virus and the bats in the cave merit further investigation and research." The thesis concludes that severe pneumonia in miners could be due to a SARS-like coronavirus from horseshoe bats.

While any sensible person would stay away from the bat caves where the miners were presumed to have contracted the virus, the potential discovery of a new coronavirus was an exciting prospect for Shi Zhengli. She designed and coordinated a study based around the cave, sending at least nine scientists to the Mojiang mine, where they collected dozens of virus samples from six species of bats.

This project began just three months after the first of the miners had died.

The scientists visited that cave four times in the 11 months from August 2012 – and would return over and over again in the years ahead. (In an addendum to another article in November 2020, they acknowledge visiting the mine again several times in 2015). In their first four visits, they took faecal samples from 276 bats. Half of them were positive for a coronavirus. They identified 150 alphacoronaviruses and two betacoronaviruses – and one of these was a SARS-like betacoronavirus. They called this SARS coronavirus BtCov/4991.

Shi Zhengli published a study on these findings in *Virologica Sinica* in February 2016, titled "Coexistence of Multiple Coronaviruses in Several Bat Colonies in an Abandoned Mineshaft." But the new

BtCov/4991 coronavirus had just a brief mention. "Our findings highlight the importance of bats as natural reservoirs of coronaviruses and the potentially zoonotic source of viral pathogens," she wrote.

The discovery of a new coronavirus should have raised alarm bells. But no one seemed to pay any attention to Shi Zhengli's scientific paper disclosing, albeit benignly, the discovery of BtCov/4991. This potentially lethal coronavirus was long forgotten. Until the pandemic hit.

Fast-forward to February 3, 2020, when Shi Zhengli published a paper with her colleague Peng Zhou and several others in *Nature*. There, they contend that SARS-CoV-2 was a virus of natural origin and float the theory that the new coronavirus originated in a bat. They say Covid-19 has a "probable bat origin" and shared a 79.6 per cent sequence identity with the SARS from the 2003 outbreak.

Dr Steven Quay, in Taiwan, said the paper was a "stake in the ground" for Shi Zhengli to say that SARS-CoV-2 originated from bats and "maybe as a distraction". That was interesting, but there was something else about this paper that was absolutely explosive. Shi Zhengli revealed for the first time the existence of a SARS-like coronavirus in her laboratory that no one had ever heard of before. She said it was called RaTG13. And she said that this virus was 96.2 per cent identical at the whole-genome level to SARS-CoV-2.

The importance of this revelation cannot be overemphasised. The closest known coronavirus to the one that causes Covid-19, with a 96.2 per cent genetic similarity, existed inside the Wuhan Institute of Virology.

To many scientists, it was astonishing – and highly troubling – that no one had ever heard of RaTG13 before this article. Shi Zhengli and her team had not mentioned it in any other scientific papers. Yet, suddenly, here it was – a virus whose genetic sequence was 96.2 per cent identical to a virus that was fast causing a global pandemic. She didn't say where it had come from, only Yunnan province "previously". It was puzzling. Where had this virus sample so similar to SARS-CoV-2 originated and how? Shi Zhengli made no mention of the abandoned mine and did not even cite her 2016 paper.

Perhaps no one would have been any wiser were it not for a group of internet sleuths, and a highly qualified scientist and mother of a young son living in Pune, India called Dr Monali Rahalkar. She is a microbiologist at the Agharkar Institute's Department of Bio-Energy, and studied in Germany.

She was reading the Wuhan Institute of Virology's scientific research and analysing the viruses they had been working with when she made a stunning discovery one rainy evening. Looking on GenBank, the genetic sequence database for every deposited virus, she realised that the virus Shi Zhengli's team had discovered in the abandoned mine – BtCov/4991 – had exactly the same genetic sequence as RaTG13. It was a 100 per cent match. BtCoV/4991 had been deposited in 2016 and RaTG13 was deposited in January 2020.

It was the same virus. For some unexplained reason the virus had been renamed in Shi Zhengli's February 2020 paper.

It was a puzzle Rahalkar set to work solving, discussing it with her husband Rahul Bahulikar, a scientist at Pune's BAIF Development and Research Foundation. Following on from crucial earlier discoveries made by Yuri Deigin, Rossana Segreto, Luigi Warren and an anonymous Twitter user in India called "The Seeker", in the weeks ahead they would piece together the story of the miners, their deaths, the team's visit to the cave and the discovery of the new SARS-like coronavirus. "It turns out RaTG13 was found in the same mine where the miners had died," Rahalkar says.

When they cracked the puzzle, Rahalkar didn't feel excited. "I felt shocked and angry because they were hiding this information in the first paper on the closest genetic virus to Covid-19," she tells me. "The pandemic was spreading globally, we had a major lockdown in India. It was a big shock for me that Shi Zhengli had hidden this information in her first paper."

As Rahalkar continued her scientific investigation, she came to believe it was a deliberate cover-up designed to hide the truth about the closest genetic relative to the virus that was causing global mayhem and loss of life. "I think they didn't want the miners' deaths to be associated with their lab directly," she said. "They were hoping no one would find out. If this was a progenitor virus, everyone would have thought they had made a genetically modified virus based on the sample they had brought home from the mine."

Rahalkar sent her paper that made all of these connections to *Nature* in May 2020 and published it on pre-print in late May. In October, it was finally published by *Frontiers in Public Health*. Rahalkar would later join a group of international scientists making headlines for calling for the WHO to conduct a new inquiry into the origins of the pandemic. After her paper was published, the scientists and researchers of DRASTIC reached out to her.

Deigin had already raised questions about where RaTG13 came from in his April 22, 2020 article on Medium, and tweeted about it a few days later. Segreto had suspected since March that BtCoV/4991 and RaTG13 could be the same virus. The miners' deaths were discovered by "The Seeker", who then passed the information on to Rahalkar. They encouraged her to join their conversation on Twitter, where they share research findings in long scientific threads that are often unintelligible without a science degree. "They introduced us to 'the Twitter' in June and I met the community of DRASTIC," Rahalkar laughs. "I had to set up a Twitter account."

DRASTIC has about 25 members who have been investigating the origins of the virus – night and day – since early in 2020, the group swelling as the months rolled on. Many choose to stay anonymous, owing to safety concerns and potential professional repercussions. At least one former member of the group lost his teaching job at a prestigious North American university. Some effectively live a double life. They have a strong online presence, on both the DRASTIC website and on Twitter, but their friends and family are unaware of their role in unearthing some of the most critical material to date on the origins of the virus.

The group started as a chat group called "Daszak's fan club", and then a Twitter user who goes by the pseudonym "Billy Bostickson" joined and renamed the group DRASTIC in May 2020. Billy, who represents himself on Twitter with the avatar of an abused experimental lab monkey, is one of those who has spent every day since early 2020 investigating the subject in incredible detail, which he shares in thousands of Twitter threads and publishes in Researchgate reports with co-author, forensic microbiologist Dr Yvette Ghannam. "In January 2020, I smelled a rat like many people did and decided to dedicate myself to uncovering the truth," he says. "What kept me going 15 hours a day, every day, for more than a year was that I felt it was a duty to do this out of respect for so many old folks who died and the terrible effect on local economies." He would reach out to others who had published interesting findings online and encourage them to join DRASTIC.

They've become a focal point for whistleblowers looking to share information. Billy says they "communicate mainly on Twitter in closed message groups and by secure email, sharing documents on drives for collaborative research work."

His and DRASTIC's work has been credited in hundreds of news stories globally. Such is his knowledge that government investigators and members of Congress have reached out to him, which is ironic because he's rather anti-authoritarian and seems to lean towards anarchy. Some of the members of DRASTIC are left-leaning, others are conservative climate-change sceptics; some are wealthy and others beg for donations or sell their discoveries to media outlets who will pay. Some hold down day jobs in universities or financial institutions, while others are unemployed. They're a maverick bunch with a common goal of investigating the origins of Covid-19. They each have their own separate view about how the pandemic started.

Having been privy to some of the private conversations among DRASTIC, I can certainly vouch that they can get fairly brutal. Billy often attempts to exert order by asking for people to sort their various issues out separately and reminding people to ignore political differences and focus on the search for the origins. To assert some order in the unwieldy bunch, Billy loosely divided it up into around 15 working groups to investigate different aspects of the origin question, such as the early cases in Wuhan, the conflicts of interest, the Chinese cover-up and translating Chinese documents.

Virologists have accused some members of DRASTIC of bullying and harassment on Twitter and, it's true, there are some who behave poorly. I have had to block one particular member for his unwarranted offensive comments. Another member is a convicted felon.

By and large, however, DRASTIC's role in unearthing information buried away has been pivotal, particularly given the lack of attention from intelligence agencies and government officials. The meticulous attention to detail has seen the group expose inconsistencies in accepted truths spouted by the WHO or leading virologists.

One member, known as "Jesse" has archived hundreds of deleted Wuhan Institute of Virology webpages and data scientist Francisco A. de Ribera specialises in the viruses the Wuhan Institute of Virology has failed to publicly disclose. Scientists already mentioned in earlier chapters, Yuri Deigin and Rossana Segreto, are also part of DRASTIC.

While still holding down a day job at a bank as their Data Science Technical Lead, Gilles Demaneuf, 52, has worked three to four hours a day, six days a week – and the odd all-nighter when he came across something particularly exciting or when working with colleagues in Europe – investigating the origins of the Covid-19 virus. "As a scientist I could not accept the lack of objectivity in the early scientific discussion on the subject. It struck me as totally absurd and suspicious that some top scientists, under the guidance of an organisation which had been funding the WIV, were dismissing any possible lab leak as a conspiracy theory," Demaneuf says. "The posturing, the choice of words, the poor logic displayed were all more consistent with a crude attempt to kill any scientific investigation than with the absolute lack of hard data on which to base any conclusion."

Demaneuf is disheartened by how the media, scientists and the intelligence community reacted to the search for answers relating to how the pandemic began. "For most of 2020, when there was not much room in the scientific debate and scientific journals for any such questioning, as a scientist you could often lose your job for taking such a position," he says. "For me, the most important thing that DRASTIC has achieved is simply that we did not buckle, we did not give up. We just kept building the case. Science should not be censored – but I hope that people will realise how close it got to be[ing] censored for good. This is actually very upsetting and frightening."

Demaneuf, who also has a background in start-ups, says his girlfriend has been "very patient" and his family "is not particularly surprised" by his dedication to the cause. "They know me. By the way I am Asperger – that may explain my capacity to focus, to work with numbers and to pick up patterns," he said.

With greater manpower, the group continued to investigate RaTG13. Together, they made even more remarkable discoveries. RaTG13, which was meant to have come from a bat faecal sample in the abandoned mineshaft, could not infect bats.

In March 2020, when Nikolai Petrovsky analysed the receptor-binding domain and found that the SARS-CoV-2 spike proteins would bind more tightly to the ACE2 receptor in humans than any other animal? Well, RaTG13 did not have a high-binding affinity with the bat ACE2 receptor. Instead, it was able to infect mice and rats.

This was very peculiar, given the virus was meant to have come from a bat sample. "If it's a bat coronavirus, it should bind to bats," Rahalkar says, matter-of-factly.

Further analysis showed that the SARS-CoV-2 receptor binding domain (RBD) was highly unusual. It was almost identical at an amino-acid level to an RBD from a pangolin sample called MP789 that the Guangdong Institute of Applied Biological Resources had deposited to GenBank. "The pangolins are from Malaysia. They were confiscated by Guangdong customs and sent to a wildlife refuge centre," Deigin says.

Like Petrovsky, Rahalkar says she doubts the viruses recombined naturally from pangolins and bats, adding that pangolins are very shy animals. "My guess is they used this because the bat coronaviruses would have receptor binding domains that would not immediately match to human beings. Pangolins were similar to humans."

The mystery remains: What exactly had the scientists done with RaTG13 from the time they brought it back from the mine on their fourth trip there in July 2013? What happened to the virus when it was back at the laboratory? Was it the subject of gain-of-function research? And was it used to create SARS-CoV-2? Given the Wuhan Institute of Virology was engaging in gain-of-function research, where one of the techniques is to combine existing viruses to create deadly new viruses, these are reasonable questions to ask.

We don't have all the answers, but there are some clues as to what the Wuhan Institute of Virology did with that sample. Francisco A. de Ribera, 40, a data scientist now completing a PhD in economics at Comillas Pontifical University in Madrid, Spain discovered that the virus had been removed from storage at −80 degrees Celsius (−112 degrees Fahrenheit) freezer in 2017, again in 2018 and then, as we already know, in 2020.

Ribera knows this because he found in a database for meta-genomes (called NCBI SRA) that some "amplicons" or long sequences used for helping the sequencing process of RaTG13 had dates of 2017 and 2018. This contradicted Shi Zhengli's claim in her February 2020 paper that this was a new virus only fully sequenced for the first time. A month after Ribera's discovery, Shi Zhengli conceded in an interview that they had sequenced it back in 2018. A correction was also later included in the paper's addendum in November 2020.

There was another unusual element. The RaTG13 virus deposit was only made after the pandemic, even though it was ostensibly found back in 2012. Shi Zhengli was then unable to produce the virus sample for RaTG13. She said it no longer existed and that it had disintegrated.

She was asked about the cave at Mojiang in a question-and-answer with *Science* in July 2020. In her response she simultaneously argues that she didn't pay much attention to the virus and that she used it so much that the virus had disintegrated and there was no sample left.

The *Science* interviewer asked her, "What about the cave at Mojiang in 2013? When did you first isolate RaTG13? When did you complete the full sequencing of it?"

This is her answer in full: "We detected the virus by pan-coronavirus RT-PCR in a bat faecal sample collected from Tongguan town, Mojiang county in Yunnan province in 2013, and obtained its partial RdRp sequence. Because the low similarity [sic] of this virus to SARS-CoV, we did not pay special attention to this sequence. In 2018, as the NGS sequencing technology and capability in our lab was improved, we did further sequencing of the virus using our remaining samples, and obtained the full-length genome sequence of RaTG13 except the 15 nucleotides at the 5' end. As the sample was used many times for the purpose of viral nucleic acid extraction, there was no more sample after we finished genome sequencing, and we did not do virus isolation and other studies on it. Among all the bat samples we collected, the RaTG13 virus was detected in only one single sample. In 2020, we compared the sequence of SARS-CoV-2 and our unpublished bat coronavirus sequences and found it shared a 96.2 per cent similarity with RaTG13. RaTG13 has never been isolated or cultured."

This story is highly improbable. Remember how Shi Zhengli's researchers visited the abandoned mine four times in the space of 11 months, sampling 276 bats? Out of all of this they found just two SARS-like coronavirus – the gold in the mine they were searching for. Is it really likely that they would not have sequenced it in full?

It's a point Nikolai Petrovsky made to *The Sunday Times*, saying it was "simply not credible" that they wouldn't have carried out analysis on it before 2020. "If you really thought you had a novel virus that had caused an outbreak that killed humans then there is nothing you wouldn't do – given that was their whole reason for being [there] – to get to the bottom of that, even if that meant exhausting the sample and then going back to get more," he said.

The other element potentially lacking plausibility is that the virus sample disintegrated and vanished, to exist no more. Asked if it is possible to use up a virus sample, Dr Quay said its "pretty unlikely" but "it's possible". "It's not good practice and 90 per cent of scientists wouldn't do it. Because this is an amplification process, you can literally have one molecule and get as much as you want," he explains. "Pretty unlikely to have used it up, but you can give her the benefit of the doubt on that particular fact."

Deigin said, "Theoretically, the faecal swab sample that was used to extract RNA for sequencing could have indeed been used up, although I don't buy it. Usually viral samples are aliquoted (split up and diluted) into many vials before cryostorage and then further diluted and split up if you start running out of aliquots."

Shi Zhengli's long-term research partner Peter Daszak was also asked about the likelihood of the sample disintegrating in an interview with *The Sunday Times* investigative journalists Jonathan Calvert and George Arbuthnott in July 2020. He said the mine sample had been stored in Wuhan for six years and then scientists "went back to that sample in 2020, in early January or maybe even at the end of last year, I don't know. They tried to get full genome sequencing, which is important to find out the whole diversity of the viral genome. I think they tried to culture it but they were unable to, so that sample, I think, has gone." He downplayed the significance of RaTG13. "It was just one of the 16,000 bats we sampled. It was a faecal sample, we put it in a tube, put it in liquid nitrogen, took it back to the lab. We sequenced a short fragment," he said.

Deigin said Daszak's claim that they only went back to the sample in January 2020 is not accurate, "as Shi Zhengli later had to admit they actually had the full sequence as far back as in 2018. So Daszak now looks very silly with his assertion they only went back to that sample in 2020 and it was in the freezer until then." Deigin said it's also clear that they tried to amplify the N gene of the virus as far back as 2014, as a newly discovered Wuhan Institute of Virology doctoral thesis shows.

On Twitter after the article was published, Daszak claimed the three miners had died of a fungal infection. He also disputed that RaTG13 was the progenitor of SARS-CoV-2. "RaTG13 is clearly not the progenitor (ancestor) of SARS-CoV-2 – it's a completely different virus. Also, conclusion in research was that miners died of fungal pneumonia, therefore not relevant to the scientific paper on these viruses," he said.

WHO investigator Marion Koopmans had also claimed the miners' deaths "related to fungal infection". But the fungal theory did not stand up to scrutiny. Not only had the patients tested positive to SARS antibodies, but scientists at the Wuhan Institute of Virology itself admitted the miners had died of pneumonia and say it was likely from a pathogen carried by bats in scientific research papers only uncovered in May 2021 by DRASTIC.

The doctoral thesis, by Wuhan Institute of Virology scientist Wang Ning, dated May 2014, states: "Three miners died from pneumonia in Mojiang, Yunnan province in 2011. After investigation, these miners had worked in an abandoned mine cave. A large number of bats were present in the cave, so we investigated the virus carried by bats in this cave."

Involved in the miners' case was Dr Zhong Nanshan, whom Deigin describes as "the most famous Chinese SARS academician, sort of like Fauci and Collins combined". "The fact he was closely monitoring this case tells you a lot already. The Mojiang outbreak was a big deal," he says. Zhong Nanshan's view was that the fungal infection one or two of them had was secondary.

Professor Ebright disagreed with Daszak about RaTG13 being a potential ancestor as well, saying: "The genome sequence of the outbreak virus indicates that its progenitor was either the horseshoe bat coronavirus RaTG13 or a closely related bat coronavirus." But some scientists who suspect a lab leak, like Dr Quay, question whether RaTG13 would have been a direct ancestor because the evolutionary divergence is too great.

"I don't believe it is. There's 1100 nucleotide changes you have to make to get from RaTG13 to get to SARS-CoV-2. It gets very convoluted, it doesn't mean it didn't happen but .. it's subject to a lot of criticism because it takes so many steps to get those nucleotide changes," he said.

Dr Quay views the name change from BtCoV/4991 to RaTG13 as "very sketchy" and says there are "so many strange things about it". "In that nature paper Dr Shi Zhengli says we looked in our database, lo and behold and there was this RNA dependent, RNA polymerase [RdRp] gene that looked really close to SARS2, only 2 or 3 nucleotides different and then we sequenced the whole specimen, and it was 96% similar," he says.

RaTG13 wasn't the only virus the Wuhan Institute of Virology had failed to disclose. "Live virus isolates" are the actual virus samples scientists experiment on, as opposed to genetic sequences they can model on a computer. Ribera noticed that the Institute had assigned a number to each new live virus isolate, so he decided to compile a list of them all. He found that there are two live virus isolates the Wuhan Institute of Virology has never disclosed: WIV6 and WIV15. "This is important because these are real viruses that you need to use for experiments. You can't work just with a sequence in a lab," he says. WIV6 was finally disclosed in June 2021, but, as of going to print, WIV15 was still missing.

The virus sample RaTG13 is 96.2 per cent identical TO SARS-CoV-2 – as Shi Zhengli said in her February 2020 article. But if you look at the original, shorter RdRp segment of RaTG13 that was published back in 2016, it is 98.65 per cent identical to that of SARS-CoV-2.

The first scientists to notice this were Chinese scientists at the Wuhan University, Liangjun Chen and colleagues, who released a paper in early 2020 titled "RNA Based mNGS Approach Identifies a Novel Human Coronavirus from Two Individual Pneumonia Cases in 2019 Wuhan Outbreak". Ribera says Shi Zhengli clearly chose not to mention this higher genetic percentage of the RdRp in her paper that laid the stake in the ground for the natural-origin argument. "Shi Zhengli skilfully avoided admitting this in her *Nature* article by saying that it has a 'high sequence identity' and then moving quickly to talk about the complete genome and the 96.2 per cent ," he says. He adds that although the complete genome's percentage is expected to be lower because other parts of the genome mutate faster than the RdRp, this figure is still revealing.

A second reason for the lower genetic similarity of the whole genome could be due to laboratory experiments or recombinations, as Petrovsky and others suggest. The sections of the genome that have been swapped with another virus will be very different, thus lowering the percentage. "RaTG13 could have been manipulated 'in silico', in a computer, to appear less similar to SARS-CoV-2," Ribera speculates. "The only part that they could not fabricate is the partial RdRp because it was already published in 2016, but they may have retouched a little the other 99 per cent of the genome, although not unrestrictedly. One of my hypotheses is that they could have made a chimera not because they want the best of the two viruses but because they want to obtain a live virus with the spike of a virus that they were not able to isolate. It is very hard to isolate a virus. What we saw in their articles is that doing a chimera starting with another live isolate was much easier."

Letting world researchers find a virus that has a partial 98.65 per cent genetic match to SARS-CoV-2 while the sequence of the next virus is only 89 per cent identical would have been very suspicious, Ribera says. "I think the Wuhan Institute of Virology wanted to avoid having people consolidate that anchor of 98.65 per cent, which is what would have happened if the Chen et al. paper was not eclipsed by the WIV's article," he speculates. "So they needed to have this article out ASAP. This could also be another reason the Chinese delayed the publication of the first genome sequence."

Now here is where this all gets really fascinating. Rahalkar has already explained how RaTG13 can't infect bats. Despite its RdRp being more than 98 per cent similar to SARS-CoV-2, RaTG13 can't infect humans either. A paper published in *Nature Structural and Molecular Biology* by the esteemed Francis Crick Institute in London confirms this. "Together, our structural and biochemical data indicate that a bat virus, similar to RaTG13, would not be able to bind effectively to human ACE2 receptor and would be unlikely to infect humans directly," it states.

They suspect a recombination event has occurred to "generate" Covid-19. "Given the modular nature of the human and bat S glycoproteins, and the number and structural locations of the amino-acid-sequence differences between them, our observations support the involvement of recombination between distinct coronavirus genomes in the generation of SARS-CoV-2," the paper concludes. "Furthermore, our study suggests that the presence of the furin-cleavage site in the S protein of SARS-CoV-2 facilitates the conformational change required for RBD exposure and binding to surface receptors."

So which part of the virus specifically is different between RaTG13 and Covid-19? The RBD in the spike protein – precisely the area with which Shi Zhengli had been experimenting for more than a decade. In other words, it is the part that makes the virus infectious to humans.

You can see on the first SimPlot analysis graph below (which tracks the virus genome) that this is where the difference in the genome sequence identity lies. Within the genome of a virus, the spike gene runs approximately from base pairs 20,000 to 25,000. In this first SimPlot comparing the genome of RaTG13 and the SARS-CoV-2 virus, you can very clearly see the circled divergence where the spike protein is.

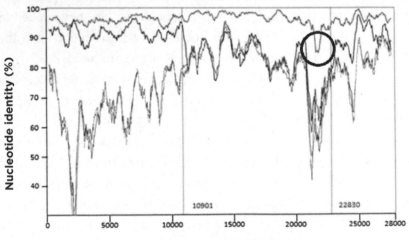

But in Shi Zhengli's February 2020 *Nature* paper, she took a wide window size of the graph (below), over-smoothing it to hide the huge drop in the spike specifically in the RBD, which then led her to claim there had been no recombination – a fact already disputed by too many scientists, including those who promote a natural origin.

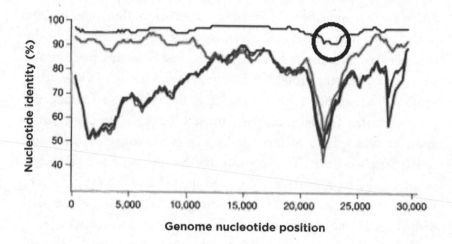

Some scientists suspect that while BtCoV/4991 was a genuine sample, RaTG13 may not be a real virus sample. They question whether it may be a partially fake or invented genetic sequence. "There are several anomalies in the RaTG13. It doesn't look completely original. They deposited everything after the pandemic so they could fake a sequence," Rahalkar hypothesises.

Deigin adds, "This was questioned pretty early on by pretty much everyone as soon as we realized Shi Zhengli used a different name for RaTG13; we wondered why. Is it because it really is different from 4991 and she is hedging her bets in case this is later proven? I mean, we now have circumstantial evidence the two really are different, as The Seeker has found a new 2019 WIV doctoral thesis that has a different genome match percentage between SARS1's spike gene and 4991's spike than between SARS1 and RaTG13 spike genes."

Ribera says, "It's fine to not trust the RaTG13 full genome, but I do not think they fabricated Ra4991 RdRp back in 2016. At the moment of the outbreak, Ra4991 RdRp was – by a lot – the closest virus with a 98.65% identity and the next one came at 89%. You cannot change that."

The question then is, which virus has an identical spike protein or RBD to SARS-CoV-2? And did the Wuhan Institute of Virology have it in its freezers? Multiple scientists, including Dr Nikolai Petrovsky, say it is the pangolin spike. Petrovsky says the spike protein in SARS-CoV-2 appears to have been taken from the spike protein in the pangolin coronavirus, given they are almost identical in the relevant part that binds human ACE2. "Just how this piece of the pangolin virus spike protein ended up in the pandemic SARS-CoV-2 virus is yet another mystery. But it is impossible to exclude the possibility that Chinese scientists moved the pangolin coronavirus spike protein gene into some unknown bat coronavirus they had isolated to see if this would make the bat virus be able to infect human cells," he speculates. "If this happened and it had succeeded, then the stage would be set for the new virus to jump out of the petri dish to infect one of the lab-workers, and the rest is history."

What's also highly unusual is the number of viruses Shi Zhengli discovered at the mine whose full sequences have either never been deposited in GenBank or were withheld. On May 21, 2021 – 15 months after the start of the pandemic – Shi Zhengli released a pre-print finally disclosing a group of eight viruses she had discovered at the mine six years earlier. The full genomes for the eight viruses were almost identical, which is unusual. She also confirmed they had been discovered at the same location as RaTG13, although she avoided mentioning the mine, as usual. The eight missing viruses (known collectively as "clade 7896") had been discovered by Ribera in July 2020 after an anonymous Twitter user noted the proximity of eight viruses to SARS-CoV-2 in one of his phylogenetic trees. (Ribera found that one of them – named 7896 – appeared as a label in the amplicons of RaTG13.)

The eight missing virus samples had been collected in the Mojiang mine in May 2015 and uploaded to GenBank in October 2019, but they were embargoed from being publicly released until June 2020. Even then, they only had their partial RdRp fragments published. As already noted, their complete genome was only disclosed on May 21, 2021.

Two viruses from the clade were labelled "Mojiang Bat CoVs" in a slide presentation Shi Zhengli gave on "SARS-related CoVs" dated December 2020, but when she gave the same presentation just two months later, in February 2021, those viruses and the label had been deleted from the corresponding slide. "Not only did they lie about when they sequenced RaTG13 (2018, not 2020) and left the 7896-clade embargoed for months, but they also hide that they have sequenced the spikes of 7896-clade," Ribera says. "They accidentally leaked this fact and then removed it. It proved the 7896-clade came from the mineshaft and also that they have sequenced the spikes."

Gilles Demaneuf says the missing viruses are part of the Wuhan Institute of Virology's "pattern of obfuscation" where they "very slowly release only partial information". "That's troubling, especially if you think that these viruses are nothing special, then why would they take so much time to release proper information about them? It's a bit odd that they'd go to such lengths to obfuscate the details," he says.

Ribera points out that the best example of the Wuhan Institute of Virology keeping a virus secret was RaTG13 itself. They had fully sequenced it in 2018 but kept it under wraps until January 2020, when Shi Zhengli suddenly shocked the world with this new virus that was the closest genetically to Covid-19. Dr Quay says: "It clearly looks like she was covering up its relationship to the mine and seven or eight other viruses that were collected at the same time, which is probably where SARS-CoV-2's backbone comes from."

In total, 630 viruses obtained by the Institute have only had their partial RdRps published – they were all embargoed from October 2019 until June 2020, according to an August 2020 scientific paper by Alice Latinne and colleagues titled "Origin and Cross-species Transmission of Bat Coronaviruses in China".

A US State Department fact sheet released in January 2021 pointed out this lack of transparency over the disclosure of RaTG13. It states: "The [Wuhan Institute of Virology] has not been transparent or consistent about its record of studying viruses most similar to the COVID-19 virus, including 'RaTG13,' which it sampled from a cave in Yunnan province in 2013 after several miners died of SARS-like illness."

When under threat, pangolins roll up into a scaly impenetrable ball, which means they can fend off predators far more powerful. Videos *National Geographic* obtained from a Kenyan reserve show how even the full force of a lion's jaw is unable to pierce the scales of a pangolin. This also makes them one of the world's most easily captured and trafficked animals. Their meat is a Chinese delicacy and their scales are used in traditional medicine. Early scientific studies published by medical journals like *Nature* on the origins of Covid-19 that relied on pangolin sequences have come under scrutiny.

China's People's Liberation Army has been involved in scientific research into the origins of the coronavirus. One study, published online in *Nature* on March 26, 2020 and titled "Identifying SARS-CoV-2 Related Coronaviruses in Malayan Pangolins", was described by the University of Sydney as helping to solve the puzzle of how SARS-CoV-2 transferred from animals to humans. It relied on a key laboratory in the microbiology institute within the PLA's Academy of Military Medical Sciences to conduct its "genetic sequencing" and "virus isolation". The study was co-funded by the Australian Research Council and the Chinese government.

The Director of the microbiology institute, Professor Cao Wuchan, who is thanked in the paper's acknowledgments for his "substantial contribution", has the rank of colonel and is a Wuhan Institute of Virology board member. One of the study's co-authors, Tong Yigang, began working in the same PLA-run microbiology institute in 2005. Another co-author was Professor Eddie Holmes of the University of Sydney, who is also an Honorary Visiting Professor at Fudan University, Shanghai.

A University of Sydney spokesman said Holmes's work was academically independent and that he had not received any research or personal funding from the Chinese government or Chinese companies or institutions. "Where he has undertaken research with scientists from China, his work has been funded by the Australian Research Council, the National Health and Medical Research Council and the University of Sydney," she said. "Prof Holmes has no link with the Academy of Military Science. Their involvement with the research was declared in the acknowledgments, as is standard practice. Dr Cao coordinated the laboratory work before Prof Holmes' involvement. He did not direct or supervise the work of Prof Holmes, which was undertaken independently."

A completely separate paper published in *Nature* on May 7, 2020 claimed the RBD in pangolins was almost identical to that of SARS-CoV-2, indicating Covid-19 "may have originated in the recombination of a virus similar to pangolin CoV with one similar to RaTG13". Scientists then contacted *Nature* pointing out that the pangolin samples from several papers all seemed to come back to the one sample.

In response to questions for this book, *Nature*'s Editor-In-Chief Magdalena Skipper said, "Concerns have been raised about the identity of pangolin samples (not to the best of my knowledge about "the credibility of pangolin sequencing" as you state) in this study and the following Editor's note has been added to the paper: 'Editor's note: Readers are alerted that concerns have been raised about the identity of the pangolin samples reported in this paper and their relationship to previously published pangolin samples. Appropriate editorial action will be taken once this matter is resolved.' We are in the final stages of assessing this. We would be happy to inform you when we reach a conclusion."

One of the lead authors of this paper is Shen Yongyi from South China Agricultural University's Centre for Emerging and Zoonotic Diseases. It was the Broad Institute's Alina Chan and Shing Hei Zhan of University of British Columbia who noticed irregularities in many of the papers involving pangolin research that claimed a natural origin of the virus because pangolins could be the intermediary host. "Multiple publications have independently described pangolin CoV genomes from the same batch of smuggled pangolins confiscated in Guangdong province in March, 2019," Chan wrote in a pre-print paper published in July 2020. "This raises the question of whether pangolins are truly reservoirs or hosts of SARS-CoV-2-related coronaviruses in the wild, or whether the pangolins may have contracted the CoV from another host species during trafficking. Our observations highlight the importance of requiring authors to publish their complete genome assembly pipeline and all contributing raw sequence data, particularly those supporting epidemiological investigations, in order to empower peer review and independent analysis of the sequence data. This is necessary to ensure both the accuracy of the data and the conclusions presented by each publication."

Other scientists, such as Dr Quay, also do not trust the research that relied on pangolin data and, they fear, may boil down to just one sample. It shows just how murky and difficult the business of tracing the origin of Covid-19 is. Petrovsky describes the idea the pangolin was the source of SARS-CoV-2 as a "red herring". He says a virus found by Chinese scientists in pangolins "was in fact a completely different pangolin coronavirus that was not related to SARS-CoV-2". "The pangolins were exonerated. Nevertheless, every so often the pangolin gets dragged back into the frame by Chinese authorities trying to find a scapegoat for the source of the virus."

Journalists are now strictly forbidden from visiting that abandoned mineshaft. A *Wall Street Journal* reporter finally arrived there on a mountain bike in 2021, but was detained and questioned for five hours by police and a photograph of the mine was deleted. AP journalists who tried to visit the Jinning cave were tailed by plainclothes police in multiple cars who blocked access to roads. Their article reported: "More than a year since the first known person was infected with the coronavirus, an AP investigation shows the Chinese government is strictly controlling all research into its origins, clamping down on some while actively promoting fringe theories that it could have come from outside China."

AP reported that bat researchers who had visited the site had samples confiscated and that all scientific findings were first vetted by the Communist Party. "The government is handing out hundreds of thousands of dollars in grants to scientists researching the virus' origins in southern China and affiliated with the military, the AP has found. But it is monitoring their findings and mandating that the publication of any data or research must be approved by a new task force managed by China's cabinet, under direct orders from President Xi Jinping."

To sum up, we know already from the previous chapter that the Wuhan Institute of Virology had done risky research on many viral spike proteins since 2006. They were changing the spike proteins and then passaging the resulting viral constructs to assess the effects the changes might have on the ability of the viruses to infect humans.

We also know that despite Shi Zhengli presenting RaTG13 as a new virus in February 2020, as she tried to convince the world Covid-19 had a natural origin, RaTG13 had in fact been taken out of her laboratory freezers several times over the years. We don't know what experiments her team did with the virus sample – only that it was taken out of the freezer, thanks to Ribera's discovery.

In her February 2020 paper, Shi made no mention of a cave or the virus's history. No mention of the fact it had been collected seven years earlier in an abandoned mine where miners had died from a Covid 19-like disease back in 2012. She then tried to hide the fact the miners had been ill with a coronavirus, making it seem like they had died of a fungal infection, even convincing the WHO team of this.

And now we know that Shi Zhengli says RaTG13 no longer exists. Shi Zhengli, who has fudged the truth on so much about that virus and its history, says it has "disintegrated".

CHAPTER TWENTY

Conflicted

Gary Ruskin is an old-time investigative public interest researcher. The grey-haired, bespectacled father ran a group against corruption in Congress for 14 years and has more recently dedicated his time to focus on pesticides and genetically modified foods. In 2014, Ruskin set up an organisation called US Right to Know, a non-profit investigative public health group. He led a campaign for GMO foods to be labelled.

A topic like the origins of Covid-19 wasn't exactly on his hit list when 2020 rolled in. "If you'd have told me I'd be working on this I would have said, not a chance in hell because we mostly do work on food and agriculture issues," he says. But Ruskin sat back and watched as there was no satisfactory investigation into the origins of the virus by either world health authorities or the media through the start of 2020. By April, Ruskin wondered if it might be time to turn his attention to the origins of the pandemic. To do his small part, as he puts it.

In fact, his role in exposing shocking conflicts of interest among some of the scientists who promulgated the natural-origin theory would turn out to be crucial. He began filing dozens of Freedom of Information (FOI) requests for documents relating to the origins of the virus. "We didn't know what we would get or if there would be anything useful in it at all. And I was ready to file six months of requests and get nothing and think, 'Well, you know, it was worth a try,'" Ruskin says.

It wasn't long before he had a breakthrough. In November 2020, a batch of 466 pages of emails from the University of Maryland came through from an FOI request. Those documents exposed for the first time EcoHealth Alliance President Peter Daszak's conflicts of interest. The emails dated back to February 2020, when the gravity of the virus was on the cusp of beginning to be understood.

That month, the esteemed medical journal *The Lancet* published a letter signed by 27 leading scientists saying that this virus originated from animals. It then accused those questioning whether the virus was from a laboratory of spreading "misinformation".

The letter said: "We are public health scientists who have closely followed the emergence of 2019 novel coronavirus disease (COVID-19) and are deeply concerned about its impact on global health and wellbeing ... The rapid, open, and transparent sharing of data on this outbreak is now being threatened by rumours and misinformation around its origins. We stand together to strongly condemn conspiracy theories suggesting that COVID-19 does not have a natural origin." The letter went on: "Conspiracy theories do nothing but create fear, rumours, and prejudice that jeopardise our global collaboration in the fight against this virus. We support the call from the Director-General of WHO to promote scientific evidence and unity over misinformation and conjecture."

The emails Ruskin obtained showed this letter was organised by a group called the EcoHealth Alliance, which, as you already know from Chapter 16, was funnelling NIH grant money to the Wuhan Institute of Virology. Daszak was the co-author on many of Shi Zhengli's research papers, and his group, EcoHealth Alliance, funded and participated in her bat-sampling research.

The emails released under FOI show Daszak wrote the first draft of the *Lancet* statement. Two of the other scientists who signed the letter, Rita Colwell and James Hughes, are members of the EcoHealth Alliance board of directors, while William Karesh is the group's Executive Vice President for Health and Policy, and Hume Field, an Honorary Professor of the University of Queensland in Australia, is Science and Policy Advisor. In total, of the 27 who signed the statement, seven were affiliated with EcoHealth Alliance, four had current or previous affiliations with the Wellcome Trust, Ralph Baric had conducted gain-of-function experiments with Shi Zhengli and four other authors had worked with Baric. Yet no conflicts at all were disclosed. Instead it said: "We declare no competing interests."

In one email, Daszak wrote, "Please note that this statement will not have EcoHealth Alliance logo on it and will not be identifiable as coming from any one organisation or person, the idea is to have this as a community supporting our colleagues."

There was no evidence presented by the scientists in their letter to refute the possibility the virus originated in a lab. One signatory, Linda Saif, asked via email on February 6 whether there should be an addition. She wrote: "I concur with this draft! One question is whether it would be useful to add just one or 2 statements in support of why nCOV is not a lab generated virus and is naturally occurring? Seems critical to scientifically refute such claims!" Daszak replied: "You're right it would be good to be specific about the bioengineered virus conspiracy theory, but I think we should probably stick to a broad statement."

Emails show that Daszak deliberately tried to obscure his involvement. In an email dated February 6, 2020 he wrote that he had spoken with Linfa Wang, who has affiliations with the CSIRO, the Duke University and the Wuhan Institute of Virology: "I spoke with Linfa last night about the statement we sent around. He thinks, and I agree with him, that you, me and him should not sign this statement, so it has some distance from us and therefore doesn't work in a counterproductive way.

"Jim Hughes, Linda Saif, Hume Field, and I believe Rita Colwell will sign it, then I'll send it round some other key people tonight. We'll then put it out in a way that doesn't link it back to our collaboration so we maximize an independent voice."

Baric, who had done the 2015 gain-of-function experiment with Shi Zhengli, replied to say, "I also think this is a good decision. Otherwise it looks self-serving and we lose impact."

The Lancet's complicity in allowing a group of scientists, some with a clear conflict of interest, including financial ties with Shi Zhengli, to dismiss a laboratory origin is shameful. *The Lancet* did not include any disclosure of the conflicts, as the journal is required to do. "When I was reading them [the emails], the importance of them was immediately very apparent," Ruskin says. "It shows that Peter Daszak was conducting a political effort to tarnish the notion that this could be a lab origin for SARS-COV-2 and he did it in such a way as to make it look like this was a bunch of scientists making a statement when this was run by him and the EcoHealth Alliance," he said. "Daszak does a lot of PR that's dressed up as science. *The Lancet* fell for it hook, line and sinker."

Ruskin says that what is frustrating is that the *Lancet* letter set the narrative in the Western media that the virus had a natural origin – something that continues to this day. "In fact, when I read the key ones, I almost fell out of my chair, because I thought, 'Wait a second, this is a public relations deception.' It's a sad story to see that kind of deception work. In essence, it's still working."

The *Lancet* letter was extremely effective. From that moment forward, anyone who dared suggest a non-natural origin of the virus was labelled a conspiracy theorist in the media. It worked to dissuade other reputable scientists from speaking out.

Daszak was backed up by acolytes of China around the world, who shaped coverage of this issue. At the time, their roles or their links to China were often unknown. The world was none the wiser. Trusting our scientists and our scientific publications, most people believed that the scientific consensus was that Covid-19 was a naturally occurring virus. Instead, it was Peter Daszak and the EcoHealth Alliance, who had worked closely for years with the very scientists suspected of leaking the virus and causing the pandemic, that were branding a laboratory origin a conspiracy theory.

Looking back, Daszak had played a role in shaping the narrative from day one. When the outbreak happened – before CDC Director Robert Redfield had been contacted on January 3 and before even the newspapers had reported it – Daszak was already insisting China was being transparent. "Note that the market is called a 'seafood market' but also sells butchered mammal meat. SARS has not been ruled out, and we've heard that Chinese labs are using a range of tools to test for SARS & SARS-related CoVs, as well as to rule out usual suspects of pneumonia," Daszak tweeted on January 1, with a link to the ProMED post about the new virus.

"Putting this into context – there's concern about another SARS-like outbreak, but having worked with Chinese collaborators for >15 years on SARS-related CoVs, the labs in China are far more efficient now than they were in 2003, and the clinics are more numerous and better equipped," his tweet went on. "The China CDC and Provincial CDCs are working effectively already, and there is an openness and transparency right now that wasn't there during the first SARS cases." NSW Scientist of the Year Eddie Holmes, from the University of Sydney, replied to his tweet on January 1: "Agreed. China CDC are excellent. They will handle this well."

When Anthony Fauci publicly said the virus had a natural origin in April 2020, Daszak emailed to thank him. "I just wanted to say a personal thank you on behalf of our staff and collaborators, for publicly standing up and stating that the scientific evidence supports a natural origin for Covid-19 from a bat-to-human spillover, not a lab release from the Wuhan Institute of Virology." He continued, "From my perspective, your comments are brave, and coming from your trusted voice, will help dispel the myths being spun around the virus' origin."

Fauci replied on Sunday 19 April, "Many thanks for your kind note."

While Daszak's role in *The Lancet* letter would not be publicly known until the US Right to Know FOI came through in November 2020, in public interviews Daszak repeatedly reiterated the claim that anyone who pointed the finger at the laboratory was a conspiracy theorist. He told *The Guardian* that questions about a possible laboratory origin of the coronavirus are "crackpot theories that need to be addressed". His comments encouraged trust in the Wuhan scientists, who he said were open and transparent. "We work very closely with the Chinese scientists. We have had incredible openness with the labs in China for the last 15 years, since SARS," he said in February 2020.

He continued his conspiracy theme in an interview that same month with ScienceInsider: "We're in the midst of the social media misinformation age, and these rumors and conspiracy theories have real consequences, including threats of violence that have occurred to our colleagues in China. We have a choice whether to stand up and support colleagues who are being attacked and threatened daily by conspiracy theorists or to just turn a blind eye."

Daszak would continue to tweet throughout the months of the pandemic, constantly attempting to discredit anyone, including politicians who were calling for inquiries into all possible origins. "Here's that guy again who pushes the conspiracy theories on COVID-19. His earlier statements were shown to be completely false and egregious," he said on Twitter, referring to Secretary of State Mike Pompeo in August 2020.

In his 3196 tweets from July 2020 to May 2021, Daszak used the word "conspiracy", "conspire" or "conspired" 97 times. He tweeted in July 2020: "Incredible to see anti-China rhetoric, conspiracy theories & politicization launched against @DrTedros & @WHO purely as a political campaign strategy to dream up villains that might make our current president look stronger to his base. Damaging & blatant. I stand with @WHO!" In another September 2020 tweet, Daszak said: "Conspiracy theorists usually complain I'm being too 'defensive' or that I'm 'ranting' when I simply point out the logic that COVID emerged naturally & that it's a waste of resources, & doesn't protect us against future pandemics to use COVID to focus on 'germ warfare.'"

When questions were asked about the Wuhan Institute of Virology's virus database, he defended the team for not making the samples public. "More or less all the bat coronavirus work that they've done there has been done in collaboration with us, almost all of it. So we know that they did not have isolates of the virus that leads to Covid-19 in the lab," he told NBC news in August 2020. In another tweet, Daszak spoke about doing karaoke with Shi Zhengli, indicating his friendship with her. When Biden won the election on November 8, 2020, Daszak tweeted "We're drinking it all – 4 years worth of champagne tonight!" with a photograph of Perrier-Jouët Champagne. Author and journalist David Quammen replied saying: "Peter, Brut and martinis toasting back! Next year in Wuhan." To this, Daszak responded: "Amen to that. Looking forward to that special moment when we hit the baiju and the karaoke with Zhengli and Linfa."

It's extraordinary that a scientist who had partnered with the Wuhan Institute of Virology, which was genetically manipulating coronaviruses at times to make them more transmissible to humans, was repeatedly calling a laboratory origin a conspiracy theory.

In a further incomprehensible conflict of interest, Daszak was then appointed to the WHO investigation into the origins of the virus, flying into Wuhan in February 2021. Daszak had worked for 15 years with the Wuhan Institute of Virology, sampling more than 5370 bats with them by 2018. When he visited the institute as part of the investigation, he was questioning his colleagues and even friends.

The United States had recommended three health officials participate, but former American Ambassador to Geneva Andrew Bremberg said they weren't chosen. The US names put forward to the WHO were CDC epidemiologist Matt Moore, FDA Senior Regulatory Veterinarian Brianna Skinner and Dr Heinz Feldman who works with NIH and NIAID at the Rocky Mountain Laboratories. Instead, Daszak appeared on the list. *The Daily Mail* in the UK reported in 2020 that the WHO allowed China to vet scientists taking part in the inquiry. Bremberg tells me ultimately it was up to China to approve visas for each of the WHO members visiting.

Despite almost a hundred tweets calling the lab-origin possibility a conspiracy, Daszak claimed he would investigate every angle. "Any hypothesis we'll follow the data, we'll follow the evidence where it leads us," he told CNBC. Arriving at the Wuhan Institute of Virology on February 3, 2021, Daszak's car slowed down for the many reporters covering the moment. "We're looking forward to meeting with all the key people here," he said.

Out of the two weeks that WHO investigators spent in Wuhan, they only spent three hours at the Wuhan Institute of Virology. Daszak tweeted on February 9, 2021: "We had detailed discussion with people there about all aspects of lab leak hypothesis and received satisfactory answers." At a March 10 virtual panel at the Chatham House think tank in London, Daszak confirmed the WHO mission "did not" ask to see the missing virus database. He explained how Shi Zhengli told the WHO team that the database had been taken down after more than 3000 "hacking attempts". He followed up by saying "a lot of this work is conducted with EcoHealth Alliance … and we do basically know what's in those databases". Yet the database was not made available for other investigators.

In an interview with CNN after his visit to the Wuhan Institute of Virology, Daszak said there was no evidence that the virus originated from the lab and spoke of "conspiracies around lab leaks". "It is something that we talked about with people at the Wuhan lab, and got really honest and frank and good informative answers to," he said. The WHO report concluded it was extremely unlikely that the virus had come from a laboratory but found other pathways plausible, including that it was imported into China in frozen food, with the most likely scenario that it was a natural zoonosis transfer to humans.

Daszak was also appointed as the lead on *The Lancet* COVID Commission Task Force on the Origins of SARS-CoV-2, a group of 12 scientists from around the world intended to investigate where the virus came from, how it escaped control and how future pandemics can be prevented. "We intend to conduct a thorough and rigorous investigation into the origins and early spread of SARS-CoV-2," Daszak said in November 2020.

While investigating this book I sent a series of questions to *The Lancet* asking why it had declined to publish papers from scientists that suggested a non-natural origin of Covid-19. I also asked, "Why weren't the conflicts of interest that Peter Daszak has with the Wuhan Institute of Virology (a substantial financial and working relationship) disclosed to the readers of *The Lancet*?" And "Have you misled readers by not disclosing this clear conflict of interest?" I also asked why they had not added an Editor's note to the article notifying readers of his conflicts. "Does *Lancet* acknowledge that any legitimate 'Covid-19 Commission' would not involve Daszak or others with conflicts of interest? Will you be asking Peter Daszak to step down as commissioner of *The Lancet*'s 'Covid-19 Commission'?"

The Lancet finally responded on June 22, 2021 by publishing an updated declaration of interest statement for Daszak that noted EcoHealth Alliance's work in China. They also recused him from their Commission on the origins of the pandemic.

EcoHealth Alliance, which as we saw in Chapter 16 has received US$60 million in funding from American taxpayers, has not been transparent. Far from it. Daszak has actively mocked requests for information from the NIH, the very body giving him so much funding. When the NIH stopped funding EcoHealth Alliance in April 2020, and said it would only resume funding once the organisation cooperated with questions related to the Wuhan Institute of Virology and the suspicious events that unfolded around the time of the outbreak, Daszak tweeted that the requests were "straight out of the conspiracy theory playbook". He also said in an interview with *Nature* that the demands were "heinous" and "absurd" and outside his remit. When *The New York Times* published an article shedding light on the fact that China had not shared crucial data with the investigative team, Peter Daszak tweeted: "Shame on you @nytimes!"

On February 10, 2021, responding to a *South China Morning Post* report that said the US will not accept the WHO findings without verification, Peter Daszak tweeted: "Joe Biden has to look tough on China. Please don't rely too much on US intel: increasingly disengaged under Trump and frankly wrong on many aspects. Happy to help (White House with) their quest to verify, but don't forget it's 'TRUST' then 'VERIFY'!"

What kind of independent investigator dismisses US intelligence and is outraged at *The New York Times* for criticising the Chinese government for withholding data, but then immediately trusts answers given by the Wuhan Institute of Virology? As former head of intelligence agency ASIO, Dennis Richardson told *The Australian*, "The way [China] has handled the COVID-19 matter should make people worry. This is a classic authoritarian power response, which simply tells lies."

This is more than a conflict of interest. It is beyond comprehension to appoint someone to investigate the origins of Covid-19 who has personally worked, for 15 years, with the very people whose laboratory may be responsible for leaking the virus. That is clearly not an independent or reliable approach. An individual sent in by the WHO to investigate how the virus started already had a very strong view on this back in February 2020 – before the world was even coming to terms with the pandemic itself.

Mike Pompeo tells me the fact Peter Daszak was put in charge of investigating the origins of the virus through the WHO was astounding: "Breathtakingly, breathtakingly dangerous, incompetent and a conflict of interest of the most extraordinary proportions."

Ruskin says: "China is trying to control the information flow very closely about Covid-19 and its origins, and that fits in very well it seems with Peter Daszak's effort to do the *Lancet* statement with the 27 scientists to call the lab-origins approach a conspiracy theory."

It's absurd that a group of scientists – just a month after the virus emerged publicly – dismissed any suggestion that it did not have a natural origin as misinformation. And what's more incredible is the willingness of vast sections of the media to accept this line without question. Those who did question it were attacked by media outlets. The effect was that the media sided with the Chinese government in trying to shut down reporting of this question, just like the Chinese government has tried to shut down an inquiry into the origins.

"The Chinese government and U.S. scientists who are close associates of the Wuhan scientists doing bat coronavirus research have tarred anyone who uttered it as conspiracy theorists, or worse (in their eyes), as pro-Trump," journalist Josh Rogin wrote in *The Washington Post* in April 2021. Mary Kissel says aside from the scientists with vested interests, there is also a "naivety in the scientific community when it comes to politics and the nature of the Chinese Communist Party". "That's damaging because journalists and other commentators often turn to the scientific community for guidance on these matters. Their word is often taken as fact." When Sir Richard Dearlove, a former head of MI6, did an interview in June 2020 where he said the virus may have leaked from a laboratory, he was slammed as a conspiracy theorist, including by Daszak. "I was the first person in public [to speak out] last June and, boy, did I get a lot of stick," he tells me.

There were two reasons for this. Firstly, because Trump in April lent credence to the theory that the virus leaked from a laboratory, no one would admit he had said something correct. Secondly, some scientists were trying to protect themselves from regulation and having their research curtailed.

"What's scandalous is the suppression of the debate about the evidence. We need an atmosphere of debate," Sir Richard says. "Because of what Trump had said and done, no one wanted to associate themselves with Trump's position. The virologist position generally can be explained by their fear of international regulation. They do not want to be internationally regulated. They do not want to be treated as if this was biological warfare, and subject to international agreements."

David Stilwell says the extent to which the hatred for Trump influenced the scientific discussion around the origins of the virus has still not been properly understood. "This is something that's going to come out in spades – just how much people hated the guy," he says. "It was somehow okay for scientists to sacrifice their integrity and say a lab leak wasn't possible because Donald Trump said it was true."

Daszak wasn't the only WHO investigator with a pre-existing relationship that should have prevented him from being part of the inquiry into the origins of Covid-19. The WHO study team was divided into two groups: the international side and the Chinese side. But many of those appointed had pre-existing relationships that created real or potential conflicts of interest.

The Danish mission chief, Dr Peter Embarek, had formerly advised the Chinese government. While working in the WHO China office, he had provided "policy and technical advice to the government of China on food safety and nutrition issues". There is also a photograph of him receiving the Scientific Spirit Award of the Chinese Institute of Food Science and Technology from the Chinese government in 2017.

Another WHO investigator, Dr Marion Koopmans, was appointed in 2008 as a "scientific consultant" of the Guangdong Provincial Centre for Disease Control and Prevention. The centre's website, which is written in Chinese, says Koopmans undertakes research in infectious disease immunology and epidemiology, as well as research of molecular diagnosis technology. The website also states that Koopmans has "conducted studies on highly pathogenic avian influenza viruses". On Twitter, she shared a news story from the *South China Morning Post* that the US would not accept the WHO findings without verification, commenting: "And so it starts. No need to wait for the report, right?"

A member of the Chinese WHO team, Tong Yigang, has worked under PLA institutions and military facilities. From January 2016 to December 2019, Tong Yigang was involved in a "major logistic research project" for the PLA, for which the name was marked "secret", according to his own biography.

Another Chinese WHO member, Feng Zijian, is also the Deputy Director-General of China's Centre for Disease Control. In a clear conflict of interest, Feng Zijian was actually involved in the cover-up of the virus in the early days. He was responsible for drafting a gag order, dated February 25, 2020, that prevented researchers and institutions from sharing the results of their coronavirus research. "No one can, under their own name or in the name of their research team, provide other institutions and individuals with information related to Covid-19 epidemic on their own including data, biological specimens, pathogens, culture etc," the memo obtained by Associated Press said. The memo also came with a warning: "In case of any violation of relevant regulations, the offender and their unit will be held accountable." Interestingly, the memo was released just one day after the February 2020 WHO–China Joint Mission finished its investigations in China.

Several other WHO investigators are PLA-trained or active participants in military research. One is a bat virus researcher working with the Wuhan Institute of Virology. Another seven WHO members held official, senior positions with China's Centre for Disease Control, and several others worked for institutions that sit under the PLA. Yet these participants were given an equal say in the outcome of the WHO report.

The outcome was determined by a show of hands, where all the scientists sat in a room and voted whether they thought a laboratory leak, natural zoonosis, frozen food or other options were very likely, likely, unlikely or very unlikely. When the WHO handed down its initial findings into the origins of Covid-19, they were correctly labelled a whitewash, a farce and embarrassingly inadequate. The experts appointed found nothing, and crucial datasets were withheld by Chinese authorities. The Wuhan Institute of Virology did not open its books, and patient details for the first 70 people who fell sick with Covid-19 were denied. The report all but supported China's propaganda that Covid-19 may have arrived in Wuhan in frozen food.

Jamie Metzl, who is a current serving member of a WHO committee on genetic engineering, says truly independent investigators should have been appointed. "Four members of the international team had prior working relationships with the Wuhan Institute of Virology and one of them, Peter Daszak, had actually been a funder of questionable research at that institute," he said. "That is a clear conflict of interest that should have precluded him from participation in this process, so this was not an investigation. It was not capable of examining all of the possible hypotheses, and I don't think that we should see this report as authoritative in any way."

Former NSA Director Mike Rogers said people around the world had been counting on the WHO investigation for answers. "If you read the WHO report, it's a whitewash. They did not get enough specific information or have enough access to make a definitive conclusion as to the origin of this disease," he said. "It was clearly accommodating, is the way I would phrase it. The WHO was trying not to antagonise the Chinese." Pompeo tweeted: "The WHO report is a sham", while the Biden White House press secretary Jen Psaki criticised China's lack of transparency, saying "the report lacks crucial data, information and access" and "represents a partial and incomplete picture".

A statement signed by Australia, Canada, the Czech Republic, Denmark, Estonia, Israel, Japan, Latvia, Lithuania, Norway, the Republic of Korea, Slovenia, the United Kingdom and the United States expressed concerns about the study and said a second effort needed to be undertaken to detect and prepare for future pandemics. "It is critical for independent experts to have full access to all pertinent human, animal, and environmental data, research, and personnel involved in the early stages of the outbreak relevant to determining how this pandemic emerged," the statement said.

New Zealand was not a signatory to this statement. "New Zealand wants to make sure we conduct an independent analysis to ensure we understand the science before making any comment," a spokesperson for its Foreign Ministry said.

Japan's Chief Cabinet Secretary, Katsunobu Kato, said he was concerned the latest investigation faced delays and a lack of access to virus samples. "In order to prevent future pandemics, it is indispensable to carry out prompt, independent and expert-led investigations that are free of surveillance," he told reporters.

Professor David Relman told Yahoo News: "This report contributes almost nothing to our understanding of that hypothesis." Republican Senator Marco Rubio said no one should be surprised that the WHO report on the origins of Covid-19 is "misleading and incomplete". "Either through sheer incompetence, gross negligence or outright corruption, the WHO helped the CCP hide the truth about Covid-19's severity and transmissibility from the very beginning," he told reporters.

Even WHO's Director-General Tedros Adhanom Ghebreyesus walked away from his own inquiry and said there needed to be a more thorough investigation of a potential laboratory leak. "In my discussions with the team, they expressed the difficulties they encountered in accessing raw data," he said. "The team also visited several laboratories in Wuhan and considered the possibility that the virus entered the human population as a result of a laboratory incident. However, I do not believe that this assessment was extensive enough. Further data and studies will be needed to reach more robust conclusions. Although the team has concluded that a laboratory leak is the least likely hypothesis, this requires further investigation, potentially with additional missions involving specialist experts, which I am ready to deploy."

He added: "Let me say clearly that as far as WHO is concerned all hypotheses remain on the table." Now that *The Lancet* has recused Daszak from its Covid-19 Commission, the WHO report should be set aside, given the conflicts of interest of many of its investigators.

In July 2021, Tedros went even further and said there had been a premature push to rule out the possibility of a lab-leak as the cause of Covid-19. In comments that angered the Chinese Communist Party, Tedros demanded China be "transparent" and cooperate by providing the raw data he had asked for in the early days of the outbreak. "I was a lab technician myself. I'm an immunologist and I have worked in the lab, and lab accidents happen. It's common," he said. "We need information, direct information, on what the situation of this lab was before and at the start of the pandemic."

Emboldened by the success of the Daszak emails, Ruskin forged on. He also uncovered evidence of the intermingling of science and politics in China. "Chinese governmental authorities first promoted the idea that the source of the causal agent for Covid-19 in humans came from a wild animal in December. Chinese government-supported scientists then backed that theory in four separate studies submitted to the journals between February 7 and 18," US Right to Know found.

By early 2021, Ruskin had filed 68 FOI requests and launched four lawsuits to gain access to documents held by United States agencies or universities, including the NIH, the State Department, the Department of Education and the FDA. To his surprise, he found that accessing the documents related to Covid-19 was far more difficult than his pursuits in other fields. "I've been doing public interest investigations for 34 years and sometimes you file a request and hit the jackpot right away, but this has really been fighting tooth and nail for every page," he says.

While the United States was attacking China for its lack of transparency, US institutions like the NIH and universities were refusing Ruskin's requests for documents relating to the outbreak. "One of the things that's interesting as a problem here is how there's so many conflicts of interest, and how they match up in such an unusual and curious fashion," he explains. "There are some federal agencies that funded the EcoHealth Alliance, and so they have conflicts of interest, too. It's not just the Chinese. It's good chunks of the US Government as well. Lots of the scientists who do this sort of gain-of-function research or store these potential pathogens have conflicts of interest too, and potentially, so did their funders."

The litigation against the NIH for information about both Covid-19 and Chinese bio-threats was launched after the agency refused Ruskin access to any documents for the blanket reason the subject is under investigation. "There were many specific points we were asking for information on. It just can't be true that it's all covered by the investigation," he said. "I have questions about why the NIH would write a blanket denial when it doesn't seem true." No one even knows who precisely is investigating the subject at the NIH. "We don't get to know that," Ruskin says.

Scientists, just weeks after we learnt about this virus, were so quick to say it was naturally occurring and that to suggest otherwise was misinformation. In fact, it was their claims that amounted to misinformation. It was illogical that 27 scientists would dismiss this possibility as a "conspiracy theory" and "misinformation". And that they would dismiss it so soon after the world was notified of the new coronavirus. But that's what happened. Daszak drafted the *Nature Medicine* letter on February 6. Australia and the United States had only banned travel from China five days earlier, and it would be another two months before Donald Trump blamed Wuhan laboratories for leaking the virus. At that early stage, no investigation had taken place, no adequate analysis of the coronavirus had occurred. It was, quite simply, too early in the piece to say whether or not the virus had a natural origin.

Furthermore, tech giants like Facebook actually censored any information that suggested Covid-19 may have leaked from a laboratory. Facebook said the decision was made after consulting with "leading health organisations, including the World Health Organization". It would remove any posts that said Covid-19 was man-made, had been bioengineered or that it was a bioweapon because these theories had been "debunked". Posts suggesting Covid-19 came from a laboratory were permitted so long as it wasn't claimed that the virus was man-made. Facebook only reversed this position after Biden announced he had directed the US intelligence agencies to redouble their efforts to investigate the origin of Covid-19.

"In light of ongoing investigations into the origin of Covid-19 and in consultation with public health experts, we will no longer remove the claim that Covid-19 is man-made or manufactured from our apps," Facebook said in a statement.

Twitter banned Zero Hedge, a financial website, in February 2020 after it published an article about Wuhan Institute of Virology scientist Peng Zhou. At the time, Twitter, Facebook and other social media companies pledged to remove accounts it said were spreading misinformation about the coronavirus amid claims it was fuelling racism.

The picture becomes murkier amid revelations by *The National Pulse* that Google's charity arm, Google.org, has actually been funding EcoHealth Alliance research since 2010.

* * *

With hindsight, when you look at how the events unfolded in early 2020, and how the natural-origin narrative took hold at the expense of any genuine inquiry into the origin of the virus, it was a masterpiece in Communist Party propaganda and disinformation.

There was a confluence of factors at play to shut down genuine inquiry: the scientific journals refused to publish science that questioned a natural origin; collaborators and funders of the Wuhan Institute of Virology failed to disclose their role in drafting a *Lancet* letter that claimed the lab leak to be a conspiracy theory; the same scientists then advised the United States government and intelligence community, and represented the WHO in investigating the laboratory they had been working with for 15 years.

The public discourse was then also shaped by these scientists, who gave vocal media interviews and ridiculed credible figures who disagreed, such as Sir Richard Dearlove, as conspiracy theorists. When you put all of this together, a clear picture emerges: the Chinese Communist Party, assisted by Western scientists with pre-existing relationships with China, shaped the global narrative that this was a virus of natural origin from day one. This has not been lost on US national security and intelligence agency leaders.

Former head of the NSC China desk Matt Turpin said China's ability to set the narrative, even in the West, is something it has actively worked towards. "You had a massive campaign from the PRC to do everything they could to discredit the whole narrative that it may have come from a lab; this is what they've spent decades since Tiananmen preparing for – a bad news story that threatens the regime, and making sure that you've got the influence and the media and propaganda apparatus to be able to control the narrative and the story," he said. "This is why they've spent billions of dollars on all those influence operations. If you're obsessed about the threat to your power, and your own malfeasance will cause a loss of legitimacy and that will cause the fall of the Communist Party, then the return on investment of why you would build all that out is exactly the payoff of what has happened over the last year."

This is such an important point Turpin makes. Richard Dearlove agrees and says it wasn't just China setting the narrative – it was a full-blown disinformation campaign. "You can bet your bottom dollar that the Ministry of State Security has been in control of the narrative from day one and the whole thing has been a global disinformation operation," he said. "I'm absolutely sure that the Chinese narrative was completely dominant and the complicity with the Chinese is bloody outrageous."

Mike Pompeo concurs: "The CCP broad influence operations and their capacity to disseminate information through their media outlets, the Global Times, *China Daily*, all the organisations, the propaganda arms that you know, their diplomats around the world sharing this with their international counterparts, all with the central message being driven from Beijing," Pompeo tells me. "It's something that they have professionalised, they are very good at it, and this was an example of their capacity to flood the zone with a storyline and have that storyline become the narrative in the Western media as well."

Pompeo speaks of his frustration that the official Chinese narrative took hold surrounding a "scientific consensus" that Covid-19 had to have a natural origin. "It took us months to knock that down. This was Chinese propaganda facilitated and put forward by some American scientists as well, and if they were professionals they had to know better and yet that was the language," he says. "You would go out to the mainstream media, the non-medical research media, and they would repeat this time and time again and it was false. The statement that it had to be, that this could only be a natural virus, and there were half a dozen reasons proffered that it could only be a natural virus, it was an illusion. It was a little bit of a game that was being played, that it could only be natural. Of course, it can be both natural in its origin and manipulated in a laboratory. Yet by saying that it has to be natural, it was fundamentally misleading. I'll leave to others whether this was intentional or not, but I can assure you that the CCP pushing this narrative, propagating this storyline was at the centre of their efforts to cover up what the actual origin was and the sequence of this virus came to be devastating for the entire world."

Retired US Air Force Brigadier General Robert Spalding says the United States focuses on preparing for traditional warfare, making it vulnerable to disinformation campaigns and influence operations. "The intelligence community operates on a set of assumptions that says the only danger is going to come from a military attack and that our society is resilient enough to defend itself against political influence, intrigue and financial influence, but in reality, we're not. In fact, the entire nation is very vulnerable," he said. "The intelligence community can't look into our country to see the impact of a campaign that the Chinese Communist Party are running on our own people, which is one vulnerability. The other vulnerability is that they're so focused on a military attack, that in many ways becomes a diversion from anybody actually looking at what's going on."

That the United States intelligence community and the Five Eyes intelligence network may have fallen victim to the CCP disinformation campaign is extremely concerning.

It is clear Daszak was pushing a narrative right from the start of the outbreak, as early as January 1, when he tweeted that the wet market sold butchered animals and that the Chinese Centre for Disease Control would do an excellent job. It's breathtaking, as Pompeo says, that he was allowed to go into Wuhan as the only American citizen to investigate the origin of Covid-19. But it gets even worse than that.

The Office of the Director of National Intelligence said, in a rare statement, on April 30, 2020, "The Intelligence Community also concurs with the wide scientific consensus that the COVID-19 virus was not manmade or genetically modified." It's clear this is a false statement. A blatant lie. As Dr Ebright says, it is impossible to tell if a virus has been subjected to genetic modification. Yet the intelligence community assured the public that this was not a man-made or genetically modified virus. Why would the intelligence community mislead the public? Why did they get it so wrong?

The intelligence agency position may have had its genesis in a meeting on February 3, 2020, well before any lockdown, organised by the National Academies of Sciences. The meeting was held in the academy's Keck Center, Room 103, in Washington DC, but international participants could also join via their laptop or phone. Attending the meeting were senior figures at the FBI, the Office of the Director of National Intelligence, the NIH and the Department of Health and Human Services.

But most significantly, who were the scientists invited to come and brief the high-level officials from the United States government? None other than the zoonotic-origin crowd: EcoHealth Alliance President Peter Daszak, the Scripps Research Institute's Professor Kristian Andersen, the University of North Carolina's Ralph Baric and the University of Iowa's Stanley Perlman were all listed on the email invitation list. The President's top medical advisor on the coronavirus, Anthony Fauci, gave a 10-minute presentation.

A prominent discussion point at the meeting was how to fight "misinformation". The meeting objective stated: "Assess what data, information and samples are needed to understand the evolutionary origins of 2019-nCoV and more effectively respond to the outbreak and resulting misinformation." The statement of task went further: "Although a widely disputed paper posted on a pre-print server last week has since been withdrawn, the response to that paper highlights the need to determine these information needs as quickly as possible. A statement from the National Academies will be prepared and published on the Web as a 'Based on Science' article that summarises the status and needs for more and what types of data."

Two months on, the intelligence community was still turning to scientists who supported a natural origin of SARS-CoV-2 for advice.

US Assistant Secretary of State for East Asia and Pacific Affairs David Stilwell asked the Bureau of Intelligence and Research to facilitate a call with scientists in April to discuss their assessment about whether the virus may have leaked from the Wuhan Institute of Virology. On the call was Andersen and the Galveston National Laboratory Director James LeDuc, whose laboratory had worked with the Wuhan Institute of Virology, among others. During the call, the scientists are understood to have advised Stilwell that Covid-19 did not originate in a Wuhan laboratory. "The call did not go over very well. There were lots of questions about how they could be so sure," Stilwell recalls.

Andersen tells me it's a gross misrepresentation to imply he said the virus could not possibly have come from a lab. He says his scientific work "concludes that it is very unlikely that the virus came from a lab".

The intelligence agency statement has still not been corrected. For this book, I asked the agency whether they would do so. They declined to comment, simply directing me to their updated statement of May 27, 2021 that says: "The US Intelligence Community does not know exactly where, when or how the Covid-19 virus was transmitted initially but has coalesced around two likely scenarios: either it emerged naturally from human contact with infected animals or it was a laboratory accident. While two elements of the IC lean toward the former scenario and one leans more toward the latter – each with low or moderate confidence – the majority of elements within the IC do not believe there is sufficient information to assess one to be more likely than the other. The IC continues to examine all available evidence, consider different perspectives, and aggressively collect and analyze new information to identify the virus's origins."

Dealing with the intelligence community through 2020, the State Department's lead investigator into the origins of Covid-19, David Asher, says it became clear they believed the science was settled, as is evident from their public statement saying the virus had not been genetically manipulated. Asher says the incredible level of confidence of the analysis from the intelligence community reminded him of the US intelligence about Saddam's weapons of mass destruction. "They were all telling us Saddam had a nuclear program and you can take these aluminium tubes that are actually pipes, they are made for plumbing and you can refit and manufacture them into P2 centrifuge casings. It was obviously total bullshit," he says. "I had a suspicion that the IC and supposed USG subject matter experts, rather than doing their homework, had turned to anonymous academic experts ... who apparently had prior connections with PRC research.

"These academic as well as USG intelligence community bio-experts failed to provide any hard evidence for their collective conclusion of natural origins. It was based on theory and analysis that judged, bizarrely, that the Covid-19 sequence was not 'optimized' for transmission. It struck us as the antithesis of the scientific method."

The intelligence community's failure to properly examine the origin of Covid-19 is one of the biggest stories of this entire catastrophe. Before Biden, in May 2021, tasked the intelligence community with taking 90 days to reinvestigate, I had already spoken to senior figures in the Five Eyes intelligence network. The Five Eyes sources admitted they had no full-time agents investigating the origin of the virus. This was also the case in Australia; literally no one was examining the origin full time. It was being treated as a cold case and governments had moved on, irrespective of the number of people who had died from Covid-19. There was no rigorous inquiry into the origin of the pandemic until Biden forced the agencies to examine it in May 2021 – 16 or so months after the outbreak first occurred.

Worse, there was intelligence just sitting there that no one had looked at. After Biden announced his inquiry, *The New York Times* reported that intelligence agencies had untapped data on their computers that they hadn't even looked at. "President Biden's call for a 90-day sprint to understand the origins of the coronavirus pandemic came after intelligence officials told the White House they had a raft of still-unexamined evidence that required additional computer analysis that might shed light on the mystery, according to senior administration officials," the *Times* reported. "But the revelation that they are hoping to apply an extraordinary amount of computer power to the question of whether the virus accidentally leaked from a Chinese laboratory suggests that the government may not have exhausted its databases of Chinese communications, the movement of lab workers and the pattern of the outbreak of the disease around the city of Wuhan."

After this revelation, Dr Richard Ebright said there may be reasons the intelligence community had been loath to examine the possibility of a laboratory leak. "When US intel and defense agencies gave $70+ million to EcoHealth Alliance for virus collection in Wuhan and elsewhere, it is unsurprising that US intel and defense agencies would be less than enthusiastic about lines of investigation that, in part, will lead back to themselves," he tweeted on May 28, 2021.

A senior Trump administration official told me: "The intelligence community from very early on categorically denied that possibility of the lab leak. The nature of intelligence is that it's very hard to go back on this kind of assumption." The source blamed politics and hatred of Trump for the agencies' irrational refusal to properly investigate the hypothesis of a lab leak. "The most unfortunate events that occurred to the Covid investigation is the politicisation of this issue because Donald Trump said that the virus had come from China and China has something to do with it. It became such a toxic topic. Anybody who even attempted to have a different opinion would have been taking a great risk," the official said.

The Director of Harvard University's Center for Communicable Disease Dynamics, Professor of Epidemiology Marc Lipsitch, said investigating a possible lab origin was not about "conspiracy theories or China-bashing". "This is about the basic principle, at least as old as Rev. Bayes and Sherlock Holmes, that when something unusual happens, you have to consider explanations that are also individually unlikely," he tweeted.

This extraordinary failure of the intelligence community to even contemplate a laboratory leak and its willingness to back a pre-determined outcome will ultimately do it severe institutional and reputational damage.

CHAPTER TWENTY-ONE

Military Games

1960S, CHINA

When Wei Jingsheng was a schoolboy in the same compound as Chinese President Xi Jinping, he would discover that Chinese military scientists were conducting depraved germ-warfare experiments on young men. The experimental research was undertaken, Wei says, by the Academy of Military Sciences, which was founded in August 1951 and is the highest medical research institute of the Chinese PLA. Wei's revelations about these human experiments are explosive.

Wei, a former Communist Party insider from one of the 500 founding families, is a seven-time nominee for the Nobel Peace Prize and the winner of the Robert F. Kennedy Memorial Human Rights Award, the European Parliament's Sakharov Prize for Freedom of Thought, the US National Endowment for Democracy Award and Sweden's Olof Palme Memorial Prize. As someone praised by Nancy Pelosi and Mike Pompeo alike, and known as the godfather of the Democracy Movement, Wei's voice is credible and he deserves to be heard.

"When I was in middle school in the early 1960s, the father of my best friend in my class was the Deputy Dean of the Academy of Military Medical Sciences," he said in an interview for this book. "When I was playing with my schoolmates in their compound, and drank alcohol with the children of high-level officials of that academy, I learned the main work of that academy was to study nuclear war and germ/bacteria warfare. There was an 'exercise platoon' of soldiers composed of strong and healthy young men who ate the best food, for the results of human body experiments. To use large number of soldiers as guinea pigs in the field of military medical research is a well-known thing in China."

It's eerily reminiscent of Nazi Germany, where during World War II physicians used Jews and other prisoners of war for inhumane, painful and often deadly experiments. In the Holocaust concentration camps, Jews were used to test immunisation compounds and antibodies for contagious diseases such as malaria, typhus, tuberculosis and typhoid fever. There were also horrible experiments on how different races withstood diseases.

Wei says China's experimentation only got more dangerous as the years went on.

Even after his defection to America in 1997, he continued to hear from high-level contacts about the classified research the Communist Party was undertaking. "After I came to the USA, there was an offspring of a high-level Communist leader who came to visit me," he said. "He was a military fan who supported the CCP rule in China. When we talked about the book *Unrestricted Warfare* published in China, and I considered some of it as bragging, he was upset and said what was described in that book was not a secret and even more advanced. He also talked about the level of research having far surpassed that of the United States, and some of it was even with the help of the United States.

"Some scientists who were not allowed to do research in the USA, due to moral issues, would go to China to study, or help China to train students to study, so their level is definitely better than the United States. When I asked him why such experiments were not conducted quietly in some other countries, he said that the authorities might be afraid of affecting foreign relationships, as at that time Sino-US relationships were still in the honeymoon period. Moreover, there are conditions in China to conduct various experiments that are not permitted by foreign countries." Wei says this is all officially covered by "national secrets" of the Chinese government, but the truth had leaked out.

Wei says some young men who survived germ-warfare and nuclear experiments have in recent years demanded compensation for the effects of these dangerous experiments. "According to these angry petitioners who underwent experiments, many of their comrades died young of radiation sickness, and there were only a few who survived," he said. "A few years ago, there were a lot of retired soldiers [who] petitioned because they did not receive the subsidy promised to compensate their long-term health. There were related reports in Chinese, although I am not sure of English. The petition leader is the guinea pig who was irradiated in the nuclear tests. Not only on social media, but there were also reports on traditional news media, with many people calling for [recognition of] their grievances and [to] support them."

One of those he mentions is Yuan Gongpu, now 85, who made headlines in China in April 2019 when he couldn't afford to pay for his cancer drugs. According to a report in the Global Times, Yuan Gongpu "took part in 10 atom bomb tests and processed the uranium ball that is the key part of an atom bomb in 1964". In an interview from 2018 in the *Shanghai Daily*, Yuan Gongpu spoke about his involvement in building China's first nuclear bomb test in 1954 under Chairman Mao Zedong. They were working in the desert, filled with patriotism, according to the article. "Two people stood beside me while I was working on the uranium ball – one was writing down the statistics and the other watched my every step," he said. "Of course, my hands were shaking." The article states: "Although the rules prohibited staff from working in radioactive areas for more than six hours, Yuan said he was often in the lab for more than 12 hours."

It is rare for a defector to have enough knowledge to shed light on the classified research of their home country. Wei Jingsheng, with his flawless memory, was one of these rare defectors. Until now, the information he brought with him from China has remained exclusively in the CIA files, unable to be spoken about by any official. For the first time he has lifted the lid on the top-secret, classified military experiments China was undertaking.

China started developing its germ-warfare program after it was attacked with biological weapons by the Japanese during World War II. The Manchu Unit was a secret biological and chemical warfare unit of the Japanese Army where bioweapons were tested in China on humans during the Sino-Japanese War. "Unit 731 from Japan terrorised the Chinese PLA and hundreds of thousands of people did die," China–Japan expert David Asher says. "It scared the living shit out of the Chinese communist rebels, because when people start dying left, right and centre, they didn't know how they were dying or where they were dying. I don't think they were aware of how the Japanese aerosolised this and how it targeted people. It was like it came from God and people were terrorised."

Asher says that after this "bio-gassing" China started developing its own biological warfare program. "The Chinese in one of their first goals when they established the People's Republic in 1949 was to develop germ-warfare capabilities, because they had been the victims of it and they wanted to harness that capability. They'd seen what it could do," he told me. Asher is well aware of the live human experiments Wei had told me about. He says the experiments have also been conducted on Uighurs and other minority groups and dissidents. "We've said publicly that Uighurs have been subject to these experiments as well, even right now," he said.

Sir Richard Dearlove, the former head of MI6, has not heard of these depraved experiments. "I can honestly say I haven't seen any intelligence that records that. But put it like this: what I have seen about China would make me think that is probably true," he said.

What else had he seen that would indicate this would probably be true? What else had China done? Sir Richard said this information is classified. He then chose his words carefully and added: "The Chinese do not feel morally constrained. It's an extraordinary regime. It doesn't behave in a way that Western governments try to behave."

* * *

No one currently in government or intelligence I interviewed for this book holds the view the coronavirus was a deliberate release. Not one person. Wei's personal view, however, is that it would be within the realm of CCP conduct to release this virus, although he has no evidence to support his theory.

Wei says that before the Covid-19 outbreak there were rumours that a biological attack would be committed by terrorists against China and there needed to be training exercises for it. "In September 2019, the Chinese government held a large-scale 'anti-coronavirus exercise' in the airport and hospitals in Wuhan, which was equivalent to a military exercise," he says. "The reason is that the upcoming 2019 Military World Games may bring in the SARS and MERS like epidemic. Such a large-scale exercise was far beyond the norm and aroused my vigilance. It was when I was chatting with visiting friends, they told me that the hype in the media was very hot, and some people mentioned that foreign countries might engage in biological warfare against China. According to the custom of the Chinese Communist Party, this was in preparation of public opinion for a certain action – planting in advance is their traditional method."

There is no evidence that China was planning an attack or that Covid-19 was a deliberate release and no experts support this theory. It is true, however, that on September 18, 2019, there was a coronavirus drill at the Wuhan airport. The Wuhan Military Games executive committee held an emergency exercise where it simulated the responses to a new coronavirus infection found at the airport and a case of nuclear radiation discovered in luggage. "The exercise included epidemiological investigation, medical investigation, and temporary quarantine. There are multiple links such as regional setting, quarantine, case transfer, and sanitation treatment," a Chinese-language article on the Xinhua news site about the drill states. It's quite a bizarre coincidence that in September 2019, right before the coronavirus outbreak in Wuhan occurred, there was a test-drill for this exact situation at the airport.

After the 2019 Military World Games, Wei claims that a Chinese doctor warned his colleagues in Hong Kong about an outbreak of an infectious disease and "Taiwan arranged anti-epidemic measures in advance". He spoke about athletes who were allegedly hospitalised in Wuhan and could not participate in the competition.

In Wei's opinion, it's possible there was a deliberate release of the coronavirus during the Military World Games to test the biological warfare, and send the virus back around the world through the visiting athletes. He theorises the military games was "convenient" because it was under the control of the CCP and would be easy to "spread the virus to the world". "The participants were all physically strong athletes, similar to 'exercise platoons', and the after effects can be observed," Wei says.

What would the motive be for such an attack? "If everything goes well without being discovered, then in the future, they can engage in vaccine diplomacy, expand the circle of friends and fight against the West," Wei speculates.

When Wei first heard about the virus in October 2019, he wondered if it was a small-scale experiment. "When I learned that there was a strange illness during the 2019 Military World Games in Wuhan, my first reaction was: they have found a compromise method, to conduct social-scale experiments in China with foreigners," he said. "My reaction was why is this biological war starting at this time, and I could even hardly believe why it was in the Chinese Communist Party's own country."

I put to Wei specifically that no one I have interviewed thinks the virus was an intentional release. What makes him think this is a possibility? "The kindness of Western scientists is worthy of respect. Therefore, they cannot understand the evil way of thinking and cannot understand the extent to which Chinese scientists exaggerate their achievements," he said. "In the past several decades, the CCP's capacity to seal information is hard to be understood by you Westerners. There are things that are knowledge to everyone in a small circle, that the outside world would not know even decades later. That is because anyone who releases information to the outside, even just out of that small circle, would soon be severely punished."

Wei also thinks a vaccine had been developed at the Wuhan Institute of Virology, and says his information suggests that General Chen Wei took the Chinese vaccine as early as February 2020, although news reports record her taking it in March. (China's first Covid-19 patent was lodged February 24, 2020.) "Since there was already a vaccine, then using the Military World Games in Wuhan to spread the virus can harm others but not oneself." As Wei told Dimon at her dinner in November 2019, "The Chinese do not eat bats and it is impossible to sell bats in the seafood market in Wuhan". "This lie by the Chinese government was too low-level. This shows that the CCP planned carefully, were confident, have no expectation that the vaccine will be ineffective, had not figured out how to lie," he said.

Sir Richard Dearlove finds the notion of an intentional leak "out of the question" and extremely, extremely unlikely. "I suppose one has to say there is a minute possibility that it might have been, because I wouldn't like to say it's out of the question, but my feeling is it is out of the question," he said.

Wei's position is precisely the reverse. His opinion – with no evidence – is that it was most likely an intentional release but could be an accident because of poor laboratory safety practices. "I don't rule out the possibility of unintentional disclosure. The CCP only care about the results, and their security has always been really bad," he said. "I also guess the CCP may have had the experiments in mind and not necessarily had plans to launch biological warfare."

That Wei holds this opinion is an indication of his very real lived experience, the brutality of the regime that imprisoned him for such a large part of his adult life.

It is highly possible, however, that Covid-19 may have been circulating during the Military World Games. Almost 10,000 athletes from 110 countries attended, including from Germany, Qatar, Vietnam, Switzerland, India, Iran, Colombia and Sweden, with the event kicking off on October 18 and closing on the 27th. This was

21 days before the *South China Morning Post* reported the first case of Covid-19 on November 17. China had spent a lot of money on renovations and construction in Wuhan for the Military World Games, building some 30 facilities. There was even a PLA early-air warning system as part of the refurbishments. They constructed a "military athletes' village" with accommodation, located about 10.5 kilometres (6.5 miles or a 20-minute drive) from the Wuhan Institute of Virology. The 17 sports at the games included volleyball, judo, fencing, archery, taekwondo, table tennis, wrestling and golf.

But during the games, many international athletes came down with a severe flu. In May 2020, French newspaper *Le Parisien* reported that pentathlete Elodie Clouvel, 31, fell sick along with a teammate. "We were in Wuhan for the Military World Games at the end of October," she told the newspaper. She says that after the Games they all became sick and one teammate missed three days of training. "I was sick too," she said. "I had things that I hadn't had before. There are a lot of Military World Games athletes who were very sick. We recently had contact with the military doctor who told us: I think you had it because there are a lot of people from this delegation who were sick."

German volleyball player Linda Bock told the *Daily Mail* that many in her team were sick and even her father fell ill a few weeks after her return to Germany. "I got sick in the last two days," she said. "I have never felt so sick. Either it was a very bad cold or Covid-19. I think it was Covid-19." Italian fencer Matteo Tagliariol also told the *Daily Mail* that everybody in his Wuhan apartment became sick with symptoms similar to Covid-19. His son and girlfriend later got sick.

Another athlete, Luxembourg swimmer Julien Henx claims that when he landed in Wuhan there was a non-contact body-temperature scanner at the airport. He told media that two of his teammates were sick during the competition. Another in the Luxembourg team, triathlete Oliver Gorges, who also fell sick, claimed Wuhan was a "ghost town" when he went for a cycle in the city, and also said his temperature was recorded on arrival at the airport. Luxembourg swimmers Raphaël Stacchiotti and Pit Brandenburger also fell ill, while their teammate Michel Erpelding, a boxer, said a cafe owner had been advised to keep track of who had visited his house. When journalists jumped on the story, they found many athletes had been gagged from speaking to the media about the illness.

As already noted, the Military World Games finished just 20 days before the first recorded case of Covid-19 in Wuhan. "If more evidence were discovered, it would add to the growing body of evidence that the virus was circulating in Wuhan as early as October 2019, months before the Chinese government acknowledged it to the rest of the world," Josh Rogin wrote in a June 2021 column, revealing US politician Mike Gallagher was demanding an official investigation.

Even when news broke of a new coronavirus in Wuhan, no government officials thought to test the athletes who had participated in the games for antibodies. It may have very well been a super-spreader event, taking Covid-19 around the globe.

The Pentagon told news outlet *The American Prospect* in June 2020 that there was no reason to test or screen the 300 Americans who had travelled to Wuhan for the Military World Games, returning home to 25 states because it "was prior to the reported outbreak".

If the virus was circulating at this time, Miles Yu said it explains why the Chinese Communist Party tried to keep it under wraps. "The Military [World] Games were so important for the CCP so if there was an outbreak there is motive for them to cover-up," he says. Yu was the only United States Government official who tried to investigate why the athletes had fallen sick. He looked at the traffic patterns via the Wuhan Traffic Control Bureau, and noticed certain roads were closed around the Wuhan Institute of Virology. He also noticed how close the athletes' village was to the Institute. "There was something weird going on, but my investigations were not conclusive enough," he says.

In the weeks after the military games, a British schoolteacher Connor Reed, who was working in Wuhan at the time, fell ill with what he later suspected was Covid-19. From November 25, 2020 he became extremely sick with a fever, cough and pneumonia, giving an account of his symptoms to multiple media outlets after he recovered. Tragically, he died just under a year later while in lockdown in Britain. His parents in Queensland, Australia watched his funeral remotely via a live-feed.

The illness during the Military World Games gave rise to conspiracies in China that America was responsible for the outbreak. The Chinese Ministry of Foreign Affairs Director claimed that it could have been the US Army who brought the virus into Wuhan. "When did patient zero begin in US? How many people are infected?" he asked on Twitter on March 13, 2020. "What are the names of the hospitals? It might be US army who brought the epidemic to Wuhan. Be transparent! Make public your data! US owe us an explanation!"

Meanwhile, other conspiracy theories claiming the virus was released during the Military World Games point to YouTube footage where Xi Jinping gives a speech at the opening ceremony. It does not include a wide shot to place him in the city or at the venue. Instead he is speaking against a red screen. The broadcast then flashes to photographs of the crowd. Conspiracy theorists say perhaps he wasn't actually at the Military World Games and this is when the virus was released. Of course, there is no evidence for this.

David Asher, who has had experience leading task forces into North Korea and Iran to investigate nuclear weapons programs, retains an open mind that the virus potentially could have been deliberately released. But he thinks it's extremely likely it was an accidental release based on the fact that "Beijing authorities seemed surprised in the fall of 2019 and totally caught off-guard." Even with an accidental release, Asher says the possibility could not be ruled out that the "Wuhan Institute of Virology coronavirus super-virus research" was directly related to vaccine research done by a laboratory on the same compound called the Wuhan Institute of Biological Products. "That pan betacoronavirus vaccine may have been developed as 'antidote' to a future bioweapon including involving Covid-19," Asher hypothesises. Asher says one theory on the table is that Covid-19 actually leaked during vaccine development. This may explain, he says, "how on earth Major General Chen Wei, the PLA leader who took over the Wuhan Institute of Virology on January 23, and six military scientist on her team stood in front of a Chinese Communist Party flag in March and received injections of an experimental Covid-19 vaccine. There's also some published evidence certain scientists have found that there was adenovirus present in the sequences posted publicly," Mr Asher said. "Adenovirus means that there was a vaccine present for Covid-19; that could indicate that this was a bio-defence project putting a vaccine together. People don't normally develop a vaccine for something they are working on that is many evolutionary turns away from a naturally occurring virus. That doesn't make any sense, to develop a vaccine in advance for something that would never see the light of day makes it sort of ridiculous, but is totally consistent with a biological weapons program. An offensive biological weapons program would logically have to develop an antidote."

In two of the Wuhan Institute of Virology's earliest samples from Covid-19 patients, the raw-reads (basic sequencing output) of deep sequences (multiple sequences of the same genetic region) showed extensive contamination. This could indicate a dirty laboratory environment, Dr Steven Quay says. "The one thing other than SARS-CoV-2 that stands out is an influenza vaccine that's never been published," he said. "In one sample, it's even higher than the SARS-CoV-2 level." This could potentially indicate that while the patient was sick in hospital with Covid-19 they were given a flu vaccine. This would be unusual.

US physicist Professor Richard Muller has another theory. Professor Muller is a brilliant scientist. He has published more than 120 scientific papers including on the origin of comets and the nature of time, and written 10 books, including one called *Now: The Physics of Time*. Famous for his work in astrophysics and geophysics, he founded and led two major projects for which Nobel Prizes were awarded, and has won a dozen other awards and prizes. He's the principal author of the Nemesis theory, which postulates that there is a distant dwarf star orbiting the sun.

Over three decades, Professor Muller has been a high-level advisor to the US government, including the Department of Energy, NASA, Department of Defense and other bodies, on science and technology issues relating to energy, intelligence analysis, counter-terrorism and national security. He holds the highest level of security clearance and has advised on such top-secret issues as weapons of mass destruction.

He points to the first coronavirus samples taken at the end of December, which arrived at the Wuhan Institute of Virology on December 30 for analysis. The genetic sequence of these earliest samples were then published by *Nature* magazine, "so the Chinese scientists could not pull them back," Muller says. "Virologists can see that two samples measured were heavily contaminated and may actually have a vaccine in them," he said. Muller says it's possible the sample was contaminated, "But to me, as someone who has worked in national security for a long time, the more obvious explanation is someone in the Wuhan laboratory was a whistleblower," he says.

Muller then pauses. "Have you read *The Da Vinci Code*?" he asks. Who hasn't? "In it, someone leaves a clue behind that can only be read by the right expert. Here's my fantasy. Someone at the Wuhan Institute of Virology was really upset they were developing a bioweapon. They went into virology because they wanted to save lives, to stop pandemics, but now the military had taken control of part of the laboratory and they were weaponising viruses. That person has no direct way to get the word out. If you have a sample of the vaccine and you happen just for 10 seconds to get access to the patient's sample, you put a little bit of the vaccine in there hoping that someone in the West will notice. It went unnoticed until Steven Quay looked for it. If a vaccine was in there it indicates this was being weaponised. It's a great way to spike the sample in a way the process of publication would bring the message to the West but it would only be read by the right person. That someone would say, 'Oh my god, there's a vaccine in there.'"

It's a wonderful fantasy. Dr Quay says he hadn't considered the possibility of a whistleblower contaminating the sample until Professor Muller raised it. He says the vaccine appears to be for an unpublished influenza virus. This could simply indicate the laboratory was working on a vaccine unrelated to Covid-19, which you would expect it to do. He said he is still analysing the virus samples in collaboration with other scientists.

CHAPTER TWENTY-TWO

A Latent Threat to Mankind

One discovery Miles Yu made while investigating the Wuhan laboratories was more eye-opening than any other. Hard at work preparing his report for Pompeo, he happened upon documents relating to the United Nations Biological and Toxin Weapons Convention. It's a conference held every five years, dating back to the 1980s, to ensure the international biological weapons treaty is upheld globally.

Yu stumbled across a document that had some details from China's submission to the 2011 Convention. It wasn't China's entire submission but it included the research fields China had featured in it. They were "Creation of Man-Made Pathogens", "Population-specific Genetic Markers" and, astonishingly, "Targeted Drug-delivery Technology Making it Easier to Spread Pathogens", among others.

That the Chinese government included, in an official submission, research in the field of "man-made pathogens" was exceptional, Yu thought. It was disconcerting that the gain-of-function research underway at the Wuhan Institute of Virology fell under a category China was disclosing at a biological weapons convention. Shocked, Yu reached out to Ottawa, the host, to try to obtain China's official submission. He never received it, but he felt the fields of research alone were damning enough and he included them in his report, marked "Sensitive but unclassified", for Pompeo and others at the White House to read.

"China has been conducting research on dangerous dual-use biological and genetic technologies that are prone to causing global pandemics," his internal State Department report stated. "China's submissions are a chilling display of what its scientists are doing." The *Wall Street Journal* op-ed he co-authored with Pompeo in February 2021 featured a line summarising the research fields as well.

Yu mentioned the document to Asher and the AVC team in December 2020, but they were unable to locate it before the unit was disbanded with the incoming Biden administration. The investigation for this book led to the discovery of China's original and full submission. The document raises terrifying areas of viral research. It cannot be explained away by CCP defenders – this is the official Chinese government submission to the United Nations Biological Weapons convention. It is their last detailed submission, with China only providing a scaled-back document at the next conference five years later.

It starts by noting that modern biological sciences play an "important role in helping mankind combat disease". In the sentences that follow, China makes two unnerving admissions. Firstly, that it can't comply with the international treaty and secondly, that new biological technology poses a threat to the very existence of mankind. "At the same time, the use of new kinds of biotechnology for hostile purposes, posing a latent threat to human society, is also growing," it states. "The 'dual use' nature of biotechnology enables it, on the one hand, to pose many challenges to full and strict compliance with the Biological Weapons Convention."

In its submission, the Chinese government says that since the sixth conference, held five years earlier in 2006, "there have been almost daily developments in biotechnology – rapid advances in synthetic biology, genomics, systems biology, drug targeting technology and microbial forensics, for instance – throwing up fresh challenges and opportunities for compliance with the Convention".

The document then discusses "synthetic biology enabling the creation of man-made pathogens". Man-made pathogens are created through gain-of-function research, in which the Wuhan Institute of Virology was engaging in and the United States was at times funding. The document states that these "have the potential to be used for evil ends". "Theoretically speaking, synthetic biotechnology poses a huge latent threat to mankind, as it could be used in the future to create pathogens of even greater toxicity and infectiousness than those currently known, and which are resistant to traditional vaccines and drugs as well as hard to isolate and identify with present day technology," it states.

In another section, it speaks about how the sequencing of pathogen DNA has helped develop new drugs and vaccines. But the same data can also be used to synthesise new pathogens and modify pathogen antigenicity, infection specificity, toxicity, and resistance to drugs, causing traditional means of dealing with infectious disease to fail and rendering the prevention and control of such disease even harder," it states.

China's submission to the convention then gets even more terrifying. Its third subheading is "Systems biology further revealing population-specific genetic markers". This is about targeting viruses to specific races as weapons. A shocking and grotesque area of bio-research. It states that the Human Genome Project has helped "to reveal population-specific genetic variations across the genome". "Genome-wide association studies have found variations in the genes for susceptibility to infectious diseases among different populations; epigenetic studies further indicate the existence of population-specific genetic markers of susceptibility to disease," it states.

Then, alarmingly, "It can also create the potential for biological weapons based on genetic differences between races. Once hostile elements grasp that different ethnic groups harbour intrinsically different genetic susceptibilities to particular pathogens, they can put that knowledge into practice and create genetic weapons targeted at a racial group with a particular susceptibility." If this is what the Chinese government was prepared to raise in a public forum, to the United Nations, we can only imagine what race-specific virus experiments they've been conducting in their top-secret, classified defence laboratories.

Retired PLA General Zhang Shibo also made reference to "racial-specific genetic attacks" in his 2017 book discussing seven new domains of warfare. Zhang Shibo, the former President of the National Defence University, concludes "modern biotechnology development is gradually showing strong signs characteristic of an offensive capability", including the possibility that "racial-specific genetic attacks" could be deployed. This reference was uncovered by China analysts Elsa B. Kania and Wilson VornDick. They also found a textbook published by PLA National Defence University in 2017 that included a section about biology as a domain of military struggle. Kania and VornDick write that the textbook is "considered to be relatively authoritative" and mentions "the potential for new kinds of biological warfare to include specific ethnic genetic attacks".

China's Biological Weapons Convention submission then discusses the potential for bioweapons to be released as aerosols under the heading: "Targeted Drug-delivery Technology Making it Easier to Spread Pathogens". Yes, "easier to spread pathogens". The Chinese submission states: "Thanks to incessant advances in pharmaceutical technology, targeted drug-delivery techniques such as aerosols and viral vectors have also made substantial progress. These two targeted drug-delivery technologies can also be used to spread biological agents. Aerosol technology can be used effectively to spread pathogenic microbes, infecting humans through the respiratory tract. And viral vectors can very easily carry special genes into the body, thereby causing damage. Further, there is potential for the effects of aerosol delivery, specifically targeted viral vectors, transfection and gene expression to combine, greatly increasing the overall effect. Both technologies can be used by certain States and terrorist groups for malicious purposes, efficiently spreading pathogens and disease-causing genes."

China's submission states there is an "increased threat of biological weapons" and that the "rapid development" of biological sciences may "significantly increase the destructiveness of biological weapons". "One way it may do so is by increasing the virulence of pathogenic micro-organisms. Microbial genomic research can enhance the virulence or pathogenicity of a pathogen by modifying its antigenic properties," it states. "Another way is by rendering traditional medicines and vaccines ineffective. Supergenes conferring resistance to antibiotics can be synthesised by DNA recombination technology, making pathogens highly drug-resistant. Pathogens with detoxifying genes can also be produced, as can pathogens that can evade recognition and attack by the immune system, rendering vaccines and medicines useless.

"A third way is by making the target population more susceptible to pathogenic microbes. RNA interference can inactivate specific genes in the body, inhibit expression of important bodily proteins, disrupt physiological function and heighten the effects of a bioweapon attack. And a fourth way is by making biological attacks more stealthy. Foreign genes or viruses can be introduced into the target population asymptomatically by means of gene-therapy vectors, enabling a biological weapon attack to be mounted covertly."

China could, of course, argue that any research they were conducting in this field was for defensive, not offensive, purposes. But as its own admission states, new technological developments in synthetic biology create challenges with the treaty compliance. China's submission concludes with a section on the extreme risks of laboratories researching these pathogens. "Accidental mistakes in biotech laboratories can place mankind in great danger," it states. "Synthetic biology in some civilian biotechnology research and applications may unintentionally give rise to new, highly hazardous man-made pathogens with unforeseeable consequences."

China then goes on to suggest that biosafety management controls and regulations should "tighten" especially around the virulent pathogens in laboratories. Five years on from this, at the next Conference, China had changed its tune, providing no information on its compliance or new information on scientific developments. Instead, it steadfastly insisted it had never pursued biological weapons at all.

But one statement from the 2016 Chinese submission stands out – and is cause for alarm. "The Chinese Academy of Sciences commissioned the Wuhan Institute of Virology to conduct an annual training course on the management of laboratory biosafety and experimentation techniques with a view to strengthening biosafety management efforts in all units of the Chinese Academy of Sciences," it states.

How could the Wuhan Institute of Virology, which had so many of its own issues with safety protocols, be in a position to conduct courses on lab biosafety? The Wuhan Institute of Virology, which didn't make it to the top 20 safest laboratories in China, was training other technicians on safety procedures.

US lead investigator David Asher says Five Eyes nations and other allies held "significant concerns" about China's biowarfare compliance, specifically related to gain-of-function research and synthetic biological techniques.

"In 2016, the US and allied governments at the Biological Weapons Convention in Geneva presented evidence and information about deep concerns that the Chinese were engaged in biological developments using gain-of-function techniques that inherently had weapon-like capabilities," Asher says. "Our governments made our concerns known. They were very significant concerns. The Chinese military and Communist Party experts, even in televised appearances, for years had made it known that synthetic biology was going to be a very dangerous potential vector for biological weapons in the future," he said.

But after this conference, the Chinese "actually stopped declaring the bio-defence research they were doing on coronaviruses. This falls into the same time period the State Department fact sheet said that secret military programs kicked off inside the Wuhan Institute of Virology – programs the Chinese systematically denied pursuing in their very same BWC 'confidence building' declarations. We knew they were doing it. They even put out papers about it," Asher says.

"But they didn't declare it as bio-defence. And when you're doing classified research, and you don't declare that, it is a violation of the Biological Weapons Convention. I'm quite confident in the assertion that the Chinese were engaged in dual-use research development of capabilities that could be offensive in nature, using viruses."

Acting Assistant Secretary of State Tom DiNanno, from the Arms Control, Verification and Compliance Bureau (AVC), says for years the United States has determined that China has an offensive biological program that it has not declared, in clear violation of the treaty. "China cheats on all their international arms control obligations, as does Russia, but they use these instruments as tools of statecraft," he said. "The dual use of weaponising gain-of-function research could be, in fact, violation of the Biological Weapons Convention [BWC]. It is something we need to run to ground and vigorously pursue and it certainly is an item of relevance for the BWC."

Intelligence agencies and Western governments have known for decades that China has a bioweapons program. It was rarely spoken about, kept to the domain of classified reports or intelligence files. But Chinese military-affiliated scientists were discussing the weaponisation of coronaviruses publicly and openly – and they did so five years before the Covid-19 pandemic.

A book written by PLA Chinese military scientists and senior Chinese public health officials in 2015, titled *The Unnatural Origin of SARS and New Species of Man-Made Viruses as Genetic Bioweapons*, was obtained by the US State Department as it conducted an investigation into the origins of Covid-19. The 263-page volume was published in 2015 by the Chinese Military Medical Science Press, a government-owned publishing house managed by the General Logistics Department of the PLA. It describes SARS coronaviruses as heralding a "new era of genetic weapons" and says they can be "artificially manipulated into an emerging human disease virus, then weaponised and unleashed in a way never seen before". Some of China's senior public health and military figures are listed among the 18 authors of the document, including the former Deputy Director of China's Bureau of Epidemic Prevention, Li Feng. Ten of the authors are scientists and weapons experts affiliated with the Air Force Medical University in Xi'an, which the Australian Strategic Policy Institute's Defence Universities Tracker ranks as "very high-risk" for its level of defence research, including its work on medical and psychological sciences.

The Air Force Medical University, previously known as the Fourth Military Medical University, was placed within the command of the PLA under President Xi Jinping's military reforms in 2017. The book's Editor-in-Chief, Xu Dezhong, reported to the top leadership of the Chinese Military Commission and Ministry of Health during the SARS epidemic of 2003, briefing them 24 times and preparing three reports, according to his online biography. He also held the position of professor and doctoral supervisor in the Air Force Medical University's Military Epidemiology Department, where he supervised 100 students, including 53 PhD candidates. One of his students went on to write a thesis about SARS 2003 being of unnatural origin. Clearly, this is a conspiracy theory and a dangerous one to be peddling.

The book offers an insight into the way senior scientists at one of the PLA's most prominent military universities were thinking about the development of biological research. It notes how a sudden surge of patients requiring hospitalisation during a bioweapon attack "could cause the enemy's medical system to collapse". It then refers to the research of Michael J. Ainscough, a former US Air Force Colonel, on modes of conflict and bioweapons and "next-generation bioweapons".

The book examines the optimum conditions under which to release a bioweapon. "Bioweapon attacks are best conducted during dawn, dusk, night or cloudy weather because intense sunlight can damage the pathogens," it states. "Biological agents should be released during dry weather. Rain or snow can cause the aerosol particles to precipitate. A stable wind direction is desirable so that the aerosol can float into the target area."

Among the most bizarre conspiracist claims by the military scientists is their theory that SARS-CoV-1, the virus that caused the SARS epidemic of 2003, was a man-made bioweapon, deliberately unleashed on China by "terrorists". Scientific consensus holds that SARS-CoV-1 was of natural origin, having crossed the xenographic barrier from Asian palm civets to humans, likely through the sale of wild animals in wet markets in Guangdong province, southern China.

Pompeo and Yu made a passing reference to the book in their *Wall Street Journal* op-ed on China's laboratories in February 2021, writing: "A 2015 PLA study treated the 2003 SARS coronavirus outbreak as a 'contemporary genetic weapon' launched by foreign forces." After this, the book circulated among Chinese dissident communities online and at one point was for sale online in China.

What's fascinating is the link between some of the scientists who wrote this book and the Wuhan Institute of Virology. One of them, Yang Ruifu, is a professor at the Key Laboratory of Zoonoses Research, Jilin University, where he focuses on pathogenic bacteriology, especially the study of *Yersinia pestis*, which causes the plague. His academic profile lists an 'army project' titled "Studies on the Genome and Comparative Genomics of *Yersinia pestis*", which ran between 2002 and 2005. According to China analyst Alex Joske's "China Defence Universities Tracker", Jilin University is "designated very high risk for its high level of defence research. It has at least two defence research labs and holds secret-level security credentials, allowing it to participate in research and production for classified weapons and defence technology projects". In 2014, Yang Ruifu was awarded a "Meritorious Service Medal" by Xi Jinping. His profile shows him in his Chinese military uniform.

Yang Ruifu visited the Wuhan Institute of Virology as an invited speaker for the Ge Hong Forum on December 7, 2016, where he was presented with an award. He also made contributions to the journal edited by Shi Zhengli, *Virological Sinica*, at the time of the Covid-19 outbreak. The editors of the journal thank him, among others, for acting as a reviewer of research they published between November 1, 2019 and October 31, 2020. "Your efforts greatly improved not only individual manuscripts but the quality of the journal and the overall research in the field of viruses," it states.

DiNanno describes the 2015 book by Chinese military scientists as "highly significant" if verified. "That would be an earth-shattering development and potentially grounds for finding them in violation of the treaty," he says. DiNanno says that as the US official in charge of determining whether or not China is in compliance with a treaty you cannot dismiss documents like this written by 18 PLA scientists at a university conducting classified defence research. "Are we going to sit here and make excuses for the Chinese potential biological weapons program? We need to take their statements seriously and run them to ground and determine their validity."

After I published details of that book in May 2021 in *The Australian* newspaper, showing Chinese military scientists had discussed weaponising coronaviruses five years before the pandemic, China's foreign ministry officials denied they had any program at all. "China has always strictly fulfilled its obligations under the Biological Weapons Convention and doesn't develop, research or produce bioweapons," China's foreign ministry spokesman said.

Most believe this statement is untrue. "China most certainly does have biological warfare programs. It's also interested, frankly, in a range of fairly esoteric DNA, gene-altering technologies which might give it a military edge," the Australian Strategic Policy Institute's Executive Director, Peter Jennings, said.

Kania, Adjunct Senior Fellow at the Center for a New American Security's Technology and National Security Program, wrote with VornDick in August 2019 that China's national strategy of military–civil fusion has highlighted biology as a priority. "The People's Liberation Army could be at the forefront of expanding and exploiting this knowledge," she wrote. "Under Beijing's civil-military fusion strategy, the PLA is sponsoring research on gene editing, human performance enhancement, and more." She refers to a book, *War of Dominance*, written by the Third Military Medical University's Professor Guo Jiwei, which she says "emphasises the impact of biology on future warfare".

Former President of the Academy of Military Medical Sciences He Fuchu had also "argued that biotechnology will become the new 'strategic commanding heights' of national defense, from biomaterials to 'brain control' weapons," Kania writes. She found an article published in 2015 in the People's Liberation Army Daily that speaks about the "biological military revolution". "As the weaponization of biological bodies will become a reality in the future, non-traditional combat styles will take the stage, and the 'biological frontier' will become a new frontier for national defense," it states.

Kania and her colleague wrote in 2019 that "it will be increasingly important to keep tabs on the Chinese military's interest in biology as an emerging domain of warfare, guided by strategists who talk about potential 'genetic weapons' and the possibility of a 'bloodless victory.'"

"There's a lot of information that military and PLA personnel were undercover and were masquerading as civilian researchers and working at the WIV," DiNanno tells me. "Shi Zhengli came out and said we have no relationship with the Chinese military. That's a blatant lie."

Declassified intelligence released by the United States in January 2021 revealed there had been "secret military activity at the WIV". "Despite the WIV presenting itself as a civilian institution, the United States has determined that the WIV has collaborated on publications and secret projects with China's military. The WIV has engaged in classified research, including laboratory animal experiments, on behalf of the Chinese military since at least 2017," it states. "The United States and other donors who funded or collaborated on civilian research at the WIV have a right and obligation to determine whether any of our research funding was diverted to secret Chinese military projects at the WIV."

The State Department alleged that "secrecy and non-disclosure are standard practice for Beijing". "For many years the United States has publicly raised concerns about China's past biological weapons work, which Beijing has neither documented nor demonstrably eliminated, despite its clear obligations under the Biological Weapons Convention," the statement says.

The investigation for this book has uncovered a swathe of evidence that supports this declassified intelligence from the United States – but the collaboration has been going on for longer than the 2017 date it cites. The Wuhan Institute of Virology has an extensive history conducting virus research with the Chinese military. To start with, the English-language brochure for the Wuhan Institute of Virology's BSL-4 laboratory made an extraordinary mention of its involvement in research for the military. It said the Wuhan Institute of Virology would play a national security role and that it "is an effective measure to improve China's availability in safeguarding national biosafety if a possible biological warfare or terrorist attack happens".

A Wuhan Institute of Virology board advisor, Professor Tong Yigang, is a senior PLA scientist. His CV states he is involved with military biosafety projects, "synthetic biology national key special projects". He graduated with a Masters degree from the PLA's Academy of Military Medical Sciences and worked at the Institute of Microbiology and Epidemiology, Academy of Military Medical Sciences and is now a Dean of Beijing University of Chemical Technology.

Another member of the Wuhan Institute of Virology's advisory board, Tu Changchun, is a military researcher at the Institute of Military Veterinary Medicine at the Academy of Military Medical Sciences. He's been focused on bat-derived viruses since the SARS outbreak of 2003. One of Tu Changchun's students, He Biao, submitted a thesis titled "Batviromics", which included the discovery of new viruses from Yunnan province. He found that some viruses had a 100 per cent lethality rate for rats.

People's Daily published an article in June 2014 that noted "a joint research group led by Tu Changchun … has detected a novel SARS-like coronavirus in bats in Yunnan." It says that whole-genome sequencing confirmed the virus has the ability to infect humans.

This indicates the level of interest by the Chinese military in bat coronaviruses and how it links with the Wuhan Institute of Virology.

Yang Ruifu also has ties to the Wuhan Institute of Virology, and reviewed research for Shi Zhengli's journal during the coronavirus outbreak.

Among the board directors at the Wuhan Institute of Virology is Cao Wuchan, who has the rank of Colonel and is a Professor at the PLA's Academy of Military Medical Sciences. Cao Wuchan joined Shi Zhengli (along with Peter Daszak and others) in a 2015 small working group of infectious disease experts who developed a "transdisciplinary approach to emerging infectious disease".

A 2019 research vaccination project involved seven scientists from the Wuhan Institute of Virology and three from the State Key Laboratory of Pathogen and Biosecurity at the Beijing Institute of Microbiology and Epidemiology, part of the PLA's Academy of Military Medical Sciences. This study on a mosquito-borne chikungunya virus, used both Petri dish and live animal experiments on mice. After developing a version of the virus whose progress they could track and giving it to the mice, it resulted in "rapid death in an age-dependent manner".

Another project in 2019 on African swine fever virus involved nine Wuhan Institute of Virology scientists, and one from the Academy of Military Medical Science's Institute of Military Veterinary Medicine. A third 2019 research project involved 10 scientists from the Wuhan Institute of Virology and two from the 154 Hospital, PLA, Xinyang, Henan, China. Another scientist was from the Academy of Military Medical Sciences' Laboratory Animal Centre. A fourth 2019 study, examining how the depletion of certain cells makes HPV deadly, involved three scientists from the Wuhan Institute of Virology and one from the Third Military Medical University's Institute of Immunology.

One 2018 joint project delved into the Zika virus, which re-emerged in South America in 2015. The scientists working on it included six from the Wuhan Institute of Virology and eight from the Academy of Military Medical Sciences' Beijing Institute of Microbiology and Epidemiology.

A study four years earlier, involving the detection of anthrax, included four scientists from the Wuhan Institute of Virology and one from the Institute of Microbiology and Epidemiology. This study clearly states that the Institute was collaborating with the military on biodefence measures. A second 2014 study included two scientists from the Institute and one from the Second Military Medical University's Department of General Surgery at Shanghai Hospital.

And on it goes.

EcoHealth Alliance appears to have had some awareness that it was dealing in an area of research with a military application. An email sent by EcoHealth Alliance's Vice President for Science and Outreach, Jonathan Epstein, states that the US Defense Advanced Research Projects Agency (DARPA) "wants a written section on communicating dual-use information".

French intelligence was also highly concerned about the Wuhan Institute of Virology's growing ties to the PLA, particularly when French scientists were not welcome as soon as the laboratory was operational in 2017. In discussing the French government's decision to build the BSL-4 laboratory with the Chinese government, a January 2020 Radio France Internationale report stated that "Some French experts worried that China would use the technology provided by France to develop bio-chemical weapons. At that time, the French intelligence service issued a stern warning to the government. But with the support of then [French] Prime Minister Jean-Pierre Raffarin, China and France signed a cooperation agreement during [French President Jacques] Chirac's visit to China in 2004. France would assist China in the construction of the P4 virus centre, but the agreement stipulates that Beijing cannot use this technology for aggressive activities."

The Wuhan laboratory was meant to be built by a French architectural design firm from Lyon, but once they got the blueprints, the Chinese side redirected the building work to an inexperienced Wuhan company with links to the PLA, the radio report revealed. "Due to the above security concerns and repeated delays in the implementation of the agreement, in addition to a diplomatic crisis between the two countries in 2008, the Wuhan P4 Virus Center was not officially operational until 2017," it stated.

Former NSA Director Mike Rogers said the NSA was aware of the Wuhan Institute of Virology during his time at the helm from 2014 to 2018. "There's always a concern about biological and chemical activities," he says. "This is an area from an intelligence perspective and a national security perspective we pay attention to and we put resources together to try to understand. It's one reason why you saw the cables coming out of the embassy in Beijing. It's an area we very much publicly acknowledge we're concerned about and pay attention to."

As a result of his State Department investigation closely examining the Wuhan Institute of Virology, Asher says, "I am confident the Chinese government was engaged in a weaponisation research and development effort at the Wuhan Institute of Virology and other institutes involving coronavirus research. Whether offence or defence, which is almost impossible to tell, it was 100 per cent undeclared and that is a serious violation of the Biological Weapons Convention and the WHO International Health Regs – to the extent it spilled out and over somehow."

A leaked State Department cable in 2009 – from a WikiLeaks dump – sent in June ahead of the Australia Group plenary session in Paris included concerns about the Wuhan Institute of Virology.

The cable, sent when Hillary Clinton was Secretary of State, said of France: "The US believes participants would benefit from hearing about your experiences assisting China in setting up a Biosafety Level 4 laboratory at the Wuhan Institute of Virology from the export control and intangible technology transfer perspectives. We are particularly interested to know how China plans to vet incoming foreign researchers from countries of biological weapons proliferation concern."

The cables also state that the US believes member states "would be interested in any information you can share related to China and North Korea, specifically information related to: China's Institutes of Biological Products (locations in Beijing and Wuhan), to include overhead imagery analysis if possible" and "your perceptions of the CBW [chemical biological warfare] proliferation activities by Chinese entities."

The Wuhan Institute of Virology's links to the military raise broader concerns about Western science funding China's military modernisation. Effectively, France, the UK, the US and other countries are funding research that could be used for nefarious purposes. These countries need to carefully revise how taxpayer funds are flowing through potentially to the advancement of the Chinese military.

While the Wuhan Institute of Virology was indisputedly conducting research with the Chinese military, there is no evidence that Covid-19 is a bioweapon. "I don't think this was a biological warfare agent but the Communist Party is doing its absolute best to turn the consequences of the virus into a weaponised strategy for itself all around the world, and that's really something that we should absolutely be resisting with our sovereignty here in Australia," the Australian Strategic Policy Institute's Executive Director, Peter Jennings, says.

Some analysts dismiss the notion that viruses would be an effective warfare strategy. But US Air Force retired Brigadier General Robert Spalding, who has written a book on the Communist Party called *Stealth War*, says bioweapons are a highly effective military technique. "We know that in military fights, often it's better to wound a soldier than it is to kill, because the wounded soldier then has to be treated by other soldiers," he says. "Warfare is not necessarily straightforward about 'Hey, I need to kill the most people.' It could be that wounding will be disruptive enough, or in this case, causing a fear to really cause this kind of social political changes that we're looking for."

A textbook published by the Bradford Disarmament Research Centre in the UK called *Preventing Biological Threats: What You Can Do*, first published in 2015, states that "viruses gained in relevance as potential biological weapons over the years; by 1983, they had become the majority of recognised potential biological weapons agents". The book says that the Biological and Toxin Weapons Convention was established to deal with the prevention of the "hostile misuse of life sciences". "The continuing debate about the potential danger of carrying out 'Gain-of-Function' experiments with highly pathogenic viruses such as avian influenza has brought the problem of biological security to the attention of many within but also beyond the life science community," it states.

The book also notes the danger of an accidental laboratory release. "It is being increasingly recognised that biosecurity and biosafety are not only relevant to activities within a laboratory, but also extend to the effects that these activities can have outside the laboratory if they result in accidental outbreaks of diseases in humans, animals or plants," it says.

With these new fields of scientific research, the Bradford team warns that the bioweapons threat has increased. "Following the advent of genetic engineering, the explosive growth in the areas of genomics, bioinformatics, synthetic biology, systems biology, nanotechnology and targeted delivery systems is, according to defence analysts, all contributing to a formidable increase in the bioweapons threat spectrum, i.e. the increase in numbers and kinds of biological agents," it says. "In particular, synthetic biology and systems biology, which both rely on the enabling technologies of genomics and bioinformatics, have contributed considerably to the threat spectrum."

The Wuhan Institute of Virology is on a compound that also houses the lesser-known Wuhan Institute of Biological Products (WIBP). They are physically located just 200 metres (650 feet) apart on the same site, separated by fencing. The two research facilities are rumoured to be linked by an underground tunnel.

Years before the pandemic, biological weapon experts claimed that the Wuhan Institute of Biological Products was part of China's bioweapon program. One expert to write about this was Eric Croddy of the Monterey Institute's Chemical and Biological Weapons Non-proliferation Program. Citing an unnamed Taiwanese intelligence professional, Croddy identifies the WIBP as involved in the "cultivation of various BW [bioweapon] agents". In 2015, Dany Shoham, a former Israeli intelligence officer, also named the WIBP as a facility "associated with the defence establishment", and noted Croddy's claim of its association with China's bioweapon program.

The WIBP collaborated on the development of Covid-19 vaccines with the Wuhan Institute of Virology, and carried out intensive research into a potential vaccine against SARS in the 2000s and 2010s. David Asher, who led the inquiry into the origins of Covid-19 at the US State Department, regards the WIBP as a potential additional source of the outbreak rather than just the Wuhan Institute of Virology.

To examine these issues, members of DRASTIC – Rodolphe de Maistre, Gilles Demaneuf and Billy Bostickson – authored a comprehensive report examining the operations of the WIBP. They found it has a history of working on coronavirus vaccines. From 2003 to 2007, the WIBP produced several studies into a potential SARS vaccine, going so far as to build a dedicated P3 lab – which also contained animals for use in experiments – to continue this research.

Demaneuf discovered and translated a reference manual produced by the Wuhan Institute of Biological Products in 2006 specifically examining biosafety issues with the presence of SARS-CoV-1 in laboratories. Titled "A Discussion on the Safety of Laboratories for Large Cultivation of SARS Virus", the manual notes: "The P3 laboratory (three zones with two light structures) of our institute was put into use in 2003 after passing the assessment of the Biosafety Level 3 Laboratory of the Science and Technology Research Group of the National Atypical Pneumonia Command Headquarters. It mainly carried out the development of SARS vaccines."

Although the WIBP's research into a vaccine against SARS had ended by 2008, DRASTIC uncovered evidence to suggest it resumed work into SARS and MERS in 2017, using pseudoviruses – genetically engineered viruses that are altered so as to not replicate. A WIBP paper notes: "In particular, an outbreak of SARS caused by

SARS-CoV could lead to mass societal panic. We constructed stable pseudoviruses using pcDNA3.1-SS and pcDNA3.1- MS containing the S genes of SARS-CoV and MERS-CoV." The research was funded by China's National Major New Drug Development Project for the purposes of "significant new drugs development" – indicating a clear intention to produce drugs effective against SARS, possibly a vaccine.

There was documented cooperation between the WIBP and the Wuhan Institute of Virology well before their collaboration on Covid-19 vaccine development after the outbreak. Animals were also being studied in the Wuhan Institute of Virology's BSL-3 laboratory based on immunology work done by the WIBP. The range of known collaborations indicates that the institutes were closely tied. Insiders who believe that a lab leak is the most viable theory for the origin of Covid-19 fear that the WIBP is as viable a potential source as the Wuhan Institute of Virology.

CHAPTER TWENTY-THREE

A Can of Worms

MAY 2020, HARRY S. TRUMAN BUILDING, WASHINGTON DC

In the historic offices of the Bureau of Arms, Control, Verification and Compliance in the US State Department, Acting Assistant Secretary of State Tom DiNanno and Dave Asher had a fight on their hands. Not against China, but against American bureaucrats and intelligence officials in their own division, who they felt were siding with the Chinese Communist state to shut down an investigation into a potential laboratory leak and any links to China's bioweapons activity.

DiNanno had been appointed Deputy Assistant Secretary of State for Defense Policy, Emerging Threats in October 2018 and promoted to Acting Assistant Secretary several months later when his predecessor resigned. He oversaw missile defence, space policy and arms control. He'd previously been at Homeland Security focusing on counterterrorism.

Sitting in his suite where former Secretary of State General George C. Marshall, the US Army Chief of Staff during World War II, once worked, DiNanno emailed Anthony Ruggiero, the NSC Senior Director for Weapons of Mass Destruction and Bio-defence in May 2020. He asked for support to investigate any potential links between Covid-19 and China's biological weapons program. US Senator

Tom Cotton had gone public on Fox News with Maria Bartiromo linking the virus to biowarfare, sparking attacks he was a conspiracy theorist, but no agency was actually examining the possibility, however remote it seemed. "Hey, is anybody looking at Covid BW (bio-warfare) compliance? It doesn't smell right to me. I'm going to look into this. Any thoughts?" DiNanno recalls emailing.

Ruggiero replied with the thumbs-up to go ahead. And thus, DiNanno, on his own initiative, set up a covert team to investigate the origins of the virus. "That was when I unleashed Asher and his analyst team onto this," DiNanno says. "I knew the bureaucracy wouldn't hand this to us. You can't sit around and wait for someone to brief you. This was a national catastrophe. There was a massive pandemic, thousands of people were dying, we had to do our due diligence to see what we could find," DiNanno says, noting he had no pre-determined outcome. Asher has led investigations into money laundering, sanction evasion, nuclear proliferation and weapons of mass destruction in Iran, Pakistan and North Korea. While a traditional Republican, Asher has worked for both sides of politics. He served in the Bush administration under Deputy Secretary of State Richard Armitage, reporting to Secretary of State Colin Powell, and also worked under the Obama administration, re-joining the State Department in 2014, where he led an interagency taskforce to hunt down Islamic State extremists and develop a strategy to destroy the terrorist group – including depriving them of finances and an economic support base. Asher supported Trump's position on China, but having dealt with him personally in New York real estate finance, decided against officially joining the administration as a political appointee. He signed on as a "senior subject matter expert" contractor for the State Department, earning double the money while functionally holding similar power and responsibilities.

Their "Covid working group" investigation relied on help from others as well. "I worked in lockstep with Miles Yu, [Assistant Secretary of State for East Asian and Pacific Affairs] David Stilwell and [his deputy] David Feith, and in effect we ran a clandestine operation in our own government to get to the bottom of where

Covid-19 originated – be it from a bat cave, a lab leak, or worse a WMD accident," Asher says. "We looked at why China had covered up its propagation and why elements of the US government appeared highly complicit."

Asher and DiNanno had spent the majority of 2020 examining China's nuclear weapons compliance (or lack thereof). As they started to investigate the origins of Covid-19 full time from September, it became clear China was potentially in breach of its obligations under the biological weapons treaty through its synthetic biological and gain-of-function research creating viruses that, if released, even accidentally, could be used as bioweapons. Around this time the team also had to complete the annual compliance report of the Biological Weapons treaty, which is a legal requirement, submitted to Congress.

Together, Asher and his wingman of 15 years, Michael Pease, uncovered a wealth of evidence showing the Wuhan Institute was heavily involved in gain-of-function research with potential links to China's bioweapons program. They led the way in uncovering the Wuhan Institute of Virology's secret work for the Chinese military. "Wars are won by soldiers not by generals," one official says of their work.

The AVC is unique in that it has the authority to "task" the intelligence community to investigate, compile and collect using all national technical means up to the highest levels of classification if needed. It also has its own classified terminals located in its bureau that gave it the same raw access to the State's own Bureau of Intelligence and Research. "We had broad authorities and extensive facilities that allowed us to conduct this inquiry," DiNanno says. Stilwell, Feith and Miles Yu spent time working from AVC offices. "We used our terminals and our access to basically let our analysts loose. It was like letting Michael Jordan loose on a union basketball court with 12-year-olds," he said of Pease. "Within days he started hoovering up information that was lying in plain sight."

The team reviewed a Bureau of Intelligence and Research report that had been produced on March 26, 2020 along with a National Intelligence Community document dated April 8, 2020.

DiNanno's team obtained a bombshell classified report prepared by the Lawrence Livermore National Laboratory America's biodefence labs, which made the case that Covid-19 may have originated in a Wuhan laboratory as a result of synthetic and "serial passage" gain-of-function biological research, while also not ruling out the zoonotic theory. Lawrence Livermore is funded by the US Department of Energy and is responsible for national security and biodefence research. The report went against the official scientific consensus within the US government and intelligence community. The Lawrence Livermore report, from their intelligence unit the Z Division, was dated May 27, 2020, yet it had remained tucked away.

After reviewing the Lawrence Livermore report, the AVC team asked the laboratory to update its May document, with a phone call on October 27, 2020 where DiNanno offered to provide funding for this.

The next day the team held a "Sensitive Tele-Video Conference" with the National Intelligence Community, the CIA, the National Center for Medical Intelligence and the Bureau of Intelligence and Research on the origins of Covid-19.

DiNanno is understood to have pressed the officials he dealt with at the Office of the Director of National Intelligence (ODNI) on why they insisted the virus could not have been genetically manipulated when the official view from America's foremost experts in the field directly contradicted this. ODNI's response was that the Livermore classified report was not a consensus document and that their own scientific advisors disagreed with its analysis, adding that it was a conspiracy theory to suggest the virus may have been genetically manipulated.

DiNanno was outraged. "We're not in the consensus business," he argued. "I'm not interested in the roundtable, collective opinion. What are the credentials of the scientists giving you alternate advice? Who are they?" He was never given an answer. DiNanno had a right to question who precisely was feeding the intelligence community the advice that SARS-CoV-2 could not be genetically manipulated. At a February 3 meeting the intelligence community sought advice from Peter Daszak and other scientists, who said it was a conspiracy to consider a laboratory leak. "Little did we know at the time that prominent *Lancet* and *Nature* [*Medicine*] authors had made the rounds in the IC to get them on board and to stifle any dissent," DiNanno says. Fed up by the lack of serious examination of a potential lab leak, DiNanno and Asher decided to issue a directive to the intelligence community to pour over its databases and sources to see if there may be unanalysed information to support either theory based on specific intelligence, instead of intelligence community conjecture. Within weeks of receiving DiNanno's official tasking to support either theory, a flood of new information started flowing in, much of it dating back to the fall of 2019.

The single most extraordinary moment during their investigation was when Pease and Asher walked into DiNanno's office, with Asher waving a classified report. "Have you seen this?" Asher asked. DiNanno had just walked out of a meeting and didn't know what the pair were talking about. Pease had found freshly issued reporting from classified intelligence that several researchers at the Wuhan Institute of Virology had fallen ill in November 2019 with Covid-19-like symptoms. The trail to some of the earliest Covid cases led back to the Wuhan Institute of Virology.

Incredibly, no one had tasked the intelligence community dissemination, let alone unearthed, flagged or understood the significance of this intelligence report until this moment. The intelligence is understood to have first come into the possession of the agencies an entire year earlier in late 2019 – before the outbreak was even known. "We have several smart, diligent analysts and data scientists. They know their way around the classified networks," DiNanno says. The team put the pieces together with some of the other unusual activity at the Wuhan Institute of Virology.

Until this point, their investigation had been underground but it was time to let the more senior officials at the State Department know what they'd uncovered. DiNanno emailed his direct boss, Assistant Secretary of State for International Security and Non-Proliferation Christopher Ford, to ask for a meeting to present the findings. They prepared for the briefing but it was cancelled. DiNanno insisted on rescheduling. "That meeting was very, very important," he says.

It was eventually held in October in Ford's office in the State Department, with around 10 senior officials packed inside. Among those present was the highly respected US government legal advisor Jeff Gibbs, who had served for 41 years, including working as Deputy Counsel at the CIA.

DiNanno kicked the meeting off by telling the group they were looking into a potential breach by China of articles 10, 5, 1 and 2 of the international Biological Weapons Convention. He then turned to Asher to present the findings in detail. Asher began to walk through the gain-of-function research, the biological weapons program and the ill scientists in Wuhan. But he didn't get very far. This was a story that made global news when it broke, such was its significance, but that was far from the reaction of his colleagues in Ford's office that day.

According to some in the room, the State Department Senior Advisor for International Security and Non-proliferation interrupted him. "This is ridiculous. It's a complete waste of time. This is a public health issue," he is alleged to have said, according to several sources present. DiNanno objected, insisting it was a weapons compliance issue, not a public health one. The advisor allegedly retorted, "There's no way you guys can do this. You're going to open up a whole can of worms."

"This was a very seminal moment," DiNanno says. "It was very clear; there were other implications beyond what we were looking at. I took that as a warning. You're getting involved in stuff that you don't understand."

Ford, at that time, did not dismiss the concept out of hand but did not endorse it either. Suffice to say, the meeting was not a success.

If DiNanno had been excited with his team's discovery about the Wuhan Institute of Virology workers who had fallen ill, that enthusiasm was not met by his colleagues in the room that day. "We walked out of that meeting and I knew full well we were going to get no cooperation from that office," DiNanno says. As he walked back to his desk, he had the odd sensation of being an outsider looking in; he wondered if there was an intel operation he was not aware of.

DiNanno, curious about the "can of worms" he would potentially be opening up, went and spoke with a senior Chemical and Biological Weapons official. DiNanno says she repeated the phrase that gain-of-function and China's bioweapons program was a "can of worms". "This was earth-shattering," he says. "What is this can of worms?" he and Asher asked each other.

DiNanno spoke with another specialist in the Office of Chemical and Biological Weapons Affairs, but says she was reluctant to look into it either. The top biological weapons experts at the State Department were refusing to even countenance the possibility that Covid-19 had emerged from a Wuhan laboratory delving into bioweapons. He felt it was effectively a tap on the shoulder to say stop doing this. "If biological weapons experts aren't going to confront this, who is?" DiNanno thought.

Asher believes the "can of worms seemed to involve the ridiculous fact that the State non-proliferation bureaucracy had cleared the US Government cooperation with the Wuhan Institute of Virology and were fearful of being held responsible for, in effect, proliferating dual-use knowledge, capabilities and money to the PRC. Material support from the US government had been used against us to ensnare the NIH, State AID, and Department of Defense folks in a Chinese Communist spider web operation."

Asher, who has many years of experience following and disrupting Chinese "honey-pot operations" notes that "it would hardly surprise anyone if the PLA ambitions at the WIV included entrapping the naive US Government gain-of-function bureaucracy so as to hold them hostage to contributing to whatever might eventually come out of China's malevolent dual-use biowarfare designs and programs."

Ford wasn't comfortable with what had transpired at the meeting either. He had been kept in the dark about DiNanno's investigation and felt that proper protocol wasn't followed. He was disturbed the AVC team had spoken about an analysis from scientist Dr Steven Quay that claimed there was a 99 per cent probability the virus had originated in a laboratory. Ford claims that towards the end of that meeting Asher made a passing comment that he personally felt SARS-CoV-2 might be a Chinese biological weapon. "According to Asher, it was possible that SARS-CoV-2 was a 'genetically selective agent' from a biowarfare program that had been designed to target Americans," Ford tells me. "He said he was concerned that Covid-19 might be a GSA because we weren't seeing reports of massive Covid deaths in Sub-Saharan Africa. To him, this suggested that the virus had been adjusted in order to hit Americans especially hard."

Asher disputes this. He says he never said a thing about a GSA and that, to his knowledge at the time, GSA merely stood for the US Government's "General Services Administration".

The State Department advisor accused of using the phrase "can of worms" says, while he can't rule out having uttered the words, the context claimed by DiNanno and Asher is false. "No one prevented the disclosure of accurate, properly contextualized information," the State Department's spokesperson Ned Price says. "No effort was made at any time to suppress or withhold information from senior policymakers or the public. Internal disagreements were about the quality of analysis and the importance of not overstating, or bending, evidence to fit preconceived narratives. This is particularly important in dealing with something complex like the origins of the pandemic."

DiNanno suggested the next step would be to convene a panel of scientists to examine Dr Quay's analysis, which said it was statistically unlikely – or even impossible – for Covid-19 to have arisen naturally. While the panel was DiNanno's suggestion, Ford alleges DiNanno dragged his feet getting it together. Behind the scenes, the Arms Control team had in fact been engaging with multiple US National Laboratory– and prominent private-sector biological scientists for months, some of whom would join the scientific panel when it was held in the first week of January. Multiple employees who reported to DiNanno then accused him of being anti-science. Deeply offended, he asked them to put their position on the record, even emailing his employees insisting on this.

DiNanno's relationship with some senior staff fractured. Asher drew their attention to a 2018 National Academy of Sciences report on the threat of synthetic biology and gain-of-function research being applied to warfare. It warned a disaster could eventuate as a result. He made the point it was worth re-examining in the context of Covid-19. "They steadfastly refused to look at what I asked them to and would refute the facts," he says. Instead, one mid-level analyst sent DiNanno the *Lancet* letter where Daszak and others said the virus had a natural origin and it was a conspiracy to suggest otherwise.

"I've read the *Lancet* article," DiNanno fumed.

Asher derided the Intelligence Community analysts for failing to understand how lethal biological viruses could be created quickly and cheaply from a laboratory anywhere in the world and which, if unleashed, could act like bioweapons.

Worse, Asher noted the threat was hiding in plain site. "You didn't need a security clearance to know that the French who led the construction of the BSL-4 lab at the new Wuhan Institute of Virology campus had been kicked out and humiliated in 2017," he says. "Our ally, France, reportedly then proceeded to warn the US Intelligence Community and Non-proliferation Community about China's sinister intention in Wuhan – warnings that were totally dismissed and ignored by the 'Dilberts, dimwits and do-nothings' who dominated the US biological weapons and intelligence community leadership."

Asher says it seemed that "getting free trips to China to go visit the Great Wall mattered more to these negacrats than penetrating its hostile interior and biological warfare ambitions and programs involving synthetic and advanced biology".

"They were being intransigent and brutally obnoxious, especially to Asher," DiNanno says.

DiNanno and Asher dug their heels in, determined to investigate the origins of the virus, and not simply take the word of officials that this was a zoonotic virus. This back and forth persisted for some time, and as DiNanno raised the issue with officials he was repeatedly told that everyone does gain-of-function research, it's not a WMD area of concern and Covid-19 is a public health issue, unrelated to biological weapons compliance.

On November 18, the AVC team emailed the Livermore Laboratories officials asking for an update of the new report, with a more concrete offer to provide funding. The team sent yet another email on November 23. Finally, they received an initial response from Lawrence Livermore National Laboratories on November 30. While the correspondence is classified, sources tell me Lawrence Livermore was prevented from updating the report, preparing a new one or conducting any official work at all for the State Department by the leadership at the US Department of Energy. "They were censored," one insider claims. On December 3, the AVC requested another update from Livermore Laboratories, while submitting a "request for information" from the intelligence community around the same time.

The team sent out even more extensive "taskings" to the intelligence community but this time received very little back compared with the initial surge of support. They weren't even able to get hold of the leaked documents CNN had obtained and published on December 1 relating to China's mishandling of the coronavirus. The CIA, but not the national intelligence community, responded to the AVC with some information on December 16, documents obtained for this book reveal. The AVC team suspected their efforts were being undermined, and said as much to their counterparts in ODNI, whose names I am unable to publish because they are in highly-classified roles. "Once we started training our guns on them it was no longer a partnership. It gradually evolved into a very adversarial relationship between ODNI and our bureau," DiNanno says.

Asher, who also has a background co-founding and investing in multibillion-dollar biotech companies, confirms the intense pushback from intelligence agencies. "I had the strong impression the experts that were advising our intelligence community were people that were highly involved with China and US cooperative programs and gain-of-function research. None of them knew about synthetic biology, China, WMD or warfare. It was us versus the rest of the government, which was buying this bullshit from the intelligence community."

Asher says it was "Trump-era bullshit" that the intelligence community "rapidly moved far away from under Biden" as their confidence in Covid-19's natural origin moved from high to "low-to-medium". "Under Biden, the intelligence community has woken up to the initial conclusions [that] our AVC-led State Department taskforce had in the fall of 2020 that there is a great deal of specific and compelling information illuminating an accident and a top-down cover-up, and the paucity of evidence supporting natural zoonosis."

DiNanno says he was repeatedly told to leave the topic alone; that Covid-19 was a public health issue and did not fall under the remit of the AVC. "We had our own people, top people, senior people, senior executives in the government, saying 'This is a public health issue' right to my face," he says. "I said, 'What's the PLA doing in the lab?' The intel was clear, we saw it. It was so compelling that we took it to our bosses." DiNanno is emphatic: "My job in the WMD directorate is to not make excuses for China's WMD programs."

With a view to holding China accountable, DiNanno also led a push to démarche the Chinese Ambassador in Geneva. A démarche is a formal diplomatic representation from one government to another. DiNanno's idea was that a senior administration official – perhaps Secretary Pompeo or himself – would stand up in a formal setting and ask China to account for potential breaches of the Biological Weapons Convention and explain the gain-of-function research they were conducting. What purpose did it serve to create new souped-up, highly infectious coronaviruses? "Tell us about your military program. The treaty says it has to be peaceful. Can you explain how it's consistent with articles in the convention?"

There was strong opposition from many in the State Department. During a terse meeting, Stilwell is alleged to have retorted, "We can legally démarche who the fuck we want." The AVC team claim Ford disagreed with the move and said it was not legal, but he denies this and says he supported it, provided the questions to China were right.

Frustrated, DiNanno wrote a memo on December 5, 2020, to

Gibbs, Asher, Pease and four senior officials in the State Department, where he outlined the case for the démarche. In it, he specified how China had potentially breached the biological weapons compliance effort through its gain-of-function research. "I spent some time yesterday and today outlining where we are in the China BW compliance effort," he wrote. "In short we have a lot of work to do to make a legal case based on the object and purpose of the treaty, the articles and historical record of negotiations. This is not an open and shut case and our leadership placed what may be an insurmountable analytic hurdle given time constraints. We have work to do."

He attached to the email a "sensitive but unclassified" document where he outlines the case to formally démarche China over its potential violation of the convention. In it, DiNanno wrote: "The research the Chinese were doing on Gain of Function (GOF) was for potential military offensive purposes, they hid it and did not/have not shared what they knew and know. We believe this behaviour violates the spirit, object, and purpose of the BWC [Biological Weapons Convention]. Moreover we have concerns China's behaviour may violate Article 1, V and X of the BWC."

DiNanno's memo went on to articulate the ways the research may have violated the Biological Weapons Convention. "I don't think this is a slam dunk by any means and Gibbs would have to prosecute the legal case as we are concerned about their compliance with a legally binding treaty," he wrote. "So if we are on record already concerned about Chinese dual-use technologies, why would these recent developments assuage our public concern? We are merely saying we don't know you're not trying to weaponise virus research and given your statements and the catastrophic global pandemic your lack of transparency gives us concerns under Article X."

In the memo, DiNanno included a proposal from Australia, Canada, France, Germany, Japan, Netherlands, New Zealand, Spain, Turkey and the US from 30 years ago demanding information "without delay" about the "unusual abnormal large-scale outbreaks of infectious diseases". DiNanno then went on to write: "So if we and others were concerned enough to raise it 30 years ago, under the auspices of the BWC, why would that position be moot in 2020 when the exact concern has come to pass?"

There was heavy internal pushback to his move to démarche China. There was a follow-up meeting to discuss China's breach of those article points a week later with one of the State Department's top weapons experts. "Can you react to the memo I sent?" DiNanno said to his BW analyst.

She told him she had not read his memo and said, "Your attitude is anti-science."

DiNanno lost his temper at the official's intransigence and admits to yelling at her in fury, "I'm the boss, and when I ask you to do something, I expect you to do it." He went ballistic, he was so furious.

The official repeatedly said, "I'm sorry, I'm sorry."

In hindsight, DiNanno says the official is a good person, but he thinks the implications were too big for her. "She didn't want China to have a biological-weapon that got out of a lab, it's too horrible a thing to contemplate," he says. "But then maybe you should work for another department. If you're in the biological weapons [agency] you have to deal with biological weapons."

Ford tells me he never blocked any démarche on Covid-19. Instead, he says, he agreed with the plan as long as the US had solid cause to do so. He directed AVC to "draw up a list of tough questions for China for a démarche". "I was determined to prevent us raising issues with the Chinese that would make us look stupid: real, serious questions only," he says. Ford disagreed with the AVC that China had violated Article X(I) by not following international health regulations early in the crisis. "This was apparently a theory that had been ginned up entirely within AVC's Front Office without involving any subject-matter experts," he adds.

He also says, "Asher's insinuations that the mere existence of classified research at Wuhan Institute of Virology made that laboratory likely to be a biological warfare facility" would pave the way for a Russian propaganda assault on the US Army's research program into infectious diseases. Ford says he suggested instead a démarche under Article V. "I insisted, however, that they get the questions properly cleared – including through me. No more working behind people's backs," Ford told me. "If we were going to surface this publicly with an adversary power, we needed to be on very solid factual and analytical ground."

On December 18, 2020, the AVC team updated State Department officials on their "efforts regarding an upcoming VCAWG [Verification and Compliance Analysis Working Group] and PRC démarche," documents state. The AVC sent around a list of proposed démarche questions at the end of December. Ford objected that it was done on the unclassified email circuit OpenNet before it had been determined that the content was unclassified. The Health and Human Services [HHS] officials were furious, Ford says, "concerned that this démarche would infuriate the PRC and thereby bollix up the pending WHO investigatory visit to Wuhan, which was a priority for HHS to ensure took place".

Ford spoke to DiNanno on the phone in the first two days of January 2021. In the conversation, he demanded to know why he had not been brought into the loop about the initial Covid-19-origin investigation. Technically, he was his superior. DiNanno told him he had been working with the Secretary's representatives and his inquiry was not an unsanctioned effort. Up until that point, it seemed Ford had perhaps not realised DiNanno had been conducting his investigation with Miles Yu and Stilwell.

On the weekend of January 2, 2021, Ford and Stilwell then spoke on the phone. Ford said during that phone call it became clear "that his [Stilwell's East Asia] bureau wanted to collapse the WHO's investigatory visit to Wuhan". "Stilwell told me that he wanted to anger Beijing and provoke China's cancellation of the WHO visit," Ford says. "The visit wouldn't produce credible results anyway, he reasoned, so it would be better for us to goad the PRC into cancelling it so we could criticise them more for hiding evidence. It is my supposition that AVC's list of questions for the démarche was intended to support this agenda."

David Stilwell denies he ever spoke to Ford about the WHO trip, and says their only conversation "dealt with the wisdom of suggesting the WIV as a possible source". In that conversation, Stilwell recalls telling Ford there was enough evidence pointing to the Wuhan Institute of Virology as a possible source of Covid-19 and that Ford was insisting on an impossible level of evidence before making this claim. "I tried to help him see my perspective that we don't need evidence beyond a reasonable doubt to make the observation that the Wuhan Institute of Virology was a likely origin of the pandemic. I told him the burden of proof that it wasn't the WIV belonged to Beijing," Stilwell tells me. "If China wants to keep us out of Xinjiang or Wuhan to prevent evidence collection, they can – and do – do that."

It was in this climate Asher and DiNanno asked Yu for help. "Their inquiry into the possible leak was fiercely opposed by Christopher Ford, who was frustrated with Trump and very woke," Yu says. "I was told that his main argument was that this can't be a lab-engineered virus and it has already been settled by the scientists, so there is no reason for you to pursue this. I went to Pompeo."

Pompeo said, "Miles you have the green light from me."

The panel of scientists was held on January 7, 2021. Its agenda was to assess the validity of the lab-leak hypothesis and of zoonosis. The question was also posed: what do we know from the sequences of SARS-CoV-2? What do they tell us about this virus? Another key element was interrogating Dr Quay's Bayesian analysis that said it was statistically unlikely for Covid to have emerged naturally.

The attending scientists included Shi Zhengli's collaborator Ralph Baric, Stanford's David Relman, Steven Quay, Penn State's Bob McCreight and Rich Muller, among others, including from the National Laboratories. It was a group of scientists with utterly divergent views. Baric had co-authored gain-of-function research with Shi Zhengli and insisted the virus had a natural origin. Relman had written a paper stating that a laboratory origin for Covid-19 was a viable prospect, while Dr Quay, based in Taiwan, put the prospect of a lab escape at 99 per cent. It was a fiery meeting.

About 10 people were physically gathered in the State Department while others joined through Microsoft Teams. Yu opened the session. "I'd like to start by relaying some words from the Secretary of State, Mike Pompeo. I spoke to the Secretary earlier today and he said: "Any research inquiry into the true origin of the virus should be encouraged and I support it. It is worth pursuing regardless of whether the result is something we'd like to see or not. We must know the truth.""

The meeting went for three hours, with Yu leaving to have dinner with the Taiwanese ambassador after his opening remarks, missing the drama that would unfold. Asher, who doesn't pause for breath, was an active and at times antagonistic participant when countering Ford's interventions. Professor Muller was chosen to moderate the discussion given his experience dealing with every WMD issue facing the United States and his scientific credentials. He allowed each scientist to speak individually before facilitating a dialogue.

But it got ugly. Dr Quay was challenged over his Bayesian analysis that had put the prospect of a lab leak at 99 per cent , which a State official from an intelligence agency said was "spectacularly wrong". "Have you ever done a Bayesian analysis before?" a Bureau of Intelligence and Research official asked him. Quay replied he had not but he'd had a prominent UCLA statistician do the analysis for him.

Baric asked Quay: "How many coronaviruses do you think there are in the world?" Quay didn't know. Baric said: "Millions!" His point was that Quay would need to change the denominator in his calculation given there were more viruses than he realised. Twelve hours later, Quay found an interview with Peter Daszak where he said there were 6000 coronaviruses in the world. He emailed the group: "So Ralph would it be ok if I used the number of 6000 rather than your off-the-cuff millions in the analysis?" Baric didn't respond to that email.

In Ford's mind, the Bayesian analysis held no weight: "Unfortunately, it turned out that Asher's argument was crap, and it collapsed like a house of cards for the reasons I described in my email to various State colleagues the next day," he tells me.

Asher asserts the Bayesian analysis was Dr Quay's, not his, but he found it more persuasive than Baric's opposing analysis presented at the same meeting that "we could never know Covid-19's origins unless every bat cave in China and South East Asia was inspected and sampled for coronaviruses."

DiNanno, meanwhile, was infuriated that the intelligence official who attacked Quay over his analysis had her own conflict of interest. Not only did she work at the State Department in intelligence but she is also an independent consultant to the WHO, sitting in high-level meetings at both organisations.

Quay then fired his own missive: "There's no evidence any of you have provided of a zoonotic origin. Where is the evidence?" He demanded to know. Baric couldn't answer. Quay fired another barb at Baric: "What possible academic purpose could your 'no-see-um' technology have? Why did you even develop it as a scientist?" The "no-see-um" technique Baric developed allows scientists to insert genetic material into viruses without leaving a mark or signature. It means no one can tell if a virus has been genetically altered. In Quay's view, this could only have a nefarious purpose or be used to try to cover your tracks. Baric was outraged. "How could you even say that, it's for the good of humanity!" he replied. "It's like putting WMD on the internet," someone else muttered.

Asher reportedly said he was "shocked" that Baric had not discussed the potential role of gain-of-function research at the Wuhan Institute of Virology in increasing the lethality of the SARS-CoV-2 virus, especially given that Baric was "connected to the WIV". "It turned into a food fight," Asher admits.

Around half the experts present said the virus was easily manufacturable and may well have been manufactured. They said it's a capability the Chinese certainly had at the Wuhan Institute of Virology and WIBP. But Baric argued that the Wuhan Institute of Virology would never do such a thing.

Quay found the way he was spoken to disrespectful, intimidating and confrontational. Baric did not respond to an interview request for this book.

At one point, Asher alleges Ford said to him: "How do you know it didn't come out of the CDC? We have a level-4 lab too." Ford refutes the accuracy of this. "I asked how the AVC team knew that the alleged laboratory of origin could not be the Wuhan Chinese CDC laboratory, which did lots of work with coronaviruses and was in fact closer to the wet market than WIV." Baric allegedly commented, "We don't really know who the first patient is in the first place so it doesn't make a lot of sense to draw conclusions about which lab was closest."

There were power plays as well. When Asher thanked the assembled scientists "on behalf of the State Department", Ford cut him down and said he did not speak for the department, he was a contractor who worked for DiNanno who reported to him. "This intervention may have upset Asher but it was necessary," Ford said. Relman, a voice of reason, who was also friends with Baric, tried to calm the tempers down.

The conversation finished with an unexpected powerful intervention from a very senior scientist working in the United States Army's biological program. "Anybody who has been involved in WMD knows this is the type of virus the Chinese have been working on," he said. "This could have been manufactured in a lab, we've been capable of doing it for decades so don't fool yourself that Covid-19 had to be zoonosis." There was dumbfounded silence.

That night, Ford stayed up until the early hours writing a four-page memo to senior officials attacking the AVC investigation, their techniques and analysis and the fact they didn't follow protocol. He resigned the next day, January 8, over Trump's handling of the storming of the US Capitol Hill, which had taken place on January 6.

DiNanno sent Yu an email on January 9, 2021 at 11.48pm, rebutting Ford's claims. He detailed the work his bureau had done over the last few months to determine the origins of Covid-19, pointing out his was one of only two State Department bureaus authorised by legislation to investigate state parties' compliance with international arms control, non-proliferation and disarmament agreements. "AVC has been closely monitoring SARS-CoV-2 for months which, until recently, had been universally attributed to animal to human transmission," he wrote in the email obtained for this book. "The IC [intelligence community] consensus has significantly evolved to where a lab release is entirely plausible. If it escaped from a lab we need to know how and what exactly this research entailed."

Yu sent an email to Pompeo the following day, January 10, 2021, knowing that he had already seen Ford's memo of complaint. "In my opinion, the small group of AVC colleagues led by SBO [Senior Bureau Official] DiNanno are American heroes who perform their duty with extraordinary due diligence, scientific prudence, and bravery to fend off constant pressure from their superior calling for stopping such worthy inquiry," Yu wrote. "They are not looking for conclusions we like or not like, but the truth, and they conducted themselves throughout in such a fashion, as witnessed by me and [Stilwell]. I took part in some of their discussions with leading scientists at our national labs (Lawrence Livermore National Lab, NCMI [National Center for Medical Intelligence], NNSA [National Nuclear Security Administration] etc.) and prestigious academic research institutes. Instead of being maligned, I think they deserve commendations from the State Department, as they are the only USG agency seriously looking at the true origin of COVID by engaging with scientists."

It seems Pompeo is in no doubt about the role the bureau played in uncovering crucial intelligence and other information related to a possible outbreak at the Wuhan Institute of Virology. When I spoke to Pompeo, he said David Stilwell, Yu and Asher were the "gang that has worked on this problem". And when it emerged the team had been disbanded by the Biden administration, Pompeo tweeted: "President Biden sides with China, WHO and the liberal media on Wuhan virus – joining the 'nothing to see here crowd' by shutting down State Department pandemic origin investigation I commenced."

In the end, the AVC did get clearance on some questions for the démarche, but they did not have the interagency support to ask specifically about the origins of Covid, which is what they had intended in the first place. The cable was scrubbed. "As far as I know, the final decision not to send the démarche occurred after the handover of power to the Biden administration," Ford says. This is one point DiNanno and Ford agree on. "Biden scrapped it. China would have been démarched with Pompeo still in charge," DiNanno said. "You either confront a tyrant or appease him. History has taught us appeasement doesn't work."

Pompeo confirmed to me he supported the plan to démarche China over the origins of Covid-19.

A sense of the pushback DiNanno and Asher were getting from Ford is conveyed in the comments he gave during an interview for this book. He saw their effort as a waste of taxpayer dollars and described their work as "shoddy" and said they were "conspiratorial yahoos". "There is good reason to suspect a WIV role in SARS-CoV-2, and it's vital to keep pressing the Chinese Communist Party for answers. Thankfully, it's now been possible to do so without this being discredited by results-driven amateur-hour skulduggery," Ford said.

Before the end of the Trump administration, the AVC team made one additional long-lasting contribution. They led a push to declassify the intelligence, to let the American public and the world know what their underground team had uncovered the secret military work at the Wuhan Institute of Virology, the sick workers and China's bioweapons program. The negotiations about whether to declassify this intelligence and discussions with the AVC team, the State Department and the intelligence agencies dragged on for around two months.

There was serious pushback among many senior figures who rejected the idea the intel should be declassified. "That decision by Pompeo to declassify the intelligence was contested, and parts of [the] US intelligence community didn't agree," a Five Eyes source tells me.

Stilwell says this was an obstacle they needed to work through. "The first hurdle was the intel community. We had to get the intel community to sign off on a level of detail in the statement that would convince people the lab leak theory had merit, without jeopardizing intel sources and methods," he says.

Ford says he agreed with the move to declassify intelligence, given the intelligence community were comfortable with it. The Secretary of State sided with the AVC team and believed the world should know the truth. But the final decision on whether to declassify was not made by Pompeo. He needed to get it cleared by intelligence agencies – the CIA, ODNI, the NSC, the FBI and others. The final call was made by the Director of National Intelligence, John Ratcliffe. A compromise position was ultimately struck to include a line in the declassified statement saying that the intelligence agencies ultimately did not know the origins of the virus. Pompeo and the AVC team could live with that.

By the time it was released, on January 15, 2021, it was the dying days of the Trump administration; the President was on his last legs, and losing credibility by the hour; and no one took notice of the powerful declassified intelligence that blew the lid on the secret workers who had fallen sick. It wasn't until much later that the world sat up and took notice of what this small unit inside the State Department had uncovered. Reflecting on this time, DiNanno says, "This was a right-leaning administration and it took every ounce of our energy, savvy and experience to get this the attention it deserved."

Mary Kissel says "there was a demonstrable lack of intellectual curiosity when it came to the lab leak theory." She adds, "This wasn't just confined to the State Department; this was true across many agencies of government and especially in the media."

In early January, as he was preparing to declassify the intelligence, Pompeo held a call with his Five Eyes partners: Australia, Canada, New Zealand and the UK. On the call, he detailed the latest intelligence on the Wuhan Institute of Virology, the sick workers and the bioweapons program that had been uncovered by Asher, DiNanno and Pease. While the intelligence had already been shared among the Five Eyes network, the specific purpose of this call was to let the ministers know he intended to make it public. It would have the dramatic effect of pointing to the Wuhan Institute of Virology as the possible, or even likely, source of the outbreak.

During the call, UK Foreign Minister Dominic Raab was profusely thankful to Pompeo for releasing this information. Australia's Foreign Minister Marise Payne also supported the declassification, advocating transparency over secrecy. "The free world expects the US to lead and not kowtow," a senior source said.

The Five Eyes call was classified but it was deliberately held on an open line, in the knowledge that the Chinese would be listening. "Anyone who had the ability to collect any communications probably knew that it was happening, especially the Chinese," a senior source said. Another source said, "That's a sophisticated intel operation. Let them hear you and then listen to their reaction. Let them know you know and see what reverberates back through the system."

The foreign ministers, expecting a major reaction from this startling new development that workers had fallen sick at the Wuhan Institute of Virology in late 2019, in the suspected first cluster of the pandemic, felt a sense of disappointment when the intelligence was eventually released. It was overshadowed by the events unfolding in the United States – the Capitol Hill riots and Trump's claims of election fraud.

The crucial intelligence was dismissed by the media and analysts alike as a political exercise by Pompeo. The gems were lost amid the noise, and very few people paid any attention to it. As the new Biden administration swept to power, the declassified intelligence was removed from the State Department's website, only to be buried in an old, archived version of releases under the Trump administration.

The officials who had led the way in declassifying it, including Asher, were warned they could be arrested for "slippage", and some State Department officials even wanted to reclassify the intelligence that had already been publicly released with the support of the Five Eyes partners. Its importance would not be rediscovered for another four months when, finally, the mood shifted, the number of deaths from Covid swelled and the public demanded answers about what, if anything, had happened in the Wuhan laboratories.

CHAPTER TWENTY-FOUR

The Window for an Outbreak

SEPTEMBER 2019, WUHAN: DELETING THE VIRUS DATABASE

It started in the autumn of 2019. Months before the first reported case of human-to-human contact, the Wuhan Institute of Virology began to go dark. Publicly available information was wiped from the internet. Staff connected with the Institute disappeared as scientists fiercely criticised its safety practices and standards. At the same time, there were burgeoning social media mentions of a new respiratory illness.

In early September 2019, Shi Zhengli spoke at a conference in Mozambique and by the 24th she was in Lyon in France. In the middle of these trips, on September 12, the Wuhan Institute of Virology's online database of samples and viral sequences, which she administered, was taken offline. It was a researcher for this book, Luke McWilliams, 24, and an open-source analyst Charles Small who made the discovery – eight months later in May 2020.

The database was an extensive catalogue of bat samples, bat coronavirus samples, mouse samples and mouse virus pathogen data. In total, the database held the details of 22,257 samples. It is believed to have held information about the more than 1500 live virus isolates stored in Wuhan Institute of Virology freezers (that figure comes from documents dating back to 2018 and it's likely that the size of the virus bank had grown significantly since then) – equivalent to a third of the virus families that have been identified worldwide. The oldest virus dates back 30 years. Some had been imported from Europe, Asia and America. There are also 60,000 'preserved strains', 20,000 of which are bat and rat samples, and pathogen data. We know this because it was recorded by the Chinese Academy of Science Database resource and service registry. Days after Charles and Luke's discovery, scientist Yuri Deigin noticed that he could not download the virus database with its 61.5 megabytes of data. Instead it amounted to an empty 1 kilobyte zip file. "Did Shi Zhengli's team's own virus database get deleted?" he tweeted on May 11. Deigin then, through an intermediary, contacted the Editorial Office of China Scientific Data, responsible for maintaining the database, to ask why it had been deleted. The response in-writing was, "We have reported this to the authors. We will inform you as soon as we get feedback". After a follow-up email, the Office responded to say, "Thanks for your advice. We reviewed the data by temporary link, and we did not keep the backup copy. As you know, data sharing is a newborn baby, we cannot push it too hurry. Our editorial office encourages them to share data which they must follow. We will follow up and let you know the progress. Hope you understand." Needless to say, the database was never provided.

A report compiled by Bostickson and scientists Deigin and Demaneuf found that the database was inactive for a week during the second half of August 2019 before it became definitely inaccessible on September 12. "It was online intermittently after this date from mid-December 2019, and occasionally until February 2020, but was not accessed from outside the WIV after 12 September 2019," they wrote. Since September 2019, China has not allowed any international or independent experts access to these databases.

Fascinatingly, Deigin, Demaneuf and Bostickson's report found that there was a password-protected section for unpublished viruses. An indication of the importance of the virus database and confirmation that not all viruses had been disclosed came from Daszak in a December 2020 tweet where he said: "Thanks to @RudyGuliani's poorly thought out interference, a grant to @ EcoHealthNYC funded under @realDonaldTrump was terminated by @NIHDirector & now we can't get access to critical samples that would help us understand the origins of COVID and could be used to improve vaccines." Shi Zhengli, pressed on the sudden removal of the information, claimed that some 3000 attempts had been made to hack the database. She said this prompted the decision to take it offline. In fact, user access records indicate there were major hacking attempts months earlier, on June 18 and 19, 2019. Yet the database was not taken offline then. Rather, "the speculation would be that they were concerned that something had gone wrong," says Internet 2.0 cybersecurity expert Robert Potter, who has done cyber-defence work for the United States and Australian governments and has helped expose secret Chinese Communist Party membership lists. "It takes a while for these viruses to percolate and spread and develop. It could have taken three or four months to really hit the general population of Wuhan and Hubei ... the implication is they did it because there were some reasons, there was something to hide, otherwise, you'd be transparent."

The US government officially called for access to the virus database: "WHO investigators must have access to the records of the WIV's work on bat and other coronaviruses before the Covid-19 outbreak. As part of a thorough inquiry, they must have a full accounting of why the WIV altered and then removed online records of its work with RaTG13 and other viruses," a State Department statement from January 2021 says.

Why was the database removed in September? Senior US government sources I've interviewed for this book link the database removal with a September incident at the laboratory. Asked how early he thinks the virus started, Pompeo says, "If you look at the dataset around folks who became sick, it's sometime in the late fall of 2019, but it's only a hypothesis, we don't know. Late September-ish."

On September 18, the coronavirus training exercise took place at Wuhan airport (see Chapter 20). It's a highly unusual coincidence, given a coronavirus outbreak would eventuate just a few months later.

October 2019, Wuhan: The Blackout at the Lab

Multiple sources of evidence then point to a series of incidents occurring at the Wuhan Institute of Virology in October. Satellite data shows a mobile phone blackout in October 2019, specifically between October 11 and 19.

This data is usually kept secret by intelligence agencies but an open-source analysis of commercial telemetry data, geospatial data and satellite images was made public. Designed to be unclassified, it comprised a "pattern of life analysis" in the Wuhan Institute of Virology and WIBP compound. The analysis reported "a large area surrounding the WIV BSL-4 was analysed and findings suggest that during 11–16 Oct, there was a noticeable drop in signals in the area when compared with the week before and the week after." Their road traffic analysis indicates "traffic closures or roadblocks" for the same time period. "Device traffic in and around the WIV in the months prior to October was consistent," it states. "Beginning on October 11th there was a substantial decrease in activity. The last time a device is active prior to October 11th is October 6th." Images show "there was absolutely no traffic in the area surrounding the WIV from October 14th–19th".

When the report surfaced, amid the climate of claiming the laboratory leak was a conspiracy theory, mainstream media discredited the analysis that accompanied the data, stating that it was not done by intelligence agencies. This is correct. But high-level intelligence and government sources in both the United States and Australian governments confirmed that the information indicating a blackout of cellular mobile phone data is credible.

The US government took evidence of a mobile phone blackout seriously enough to refer to it in an official letter to EcoHealth Alliance from NIH. The letter, by NIH Deputy Director for Extramural Research Michael Lauer, dated July 8, 2020, demanded that EcoHealth: "Disclose and explain out-of-ordinary restrictions on laboratory facilities, as suggested, for example by diminished cell-phone traffic in October 2019, and the evidence that there may have been roadblocks surrounding the facility from October 14–19, 2019."

A senior Australian government source told me: "The intelligence assessment was that the jury was still out. Some saw it as a smoking gun, it could indicate that an incident had occurred at the WIV. It's not conclusive but suggestive that something was going on." The senior official added that the intelligence assessment was the aggregate of both covert intelligence and the "open-source scrape".

Sir Richard Dearlove believes the data is "highly significant". "A lot of American analysis at the CIA would have started with overhead. They'll have a lot of material, it's just not in the public domain," he said. If there were worries about an outbreak early on in China they would have certainly stuck one of the satellites in the right place. There would be a massive amount of NSA intercepts as well. This is highly classified what it actually was but informed speculation would tell you that there was [a blackout]."

Perhaps no one knows more about this topic than David Asher, who led the State Department investigation into the origins of the pandemic, uncovering the classified intelligence of the sick Wuhan Institute of Virology workers. "There's a lot of things I can't get into, but I can tell you it looks accurate based also on things Americans living in Wuhan observed in mid- to late October," he says. "That document lays out that there was a crazy fall-off in communications at the WIV, I can't comment specifically on that but assuming it's accurate, the question is, what happened?"

Asher said advice to the US government is that the blackout is consistent with the protocol for a biological incident occurring at a laboratory. "We are pretty confident that a bad incident occurred in October and they cleaned it up. That's why everyone was kicked out, except for the security guards," he said. "When I talked to people who run BSL-4 and BSL-3 labs, they say that's exactly what the procedures are, they kick everyone out and do a mass sterilisation."

And then, right in the middle of the blackout at the Wuhan Institute of Virology, on October 18, airline flights leaving Wuhan were shut down. Analysis of flights leaving Wuhan over a six-month period from August 2019 until February 2020, commissioned for this book and done by the analyst, Charles Small, shows a mean daily flight cancellation rate of 1.2 per cent – except on the day of Friday, October 18, 2019. On that day, an unusually high number of domestic departures were cancelled – 12 per cent and all from one airline, the majority-state-owned China Eastern. The weather was calm that day, at a top of 23 degrees and sunny. It was the first day of the Military World Games.

This was an intense period of activity at the Wuhan Institute of Virology. And against the background of these events – starting in September, unfolding smack-bang in the middle of October's blackout period and continuing beyond the first reported case of Covid-19 – the Wuhan Institute of Virology embarked on a spending spree. A joint effort between Internet 2.0 cybersecurity experts David Robinson and Robert Potter, and China analyst Luke McWilliams, unearthed tenders that had been virtually expunged from the internet and that reveal the procurement history of the Wuhan Institute of Virology during, as Potter puts it, "a critical time".

Follow the money and a clear picture begins to emerge. The Institute was beefing up its security – guards and system technology – at considerable expense. There were also hundreds of thousands of dollars spent on safety and testing equipment over a remarkably condensed period of time. "Efforts to hide this data are evident, but we were able to restore the records using both historical website data and other systems accidentally spilled into the public internet," Potter explains.

Our research team for this book analysed some 136 tenders dating back to the set-up of the Wuhan Institute of Virology in 2014 and up to as recently as the time of writing. On September 12 – after the same day as the Wuhan Institute of Virology pulled its virus database offline – it put out a competitive consultation for a security service, worth around US$128,000. A week later, on September 19, it put out a follow-up "correction notice". Just six days later, the Wuhan Hengchangsheng Security Guard Service was awarded this contract. On October 18, the Wuhan Institute of Virology put out a tender for a security-monitoring system. Again, there was an extremely fast turnaround. The winning bid was announced two weeks later, on November 6. Ultimately the Wuhan Institute of Virology spent more than half a million dollars on new security.

After the blackout period, on November 6, 2019, the Wuhan Institute of Virology issued a tender for a "fluorescence quantitative PCR instrument". A polymerase chain reaction (PCR) test is a fast and inexpensive way to test samples for viruses. While not exclusively used for testing for coronaviruses, the term PCR test has, during the Covid-19 pandemic, become synonymous this purpose. The Wuhan Institute of Virology was looking for a machine to test for coronaviruses, and offering to pay up to US$52,000. The winning bid, from Wuhan Bai Lei Zhen Biological Technology, came in under budget, at US$48,000, a mere two weeks after the tender was issued on the Hubei Guohua Tendering Consulting website. The last time a PCR machine appears in the tender data was two years earlier, in 2017.

The Wuhan Institute of Virology's poor safety standards were further underscored by investigations conducted for this book. "The procurement activity increases dramatically at a macro-national level and then within the Wuhan Institute of Virology itself we see complex procurement activity including security uplift and testing equipment starting on the same day that the virus database goes offline," Potter says.

Disturbing photographs obtained from the official Wuhan Institute of Virology compliance certificate and laboratory safety records show employees wearing no protective equipment crouched inside a sewage-treatment facility to collect samples for testing. A 2018 'Wastewater Monitoring' test report for the Wuhan National Biosafety Laboratory, which includes BSL-3 and BSL-4 laboratories, features photographs labelled import and export of "sewage treatment facilities". Photographs show employees handling similar sewage samples in another location. Two other photographs show close-up detail of the sewage collection. The photographs are shocking given the staff are not even wearing gloves, which would be especially risky had there been an infection or improper disposal of infectious virus materials.

Unsurprisingly, then, are the tenders from early in 2019, and which relate to incineration and toxic wastewater disposal. The Wuhan Institute of Virology put out a tender for toxic wastewater equipment worth US$62,000 in April 2019. At the end of July 2019, a successful bid was completed for "third-party biosafety testing project of Wuhan National Biosafety Laboratory". Contact with infected wastewater that had not been properly treated is one of the many ways in which a leak of a virus could occur.

A winning bid for air incinerators and testing services worth US$43,000 – in the critical time period of December 2019 – could be seen as evidence that there were also problems with incineration. The tender went out on December 3 and was completed on the 25th. The question, of course, is: Why did the Wuhan Institute of Virology need new air incinerators and testing services in early December 2019?

In March 2019, the Wuhan Institute of Virology successfully completed a tender titled "Maintenance project of the P3 laboratory and the laboratory animal centre" for US$38,000. This is part of extensive proof the laboratory houses animals and bats in cages for its experiments. A patent filed by the Wuhan Institute of Virology on June 15, 2018, is titled: "Feeding cage for insectivorous bats". The patent even has detail on guano (bat poo) disposal mechanisms.

An official Chinese Academy of Sciences video to mark the launch of the new BSL-4 laboratory in May 2017 shows bats held in a cage at the Wuhan Institute of Virology, along with a scientist feeding a worm to a bat. This is despite Daszak calling the suggestion there were bats at the Wuhan Institute of Virology a conspiracy in a tweet he later deleted. The World Health Organization inspectors also failed to mention the bats in their report following their February 2021 visit. The video was unearthed by DRASTIC's digital archivist known as Jesse, and I then had it translated by Monash University's Kevin Carrico. The video shows a bat hanging off a researcher's hat while the narrator speaks about the work of the lab's Director of Emerging Infectious Diseases, Shi Zhengli. "Over more than a decade, Shi Zhengli's research team has collected more than 15,000 bat samples in China and many countries of Africa, searching for the origins of SARS, as well as isolating and characterising many new viruses," the narrator says.

The 10-minute video, titled "The Construction and Research Team of Wuhan P4 Laboratory of Wuhan Institute of Virology, Chinese Academy of Sciences", also speaks about the security precautions in place if "an accident" were to occur. Wuhan BSL-4 laboratory director Yuan Zhiming says, "Staff in our central control room remain in constant contact with staff in our laboratory, providing necessary technical support for their experiments as well as for any accidents." Once again, the possibility of a laboratory accident is far from a conspiracy.

The Wuhan Institute of Virology has an "Experimental Animal Centre" with 12 ferret cages, 126 white rabbit cages and 3000 cages for rodents and insects. A webpage dedicated to the Experimental Animal Centre features photographs of about 20 white rabbits in metal cages so small that it would upset any animal welfare advocate. The website describes how the Centre is involved in the "preparation of virus protein antibodies, the establishment of animal models, the gene therapy of zoonotic diseases, virus proliferation, bioassay and safety". It also describes their "artificial breeding" of insects.

Corroborating this is an interview in the state-backed media outlet Sixth Tone, which speaks about how a Wuhan Institute of Virology scientist had "collected a full rack of swabs and bagged a dozen live bats for further testing back at the lab".

And at the "Second China-US Workshop on the Challenges of Emerging Infections, Laboratory Safety and Global Health Security" in Wuhan in 2017, Shi Zhengli spoke about researching with transgenic mice and "animal models".

So, in March 2019, the Wuhan Institute of Virology was issuing a tender for maintenance of the BSL-3 laboratory, where much of Shi Zhengli's coronavirus research took place, and the laboratory's animal centre. The next month, in April, the Institute bought 20 of the positive-pressure protective clothing suits they wear in the laboratory for US$226,000.

As already canvassed earlier in this book, internal Chinese government documents trace the first recorded case of Covid-19 to November 17, 2019, according to the *South China Morning Post*. Just 10 days before this, on November 7, the National Health Commission of China formally approved the BSL-3 Wuhan National Biosafety Laboratory of Wuhan Institute of Virology to engage in "experimental activities of highly pathogenic microorganisms", according to several press releases from the Chinese Academy of Science and the Wuhan Institute.

NOVEMBER 2019, WUHAN

By November, the virus was already spreading. Chinese infectious disease specialists from the Second Affiliated Hospital of Xi'an Jiaotong University in China analysed the date when words relating to coronavirus started appearing on the most popular Chinese social media site, WeChat. The study, published in *JMIR mHealth and uHealth* (JMIR stands for *Journal of Medical Internet Research*), analysed WeChat data sent from November 17, 2019 to February 14, 2020, using the WeChat Index, a data service that shows how often a specific keyword appears in posts, subscriptions and searches. Unfortunately, when the infectious disease specialists decided to conduct their study, they could only access the data from 90 days before. On the earliest day they could access the data, November 17, 2019, the hits for "SARS" were at 100,000 mentions. In a single day. On December 1, there was a spike with more than 200,000 mentions. And the hits for "Feidian", which means Severe Acute Respiratory Syndrome, were at about 65,000 on November 17, climbing to 150,000 on December 15, according to a graph included in the report.

"From November 17, 2019, to December 30, 2019 (44 days), the WeChat Index results also spiked or increased for 'novel coronavirus,' 'shortness of breath,' 'dyspnea' and 'diarrhea,' although these terms were not as meaningful for the early detection of the outbreak as 'Feidian',' the report states. "The WeChat Index results for the word 'Feidian' offered a strong warning sign of the developing SARS-CoV-2 outbreak." The Chinese infectious disease specialists recommend paying closer attention to social media sites for earlier detection of serious outbreaks in the future.

A paper published in *Science* in April 2021, titled "Timing the SARS CoV-2 Index Case in Hubei Province", tried to calculate when the first case would have emerged in Wuhan and decided that it could have been closer to mid-October. "We used a coalescent framework to combine retrospective molecular clock inference with forward epidemiological simulations to determine how long SARS-CoV-2 could have circulated before the time of the most recent common ancestor," it states. "Our results define the period between mid-October and mid-November 2019 as the plausible interval when the first case of SARS-CoV-2 emerged in Hubei province." This all, of course, coincides with the first-hand experience of doctors on the ground, such as Dr Wang (see Chapter 2).

On December 30, around the same time Shi Zhengli was on a train back to Wuhan from a conference in Shanghai to deal with the outbreak, the database containing genetic sequences was altered. It was at this time that Shi said she heard news about the outbreak and suffered sleepless nights worrying whether it was her lab that was responsible for the outbreak.

As she told *Scientific American* in an article published in May 2020, "Could they have come from our lab?" Since her initial fears, Shi Zhengli claims to have satisfied herself the genetic sequence of Covid-19 did not match any her lab was studying. It's worth remembering, of course, that there were some 300 scientists at the Wuhan Institute of Virology, and at least four major laboratories and their virus databases have been hidden from investigators and kept secret.

But on December 30 there were alterations in her database. The name of the database changed from "Wildlife-borne viral pathogen database" to "Bat and rodent-borne viral pathogen database". Keywords including "wildlife" and "wild animals" were deleted, along with "wild animal samples", "emerging infectious diseases", "viral pathogen data" and "cross-species infection". This censorship was revealed by Miranda Devine in the *New York Post* in May 2020. The British open-source analyst Charles Small, who made the discovery, told Devine it appeared the Wuhan Institute of Virology was trying to distance itself from the outbreak. "It looks like a rushed, inconsistent effort to disassociate the project from the outbreak by rebranding it," he said. "It's a strange thing to do within hours of being informed of a novel-coronavirus outbreak."

Deigin says, "The observations that the Wuhan Institute of Virology has scrubbed the description of their internal virus database and then deleted the database itself are pretty significant. For some reason, in December 2019, all of a sudden they decided to distance themselves from what they have been doing for years, namely studying 'cross-species infection', i.e. having viruses jump from one species to another. Plus obviously they didn't want the world to know what unpublished viral genomes or parts of genomes – say a pangolin CoV spike RBD, maybe? – they had in that internal database."

It wasn't the only thing to be deleted from the Institute's website. Using archive websites that capture a webpage at a specific time, researchers have been able to preserve some of the Wuhan Institute of Virology website before it was cleaned out. Most of the website was wiped entirely. Blog posts of foreign visits, project pages, committee details and old newsletters were all deleted from the website. A BSL-4 "Biosafety Laboratory Management" training course held in November 2019 was also deleted. Almost no reference to the course remains on the Institute's website.

On January 2, 2020, at 10.28am, the Wuhan Institute of Virology's Director-General, Yan-Yi Wang, silenced the staff. She sent an email to her employees titled: "Regarding the prohibition of disclosing information concerning the unexplained pneumonia in Wuhan". It was a gag order, preventing any of the researchers or employees from saying a word about the outbreak – or any of their research. "By order of the National Health Commission, all relevant information concerning the outbreak, testing, as well as data, results and conclusions from experimental treatments should not be published on social media, and should not be disclosed to the media (including official media), partner organisations (including technical service companies)," it states. PLA Major General Chen Wei, China's chief biochemical weapons defence expert, led a team to Wuhan on January 26, where she took over the BSL-4 laboratory. Under military control, staff members were silenced and subject to even greater surveillance than before. Chen Wei has worked for the Chinese military since she was 25 and specialises in researching deadly viruses such as the plague, anthrax and Ebola. According to the *Global Times*: "Chen said she believes pathogenic microbial could be used by others as lethal weapons during a war, and trigger a large-scale epidemic. 'I feel obliged to find a bio shield for the country and people,' said Chen."

She was one of the first people to receive a Covid-19 vaccine. "The world's first new coronavirus vaccine was injected into the left arm of the researcher and academician Major General Chen Wei today," a news report stated on March 4, 2020.

Miles Yu believes the military takeover of the Wuhan Institute of Virology is highly significant. "The negligence at China's biolabs, especially the WIV, was so dangerous that the PLA dispatched a general to take over the facility soon after the outbreak in Wuhan," he said.

One strong indication that China might have known the virus was the result of a lab leak is President Xi Jinping's announcement of a new national biosafety law in his very first speech on the outbreak, on February 12, 2020. He spoke about the "lessons learned" from the outbreak. Quite extraordinarily, he admitted it had exposed "shortcomings" and "leaking holes" in China's biological material management and biological security system. He said the Chinese government would immediately enact a new biological security law to "make biological security law a part of the national security system". "It is necessary to promote the promulgation of a biosafety law as soon as possible, and accelerate the construction of a national biosafety legal and regulatory system and an institutional guarantee system."

The military take-over at the Wuhan Institute of Virology came shortly after reports about a mysterious disappearance at the facility went mainstream in Chinese media.

Bright young microbiology researcher Huang Yanling had worked at the Wuhan Institute of Virology since she was 24 years old. Her future was so promising, *The Beijing News* reported that she had been recommended by the Southwest Jiaotong University to join the Wuhan Institute of Virology's Masters program in 2012. She graduated from the Institute with a Masters degree in 2015. Huang Yanling didn't work with Shi Zhengli. Instead, she worked under Professor Hongping Wei at the Centre for Emerging Infectious Diseases. In the early days of the pandemic, in February 2020, social media posts claiming Huang Yanling had disappeared swept Weibo and other Chinese forums. There was speculation that she might be patient zero. So extensive were the reports of her disappearance, a reporter from *The Beijing News* decided to investigate in mid-February. When journalist Du Wenwen was unable to track her down, she asked several Wuhan Institute of Virology workers what had happened to her. Shi Zhengli said, "How is it possible? This is fake news. I can guarantee that none of us, including graduate students, has been infected with the virus, and we have zero infection." Another Institute researcher, Chen Quanjiao, was quoted as saying: "We have no cases of infection in Wuhan Virus Research Institute."

Huang Yanling's boss at the Institute, Hongping Wei, also released a statement saying Huang Yanling had not worked there since 2015. "Huang graduated from the institute in 2015 with a master's degree," he said. "She has since then been working in other provinces and has never been back to Wuhan. She's not infected by the novel coronavirus and is in good health. At a crucial time fighting against the epidemic, this rumor has greatly disrupted the Institute's research work."

A post claiming to be from the missing scientist later appeared on WeChat, informing colleagues she was alive and well. It read: "To my teachers and fellow students, how long no speak. I am Huang Yanling, still alive. If you receive any email [regarding the Covid rumour], please say it's not true." But no firm proof of life was provided – such as a video or a media interview – to quell the rumours, and they continued to swell, with one woman even photographed standing at a public train station in China holding a sign saying, "Where is Huang Yanling?"

Adding fuel to the rumours was the fact Huang's profile had been wiped from the Wuhan Institute of Virology's website. The statement from Hongping Wei was exposed as a lie by the owner of a Twitter account called "WhereisYanling" dedicated to finding Huang Yanling. The owner, who says he needs to stay anonymous to protect his safety, discovered a photograph taken in 2018 of Huang Yanling standing just behind Hongping Wei among a group of researchers from the institute's Laboratory of Diagnostic Microbiology. It was taken three years after her boss claimed she had left the institute. It was a significant find and made the papers in the UK.

A page on the official Wuhan Institute of Virology website, under the Laboratory of Diagnostic Microbiology, features the photograph with a 2018 timestamp. It states "the research group currently has 6 researchers and 13 students". The page was deleted in February 2020 but is archived on the Wayback Machine.

Little else remains of Huang Yanling on the Chinese internet. She has no social media presence at all. We were able to find a second photograph of her, undated, where she is smiling, wearing a red overcoat. "The Chinese Government decided to scrub any mention of her from WeChat and the Chinese internet, rather than produce maybe a quick picture or some similar evidence that everything was ok," the Twitter account owner said. "I feel it's one of the easiest questions for the CCP and WIV to answer yet they won't or can't."

There was broad media reporting. A mainland China news site ran an article titled "Huang Yanling, show up soon!" It concludes by toeing the government line: "I think this is purely a rumour." An

Apple Daily report, dated January 2021, examined Huang Yanling's case, reaching no conclusion as to her whereabouts.

We found that Huang Yanling is named in three patent applications filed in November 2017 by Mike Biological (aka Maccura Biotechnology), based in Chengdu in southwest China, and two in March 2018. This could indicate she was working in Chengdu after the Wuhan Institute of Virology. We made repeated attempts at contacting employees of Maccura Biotechnology in Chengdu. In most instances, we were instantly hung up on. One employee of Maccura, however, later told us via WhatsApp that they had heard of and read about Huang Yanling but did not know anyone at the company by that name. "We're a company with more than 2600 people, I cannot know everyone of them," they said. "I have zero contact with this person, and I don't know how she was and how she is. Sorry."

It was a disappearance the US State Department and intelligence agencies investigated. "That's a very suspicious case," Miles Yu says. One line of inquiry within the US government and intelligence agencies was that Huang Yanling was one of the first to fall ill with the coronavirus around October 2019. Like the Twitter account dedicated to finding Huang Yanling, Yu says it could have been an easy victory for the CCP to produce its former researcher. "She basically disappeared. What happened is people found her information totally disappeared from the Wuhan website. Then the WIV came out and said she's alive and well and she's working at a different province and a different work unit," he said. "We don't know where the heck she is. Until this day. The particular point is this would have been such a big propaganda victory for the CCP. She could have come out easily and denied that she was sick. She never did." While her disappearance was widely noticed in China in January 2020, Yu says she went missing much earlier than that. "I think she disappeared before the outbreak, as we know it in December. I think she disappeared in the fall," he said.

Asher speculates that Huang Yanling could be one of the three workers who fell sick with Covid-19 in the first outbreak in

November 2019. But other senior administration officials said Huang Yanling could be a "red herring", to distract from examining the other researchers who fell sick and disappeared. Adding another theory in the works, Sir Richard Dearlove muses that perhaps Huang Yanling was a defector speaking to the Americans.

Where is she now? Yu says it is possible she is under police surveillance, which explains why she has never reappeared. The other alternative, he says, is that she is no longer alive.

The US government took the case so seriously it demanded answers. The NIH Deputy Director for Extramural Researcher, Michael Lauer, sent EcoHealth Alliance, which as we know had been working with the Wuhan Institute of Virology for 15 years, a letter in July 2020 saying its multimillion-dollar funding would remain suspended unless it provided information from the Wuhan Institute of Virology.

This included providing a sample of the pandemic coronavirus that the institute used to determine its genetic sequence, arranging for an external inspection of the institute and its records, and providing an explanation for "diminished cell-phone traffic in October 2019" and roadblocks around the facility in October 14–19, 2019. It also related to Huang Yanling: "Explain the apparent disappearance of Huang Yanling, a scientist/technician who worked in the WIV lab but whose presence has been deleted."

EcoHealth Alliance declined to assist, releasing a statement that said: "NIH's letter cynically reinstates and instantly suspends the EcoHealth Alliance's funding, then attempts to impose impossible and irrelevant conditions that will effectively block us from continuing this critical work." Peter Daszak then tweeted on August 21, 2020: "This person has never been associated with our work at Wuhan lab. As far as I'm aware, it's pure fake news, a junior tech who left, so name removed from website. Why should EcoHealth Alliance be forced to inquire about this to continue research NIH deemed high-priority?" He continued with another tweet: "NIH should treat us appropriately as a research org. they fund to produce science, not an intelligence-gathering branch of the US Govt. forced to investigate conspiracy theories. Imagine the reverse – a Chinese org. forced by its Govt to investigate CDC based on conspiracies!" Conspiracy theory is an easy term to bandy about to diminish the credibility of a genuine matter. As we have already seen, it has been used by Daszak to great effect when it comes to the origins and outbreak of Covid-19.

The fact is within the United States agencies there was genuine concern about Huang Yanling. She has not been heard from since she inexplicably went missing at the start of the pandemic. Her biography and research history have been wiped and no one has been able to produce her. As blogger Xie Bin wrote on February 15, in a Chinese post that has been viewed more than 4 million times: "In the past 72 hours, a name, a name that no one knew before, suddenly became the number one target of all hunters on the Chinese internet, and suddenly became a person who caught the eye more than any Internet celebrity. This person is 'Huang Yanling'."

Rumours of Huang Yanling's disappearance wasn't the only suspicious activity unfolding at the Wuhan Institute of Virology in early 2020. A female researcher and group leader, Chen Quanjiao, had been working with Shi Zhengli and Peng Zhou on that first study the institute published about the new coronavirus, where it indicated it had come from a bat. That study was published on February 3, 2020. The researcher, who graduated from Huazhong Agricultural University College of Animal Sciences in 1997, had been at the institute since 2003, where she was involved in publishing at least 10 studies related to influenza infection and the adaptation process of viruses in mice.

Two weeks after her study was published saying that the virus likely had a natural origin from bats, Chen Quanjiao sent an extraordinary social media post from her personal account on Weibo in which she accused her boss at the Wuhan Institute of Virology of being responsible for leaking the virus. "Hello everyone, my name is Chen Quanjiao, a researcher at the Wuhan Institute of Virology, my national ID number is 42242819740408626," she wrote on February 17. "I hereby report that the virus was leaked by Wang

Yanyi, director of the P4 Wuhan Institute of Virology." Chen then went on to attack her boss's credentials in her post. "Wang Yanyi has little knowledge of medicine. While at Beida [Peking] University, which enrols students only of high ability, other researchers did her research for her. She often sells animals used on experiments in the lab to game meat vendors in the South China Seafood Market. She is the culprit of the epidemic and her husband has brothers/friends who have grown up playing with a certain deputy state-level official. We must not forget Wang Yanyi, how many innocent people she has killed, and the lives lost."

The post was published at 11.51am on February 17, 2020 and included a selfie of Chen Quanjiao wrapped in a green scarf. Within minutes, the post disappeared. This allegation was never going to stay on the internet for any length of time. But in that short period she managed to get her message out. Her friends and colleagues spotted it and saved it.

A few hours later, an official post denying the allegation appeared on the Wuhan Institute of Virology site purporting to be from Chen. It said: "Statement by Chen Quanjiao. Regarding the so-called reporting remarks published in my name on the Internet today, I solemnly declare: I have never released any relevant report information, and expressed great indignation at the fraudulent use of my identity to fabricate the report information. I will pursue the legal responsibility of the rumours in accordance with the law. A series of recent rumours have affected the scientific research of our front-line researchers. Please guard against relevant conspiracy and sabotage activities."

Chen never gave a televised appearance denying she had made the original post, and neither did she publish any video on her social media. Remember, at this time, the Wuhan Institute of Virology was under strict military control under the command of top PLA weapons expert Chen Wei. But the matter was far from over.

The next day, a Chinese dissident based in Hawaii, with a large online presence of more than 140,000 followers, tweeted that what Chen had said was true. "I just received a private message from a friend on Twitter claiming to be a relative of Chen Quanjiao of the Wuhan Institute of Virology, claiming that Chen's allegation is true. Chen's currently controlled official rumor statement are fake." He then published a screenshot of a private DM conversation over Twitter, which we have translated. In it, the individual introduces himself as a friend and colleague of Chen's at the Wuhan Institute of Virology. He claims the refutation that appeared on the institute's website under Chen's name was issued under duress. He said the original Weibo post was in fact from Chen.

Again, there was no on-camera testimony refuting her private post's authenticity. Chen's profile remains on the Wuhan Institute of Virology website, with a similar picture of her in a green scarf but this time standing in a beautiful Chinese garden. Since the February 2020 paper, she has only been named on one other paper, in November 2020, according to multiple Chinese academic portals.

This private social media post purportedly from a Wuhan Institute of Virology insider was extremely damaging to the institute and specifically Wang Yanyi, its Director. Wang Gaofei, Chief Executive of social media platform Weibo, condemned the posts as "fake news" and said the messages originated from an overseas IP address, according to multiple press reports.

Three months later, on May 25, 2020, Wang Yanyi herself addressed allegations that the virus had leaked from her laboratory in a televised interview broadcast on Chinese state media, CGTN. "This is pure fabrication," she said "Our institute first received the clinical sample of the unknown pneumonia on December 30 last year. After we checked the pathogen within the sample, we found it contained a new coronavirus, which is now called SARS-CoV-2. We didn't have any knowledge before that, nor had we ever encountered, researched or kept the virus. In fact, like everyone else, we didn't even know the virus existed. How could it have leaked from our lab when we never had it?"

With insiders under immense scrutiny and pressure, and under the surveillance of the military, scientists outside the laboratory tried to get the word out about what they claim had happened at the facility. A biologist named Dr Wu Xiaohua posted a series of statements on her personal WeChat account pointing the finger squarely at the Wuhan Institute of Virology. A medical doctor, she has a Masters in atmospheric physics and a double PhD in ancient climatology and anthropology. She published damaging allegations about Shi Zhengli and the institute in a series of posts written under her own name on February 3, 2020. Taking the risk of publishing such allegations, knowing the repercussions, was incredibly brave.

Dr Wu wrote that she believes the virus is one of 50 in a database Shi Zhengli manages. She also said the Wuhan Institute of Virology is managed in an extremely haphazard way, and speculated that the virus could have leaked from the laboratory. She pointed the blame squarely at Shi Zhengli and challenged her to answer questions about suspicious gene mutations in SARS-CoV-2.

In another post, Dr Wu said she was aware that Shi Zhengli oversaw the poor disposal practices of animals that had been tested on with viruses and suggests this may have been the origin of the pandemic. She says some WIV researchers had sold animals used in experiments to wet markets in Wuhan, while others had even been sold as pets. She also said that dead laboratory animals were not properly disposed of and some lab workers had even been known to boil and eat laboratory-used eggs.

What Dr Wu's connection was – if any – to the Wuhan Institute of Virology or where she was getting her information from remains unknown.

In making the allegations on her personal Weibo account, she took an extraordinary risk that may have cost her her personal freedom, or even her life. Dr Wu's whereabouts are now unknown.

Her Weibo posts in February 2020 were her last. She has not surfaced online since then.

The claims of unhygienic, unsafe or improper disposal of animals used for laboratory testing may seem very unlikely given the strict protocols in Western laboratories. But while investigating this book, we uncovered firm evidence that these bizarre and shocking practices of poor disposal of diseased animals were taking place in

Chinese laboratories. It also became common for diseased animals from laboratories to be sold to wet markets.

Professor Li Ning, a biologist with the Chinese Academy of Engineering and Director of the State Key Laboratory of Agricultural Biotechnology at China Agricultural University, was highly regarded in his field. His colleague Zhang Lei, also considered a "distinguished associate researcher" at the Key Laboratory of China Agricultural University, was in charge of several subjects under the Ministry of Science and Technology, according to a Shanghai-based news outlet The Paper. Their research had focused on transgenic animals in agriculture.

While holding these senior academic positions, the two scientists founded a company called Beijing Jifulin Biotech. Between 2008 and 2012, they used this company to sell laboratory testing animals and animal products such as milk after they had been used for experiments. The animals were purchased with research funds, but Li Ning and a colleague pocketed a massive ¥34 million (US$5.2 million) which was deposited into three bank accounts. None of the money was returned to China Agricultural University.

The case ended up in court. "These experimental materials were purchased with project funds. According to the provisions of the fund management, the realizable funds should be handed over to China Agricultural University after the sale," a witness Ou Moujia testified. The court heard evidence from several witnesses relating to falsely issuing invoices at Zhang Lei's request. There were two trials over five years before a judgment was handed down in January 2020. Li Ning was sentenced to 12 years in prison for embezzlement and corruption. This court case offers conclusive proof of the practice of selling animals that have been used in laboratory experiments, as well as the profits to be made when this is done at scale over a number of years. Pompeo said there is no question used laboratory animals are on-sold in China. "There's no doubt that there were animals that could have been sold to the wet market, that was a practice that had taken place," he said.

On January 18, 2020, the Wuhan Institute of Virology's Director-General, Wang Yanyi, denied allegations that animals used in lab experiments were resold at Huanan Seafood Market. Xu Bo, the Chinese multimillionaire Chairman of technology firm Duoyi, based in Shenzhen, referenced this court judgment when making his own allegations against the Wuhan Institute of Virology. The technology entrepreneur risked his life to write a very long post on his personal Weibo in February 2020, where he echoed Wu Xiaohua's claims that the institute was the source of the virus.

Xu's post was titled: "This time it is no pandemic, but a biological crisis". "I think this is a man-made catastrophe caused by a genetically modified virus, and the people who caused this disaster really deserve to die," he wrote. "Based on the following facts and evidence and because of the importance of epidemic prevention work, I hereby state that I suspect that the Wuhan Institute of Virology has caused the 2019 novel coronavirus pandemic through the misappropriation of laboratory animals which caused the virus to leak out," he said. "I have decided to report the Wuhan Institute of Virology to the nation, hoping that the misappropriation of laboratory animals in the institute and the research on the transformation of related bat coronaviruses into humans will be investigated. I support research into genetic modification, but I strongly believe we must be vigilant and careful in the direction it goes in. We must be particularly vigilant about research into genetic modification that may pose major risks to our nation's interests. Otherwise, if it is not well managed, it is likely to cause heavy losses to the country and great harm to the survival prospects and development of the Chinese nation." Xu Bo even went into great detail about the ACE2 receptors, synthetic biology and gain-of-function research, specifically calling out Shi Zhengli.

His post appeared on February, 2020, so it's quite extraordinary he was across this level of detail about the work that was being conducted at the institute months and months before anyone in the Western world learned about it. Xu is a very active Weibo user, and today his account shows that every single post from December 2019 to March 2020 has been deleted. It is likely he faced an incredibly strict punishment from the Public Security Bureau or another secretive state security organ, and it's possible his public profile was the only thing that stopped him from disappearing altogether.

This was a high-profile individual – not an anonymous blogger – who risked his life to alert the world to what he believed was the cause of the Covid-19 outbreak. Not only were his claims not subjected to proper examination by Western intelligence agencies and scientists, but they were shamefully dismissed as debunked conspiracy theories.

At the very least, we owe it to these brave souls to investigate the claims that somemay have given up their lives to expose.

One close research colleague of Shi Zhengli's on coronaviruses had serious military affiliations: the decorated military scientist Zhou Yusen.

Zhou Yusen worked at the Laboratory of Infection and Immunity, Beijing Institute of Microbiology and Epidemiology, which is part of the Chinese Academy of Military Medical Sciences and sits under the control of the PLA.

Born in 1966, Zhou Yusen was about 54 years old when the virus broke out in Wuhan.

His work for the Chinese military was extensive. Not only did he graduate from the Chinese Academy of Military Medical Sciences in 1998, but he won the first prize of scientific and technological progress of the army.

Like Shi Zhengli, his research focus was "new infectious disease pathogens" and immunology research. He worked under Cao Wuchan, a senior PLA colonel who sits on the board of the Wuhan Institute of Virology.

Despite his work for the PLA, Zhou Yusen's research was at times funded by the NIH and he had ties to the United States. He did his postdoctoral research at the University of Pittsburgh School of Medicine and has collaborated closely with the New York Blood Center.

On February 24, 2020 – and this is a scandal in itself – Zhou Yusen filed a patent application for a Covid-19 vaccine in China (an image from which is extracted below). Yes, China's senior military scientist is listed as the lead inventor on a patent for a SARS-CoV-2 vaccine just one month after China admitted Covid-19 was capable of human-to-human transmission. It shows China developed a vaccine for Covid-19 extremely early on and suggests it is possible they were working on it before they officially confirmed to WHO authorities there was an outbreak.

The patent abstract, unearthed for this book, states: "The invention relates to the field of biomedicine, and relates to a Covid-19 vaccine, preparation methods and applications. The fusion protein provided by the invention can be used to develop the Covid-19 protein vaccine and a drug for preventing or treating the Covid-19." The application was lodged by the "Institute of Military Medicine, Academy of Military Sciences of the PLA". That was February 24, 2020.

In an extraordinary twist, Zhou Yusen's name appears next in a December 2020 paper with an asterisk. The explanation at the end of the paper says "Deceased". He is thought to have died sometime around May 2020.

Despite being an award-winning military scientist who invented China's first Covid-19 vaccine, there were no reports paying tribute to his life. His death was only mentioned in passing in a Chinese-media report in July where it had the word "deceased" in brackets after his name.

Five Eyes intelligence agencies are aware of the death of this PLA scientist working closely with Shi Zhengli, multiple sources interviewed for this book confirmed. One source told me there is no conclusive knowledge about how and why he died, but it was treated as suspicious. A very close relative of his is understood to be working in America as a virologist. US officials tell me it is possible he was killed by the PLA out of concerns the relative had defected, but this was speculation.

Right before the outbreak of Covid-19, Zhou Yusen was working with none other than the Wuhan Institute of Virology's Shi Zhengli along with the University of Minnesota and the NY Blood Center, on a research paper about genetically manipulating coronaviruses. It was funded with three grants from the NIH via the American universities, which took the lead on the project.

They were experimenting with both MERS and SARS coronaviruses.

Their paper had some positive results: "Taken together, our results show that RBD-specific neutralising MAbs bind to the same region on coronavirus spikes as viral receptors do, trigger conformational changes of the spikes as viral receptors do, and mediate ADE through the same pathways as viral-receptor-dependent viral entry."

They found this "novel molecular mechanism for antibody-enhanced viral entry" could "guide future vaccination and antiviral strategies".

This study was conducted "in vitro". Their last paragraph indicated the next step in a future paper would be to conduct "in vivo" experiments with humanised mice or primates. A paper published in *Nature Reviews Immunology* in April 2021, 18 months later, would find that "neutralising monoclonal antibodies" could help the treatment of Covid-19.

As far back as 2004, the PLA-trained Zhou Yusen was experimenting with spike proteins in coronaviruses.

A 2004 paper Zhou Yusen co-authored and published in the *Journal of Immunology* states: "We showed that the S protein of SARS-CoV is highly immunogenic." Immunogenic is the technical term for how well a virus or vaccine provokes an immune response. Two years later, in 2006, Zhou Yusen was listed as the main author of a paper that stated the "receptor-binding domain (RBD) of SARS-CoV spike (S) protein elicits highly potent neutralizing antibody responses in the immunized animals."

The study made clear that they were looking at vaccine development. Its conclusion states: "In summary, the vaccines containing the RBD of SARS-CoV S protein may induce sufficient neutralizing antibodies and long-term protective immunity against SARS-CoV challenge in the established mouse model. Our results suggest that RBD-Fc vaccine can be further developed as an ideal subunit vaccine for prevention of SARS epidemic."

So as long ago as 2006, a military scientist was researching the very point of infectivity of coronaviruses and simultaneously working on a vaccine. He was working with Shi Zhengli and the Wuhan Institute of Virology, he would invent the first Covid-19 vaccine for the Chinese military, and then he would die mysteriously months later.

The Wuhan Institute of Virology certainly had its fair share of problems. As early as autumn 2019, three workers fell ill with Covid-19-like symptoms. They were so unwell at least one of them, and perhaps more, needed hospital treatment. It's understood they were treated at the PLA hospital just one subway ride away from the Institute.

Their illness occurred weeks – maybe months – before the coronavirus was reported to the WHO. Months before China admitted it had a contagious coronavirus on its hands. When Shi Zhengli was asked about the sick workers she denied anyone at the Wuhan Institute of Virology had been sick at all and said every staff member was tested for SARS antibodies and no one returned a positive result. This is statistically implausible given the pandemic outbreak in Wuhan.

A WHO team member who visited Wuhan on the recent study tour, Marion Koopmans, confirmed that "one or two" workers fell sick. Her view was that it was not unusual and she did not indicate any employees had been hospitalised. But the intelligence is definitive that the Wuhan Institute of Virology workers were sick. It is unassailable, multiple sources tell me.

Pompeo says "it's entirely possible" these workers were the first cluster and "its certainly reasonable to believe" that. "It is of course circumstantial, but they became sick in the fall [autumn] of 2019, so the timing works," he said. On Shi Zhengli's denial any workers were sick, Pompeo tells me, "Here was this researcher Shi Zhengli who said there was zero infection, no infection among the staff. That's the same person they send out to do obfuscation on other issues," he says. "So the fact that's the person they sent out to deny what we now have good reason to believe to be true, it all suggests there was something to this. We also know there's a pattern or practice of this in these Chinese laboratories. It's one thing to say, hey there was this group of people who became sick with symptoms consistent with Covid-19 and by the way we know this kind of thing has happened repeatedly in the Chinese Communist Party system, the Chinese Communist Party has done this before, they've tried to cover it up before. So when I stare at that set of facts it gives me more reason to lend credence to this theory."

Asher, whose team unearthed the intelligence, first revealed the workers had been hospitalised in an interview with me that I broadcast on *Sky News* and published in *The Australian* newspaper in March 2021. "There were multiple staff members who did have to go to hospital and appeared to have had conditions of Covid-19," Asher said. "You don't normally go to the hospital with influenza, especially a cluster of people. This is the most probable source of the outbreak."

It was possible, Asher said, that there were clusters of Covid-19 before this outbreak in November, pointing to a spike in influenza in China in the autumn of 2019 that he said may have included coronavirus cases. "The point of the declassified information that Secretary Pompeo provided was that we had information that there was indeed a cluster, and they worked on related coronaviruses at the Wuhan Institute of Virology, which is almost too much of a coincidence to believe," he said.

Wuhan University Professor of Biostatistics Yu Chuanhua told the *Health Times* on February 27, 2020 he had viewed records showing two cases on November 14 and 19, 2019, and one suspected case on September 29, 2019. In total, he said there were 47,000 confirmed and suspected cases on a national database by late February 2020.

Yu Chuanhua said the September 29 Covid-19 patient had died. As the gag order was issued in Wuhan, Yu Chuanhua phoned the media outlet and asked to retract the information he had given. But it was already in the public domain. Photographs of their medical records provided to the *Health Times* include information about where the patients lived and were treated. Analysing these records, journalist Ian Birrell reported in *The Daily Mail* that one patient, a 61-year-old woman named Su, lived about a mile from one of China's Centre for Disease Control laboratories studying coronaviruses in the Hongshan district.

Scientist Jesse Bloom, in June 2021, discovered SARS-CoV-2 deep sequencing data from early Wuhan patients had been uploaded to the NIH Sequence Read Archive, but was later deleted. "The deleted dataset contains sequencing of viral samples collected early in the Wuhan epidemic," Bloom wrote in his scientific paper. The metadata suggested the samples had been collected by Renmin Hospital of Wuhan University.

Bloom was unable to access any of this data from the NIH's Sequence Read Archive website, but he was able to recover the data from the cloud where it had been initially stored.

He found that the "early Wuhan samples that have been the focus of most studies including the joint WHO-China report are not fully representative of the viruses actually present in Wuhan at that time."

"Samples from early outpatients in Wuhan are a gold mine for anyone seeking to understand spread of the virus," he wrote, noting "there is no plausible scientific reason for the deletion."

Another interesting finding is that the earliest reported sequences from Wuhan are not the sequences most similar to SARS-CoV-2's bat coronavirus relatives. "This fact is perplexing because, although the proximal origin of SARS-CoV-2 remains unclear (i.e. zoonosis versus lab accident), all reasonable explanations agree that at a deeper level the SARS-CoV-2 genome is derived from bat coronaviruses," he wrote.

"One would therefore expect the first reported SARS-CoV-2 sequences to be the most similar to these bat coronaviruses relatives – but this is not the case."

At the time of going to print, no explanation from NIH leadership, including Francis Collins, had been given as to why the NIH would have agreed to delete these crucial early sequences relating to the outbreak.

Asher says, "It's incredible under the records act to allow China [to delete such data]. The NIH engaging in the withdrawal of public records that are supposed to be kept forever is borderline illegal and the fact they did it on behalf of the CCP health apparatus, which was trying to cover-up its own digital fingerprints, is astonishing, disturbing and downright unbelievable."

State Department investigators examined whether the three who fell sick may have been among the patients whose earliest genetic sequences were posted on a genomic database but were later deleted. Another piece of evidence examined by the US State Department and some intelligence analysts is that patient zero was an infected worker from the Wuhan Institute of Virology who stopped by the wet market on the way home for dinner. His wife was later infected and died. Matt Turpin explains that intelligence has high degrees of uncertainty to it. "You're trying to piece together bits and parts of what you're looking at," he said. "The US government is trying to play its cards straight. There are things we have suspicions of, but we are not omnipotent. We don't know all the answers."

A Five Eyes intelligence source tells me the three sick Wuhan Institute of Virology workers "could be constructed in such a way to lend support" to the lab leak hypothesis, "but our analysts are not saying it's proven". "You could construct a circumstantial case from those separate fragmentary pieces of information," he says. "I can't say it's definitive evidence."

But Stilwell's view is the classified report was persuasive. "The intel was pretty clear and we wanted a statement that was as compelling as the intel itself," he says. "You can imagine from the initial report to what was released publicly there were some data and details that were sensitive and that we had to dumb down or cut out."

CHAPTER TWENTY-FIVE

The Missing

NOVEMBER 2020, WASHINGTON DC

As Asher was probing the origin of the pandemic, an extraordinary thing happened. A trusted contact he had known for years offered to put him in touch with an employee at the Wuhan Institute of Virology who had been in the facility at the time of the outbreak.

Asher regarded the intermediary as reliable and contact was made. Asher interviewed the Institute employee over video.

"That person told me about the workers falling ill. This person was present in Wuhan, at the Wuhan Institute of Virology, doing research when all hell broke loose," Asher says.

The information from the foreign scientist, with direct access to the Institute and its other staff, supported and seemed to corroborate the intelligence that workers had fallen sick. Just days after the AVC investigation was shut down by the Biden administration in early 2021, Asher then had contact with another individual who claimed to have first-hand information from Wuhan.

"It was a digital walk-in," he says. This person worked with Shi Zhengli. "They said they had worked at the Wuhan Institute of Virology and they wanted to tell me some stuff about what was going on there," he said. "There were all sorts of things they had been forced to do against their will by the Chinese military, including research that they felt was hazardous. This person showed me chat messages via a video. The laboratory worker claimed to have information about what had happened." The Institute employee claimed the outbreak started with a monkey bite in October.

Asher passed the information he had obtained onto his former colleagues, but he never heard back, perhaps because the State had stood down the AVC taskforce and reassigned its members to unrelated jobs.

A month later, in March 2021, he had indirect contact with a second scientist from another Wuhan lab but who has knowledge of the Wuhan Institute of Virology's relationship to the Covid-19 outbreak. Similar claims were made, with the main line that the outbreak was not the fault of the Wuhan Institute of Virology but the PLA was to blame for making the Institute conduct the risky research. The person also illuminated some sort of internal dispute inside the Wuhan Institute of Virology leadership between Shi Zhengli and Yuan Zhiming. This informant claimed the Institute was also involved in a much larger intra–Communist Party power struggle between former Chinese President Jiang Zemin and current "President for life" Xi Jinping.

There is limited documented evidence to support the claims made by the alleged Wuhan Institute of Virology veteran researchers. While Asher could confirm and verify the identities of the three individuals who passed on information to him, he emphasises that their information cannot be verified and their motives are unclear. Asher says we cannot rule out the possibility that the information extended to him was from someone working on behalf of the PLA or the Ministry of State Security, designed to mislead or cause other interference. He worries it could even have come from exiled Chinese billionaire Miles Guo's people and amounts to misinformation. "When someone calls me up through a secondary party, even a reliable one, and starts to tell me we were forced to do this by the PLA, it wasn't our fault. I immediately think it's the PLA," Asher says.

He took the information very seriously but ultimately could not ascertain if their claims were genuine or part of a Communist Party set-up. If genuine, their lives would be at-risk.

Former senior Trump administration officials confirm there was also a defector in Europe. A senior US source told me the United States tried to reach this defector but the person refused to speak to anyone in the administration. The United States conduit even offered for Pompeo to speak with the defector, but the option was declined.

The extent of China's Covid-19 cover-up far exceeded its standard authoritarian predilection for secrecy. Human-rights groups wonder in horror at the true number of people who have disappeared while trying to expose the source of the outbreak and the events unfolding in Wuhan. But there are some names we know (see Chapter 6). And all were attempting to make secret information public.

Chen Qiushi, the young lawyer who caught the last train to Wuhan, has not been seen since he disappeared in the midst of the outbreak, although there are unverified reports that he is under house arrest in east China with his parents. His Twitter account is run by a friend, who posts a daily reminder of the number of days Chen has been missing to his 335,000 followers. "We are still waiting for Chen Qiushi's return. Until he reappears, we will keep on counting the days. Chen Qiushi has been out of contact for 477 days after covering coronavirus in Wuhan. Please remember him!" his friend posted on May 28, 2021.

Li Zehua, the television journalist who followed Chen Qiushi into Wuhan and was arrested in his hotel room, disappeared for 56 days. He resurfaced in a bizarre video that showed him standing in front of a white wall. His address to the camera appeared to be well rehearsed and scripted. In the video, he said he had been in forced "quarantine". "Throughout the process, the police followed the law. They guaranteed my rest time and diet, and also cared about me," he said in the video. "Thanks to everyone who cared about and took care of me." Those who had been following his case, waiting anxiously for news, were sceptical.

Fang Bin, the Wuhan businessman who filmed bodies of coronavirus victims inside buses and went inside hospitals, is still missing. His family have frantically been trying to find out from authorities whether he is still alive. They are too fearful to speak with journalists. Real estate tycoon and political commentator Ren Zhiqiang is serving 18 years in prison, charged with corruption, bribery and embezzlement. Lawyer Zhang Zhan is also in prison, serving a four-year term. She is the first citizen journalist to be sentenced for reporting on the pandemic. Activist and former academic Xu Zhiyong, arrested while hiding at the home of a friend, is still in detention after calling Xi Jinping "clueless". He was originally charged with "inciting subversion", but it is understood the charge has been upgraded to the more serious "subversion of state power". His girlfriend, Li Qiaochu, was also formally arrested in March 2021 and is facing the same serious charge, many believing as punishment for speaking out about Xu being tortured while in detention. After multiple delays with their case, Cai Wei and Chen Mei, who were caught archiving information the CCP was wiping from the internet, both pleaded guilty to "picking quarrels and provoking troubles" on May 11, 2021. At the time of writing, they are awaiting sentencing.

Cédric Alviani, East Asia Bureau chief for not-for-profit group Reporters Without Borders, says more than 100 people have been punished for sharing information about Covid-19. "You can censor information on a virus; it's not going to stop the virus from circulating even more," he said. "It is not acceptable that one person would be punished for circulating accurate information. This is almost a sacred principle; one should not be punished for sharing information. The only way for the public to hold the powerful accountable and to hold their representatives accountable is to be able to base their decisions on facts."

Those sentenced to so-called house arrest in China are not exactly sitting at home watching Netflix. Rather, a report by Madrid-based human rights NGO Safeguard Defenders describes residential surveillance as "mass state-sanctioned kidnapping" and "enforced disappearance". "Using data from court verdict cases posted to the Supreme Court database, we estimated that at least 28,000 to 29,000 people were placed into Residential Surveillance at a Designated Location by the end of 2019 since the system came into effect in 2013," it states. But Safeguard Defenders estimates the true number of Chinese living under residential surveillance is far higher, with the official data only capturing cases with verdicts.

Asked what happens when people go missing in China, former MI6 chief Sir Richard Dearlove says: "They're either killed or they end up in concentration camps or the equivalent of concentration camps." Asher says the extent of the disappearances and the cover-up is a "very unusual situation". "That's not how the Chinese responded in SARS in 2002–2003. I was a senior advisor for East-Asian Pacific Affairs in the State Department and I happened to be in Beijing for discussions with the Chinese government on SARS and they were much more forthcoming," he said. "They gave us access to data. It wasn't great but it wasn't this huge cover-up. This time, they responded to few of our requests for information and basically none of our myriad offers of assistance, let alone information."

CHAPTER TWENTY-SIX

The Case for a Lab Leak

Peter Daszak, Anthony Fauci and Shi Zhengli could be right. Covid-19 could be a natural virus. It is not beyond the realm of possibility that a cousin of BtCov/4991, the virus with a genetic sequence 96 per cent identical to that of SARS-CoV-2, existed in the Yunnan cave where the eight viruses genetically closest to Covid-19 were found. It's also possible Covid-19 arose from a natural recombination event when an animal such as a pangolin was infected with two viruses at the same time and they combined to create SARS-CoV-2.

It is equally possible the virus crossed the xenographic barrier between animals and humans and spread asymptomatically in the Yunnan region, where the surrounding population may have developed antibodies or immunity to coronaviruses, according to some scientific research done by Shi Zhengli and Peter Daszak before the outbreak. The coronavirus may then have been transported to Wuhan, a 20-hour drive away, through an infected but asymptomatic individual who was perhaps a seller at the Wuhan wet market.

There is a strong history of natural viruses arising in wildlife, including SARS-CoV-1, MERS, HIV and many influenza viruses responsible for pandemics. "The historical basis for pandemics evolving naturally from an animal reservoir is extremely strong and it's for that reason we felt that something similar like this has a much higher likelihood," Fauci said. This is all conceivable. Yet it's undeniably troubling that after 80,000 animal samples from wildlife farms surrounding Yunnan and Wuhan there is no evidence of Covid-19 in nature or in any intermediary host.

Alternatively, SARS-CoV-2 may have arisen naturally in the Yunnan cave where it was then collected by Wuhan Institute of Virology scientists, or their colleagues, who were crawling around in crevices on their stomachs to access remote, disease-ridden bats. The researchers taking the samples may have become infected. Contradicting Peter Daszak's insistence that staff wore head-to-toe protective equipment, there is photographic evidence of Wuhan lab samplers failing to take basic precautions. One Wuhan Centre for Disease Control scientist went into quarantine on multiple occasions after being covered in blood and urine from a bat he was sampling.

In an alternative scenario, a naturally occurring virus may have been taken back to the Wuhan laboratories for research and, through the transportation process, an accidental leak may have occurred, allowing the virus to spread in Wuhan. Or perhaps it leaked when researchers took the natural virus out of their freezers for experiments, failing to realise just how highly infectious it is.

These are all possibilities where a virus arising naturally in disease-ridden bats leaks and sparks an outbreak.

But given the concern from some eminent scientists that SARS-CoV-2 seems almost perfectly designed to infect humans, combined with an intense period of unusual and unexplained activity that points to an incident at the Wuhan Institute of Virology in the lead-up to the coronavirus pandemic, it is reasonable to suspect the virus was the subject of laboratory research.

For years, Shi Zhengli and her team have been manipulating viruses, inserting spike protein genes into coronaviruses to make them more infectious among humans. Through this process they at times created new deadly viruses that did not previously exist in nature, using techniques that hid any trace of genetic manipulation. It was deceptive for scientists throughout 2020 to assert time and time again that there was no sign of genetic manipulation in

SARS-CoV-2 and that this constituted evidence it couldn't have come from a laboratory. They know full well these experiments can leave no trace.

Dr Steven Quay asks why any scientist would want to cover their tracks, hiding that they had manipulated a virus. Indeed, how could disguising human intervention in a virus ever benefit mankind? The Wuhan scientists were playing with fire.

Even more disturbingly, there is extensive evidence that these experiments were conducted in dubious laboratories with poor safety records and a paucity of trained staff. Even the Director of the BSL-4 laboratory, Yuan Zhiming, was highly concerned about the safety protocols at the Wuhan Institute of Virology. It's something the Institute openly admitted to visiting US officials in 2017 and 2018.

And international partners were complicit in so much of this. The global scientific community not only had full knowledge of this dual-use gain-of function research, permitting it to be conducted in China's unsafe laboratories, but Australia trained leading scientists, France constructed the laboratory with China, and America funded scientific research, even after banning it within the United States.

Those whose job it was to keep us safe from pandemics and global disasters turned a blind eye when China admitted in its 2011 official submission to the Biological and Toxins Weapons Convention that it was facing compliance challenges because of its research genetically manipulating coronaviruses that had dual-use capabilities for nefarious purposes. China's official government submission warned, "Accidental mistakes in biotech laboratories can place mankind in great danger."

Political leaders, health authorities and global regulatory bodies looked the other way in the name of international collaboration and science. In reality, our national leaders lacked the courage to confront China as Xi Jinping forged ahead with his civil–military fusion, blurring the lines between civilian research and secret projects for the Chinese military. They chose not to say anything that could cause offence to an increasingly aggressive superpower or that would impose boundaries on the limitless quests of scientists.

The coronavirus research at the Wuhan Institute of Virology was often conducted in conjunction with senior military scientists. A PLA colonel even sat on the board, while military scientists at a defence university, classified as high-risk by China analysts for its level of defence research, publicly boasted coronaviruses could be weaponised, while teaching PhD students how to unleash a bioweapon.

And Anthony Fauci can't walk back from his own published words. He acknowledged in a 2012 paper published in a scientific journal that gain-of-function research is a form of "bioterrorism" and an accident could spark a pandemic. But he forged on regardless, allowing funding to flow from the NIH through to the Wuhan Institute of Virology. He knew virus research could spark a pandemic. But he took the risk anyway, claiming it was "important research" and that the chance of a pandemic was "remote". He even clumsily admitted he funded the research in China to avoid an outbreak in Hoboken, New Jersey. And so the Wuhan Institute of Virology was permitted to persist with its research, funded in part by the United States.

Supporting the likelihood of a laboratory leak is the weight of circumstantial evidence pointing to a series of incidents around October and potentially as early as mid-September 2019. The decision to wipe the Institute's virus database and take it offline is highly suspicious and significant. This discovery that the database was taken offline – never to be uploaded again – suggests an initial incident around September 12. This is followed by a series of unusual incidents in October, including a blackout period with no cell-phone or signals activity inside the building, indicating no one was on the premises except for a security guard. It's likely the Wuhan Institute of Virology shut down the facility for a mass sterilisation, as per protocol, then, thinking it was on top of the accident, moved back in, only to realise the highly infectious virus had already spread beyond their control. We know Covid-19 has a long incubation period.

Athletes visiting Wuhan for the Military World Games in October fell sick long before anyone knew there was an outbreak – some later believing they and their families had contracted Covid-19.

In early November, the Institute ordered a PCR machine to test for coronaviruses, and boosted its security systems. At the same time, three workers from the Institute fell sick, even requiring hospitalisation, with Covid-19-like symptoms. Yet Shi Zhengli lied when asked if anyone at the facility had been unwell. China's cover-up was aggressive. Multiple people who claimed to have information about the origin of the virus, including linking it to the institute's BSL-4 lab, disappeared (now feared dead), or have been silenced, under house arrest, living like tortured prisoners.

In January 2020, the military took over the Wuhan Institute of Virology, silencing, controlling and surveilling anyone in the facility.

Disturbingly, a senior PLA scientist working with Shi Zhengli filed a patent for a coronavirus vaccine on February 23, 2020 – remarkably early – only to die by May in mysterious circumstances.

The scientific evidence is equally as compelling. As many scientists have noted, SARS-CoV-2 has highly unusual features that point to a laboratory origin. The genetic code for a furin cleavage site – which has never been seen before in betacoronaviruses – appears in the precise spot in the S gene where scientists genetically tweak viruses to make them more infectious to humans. And the spike protein the S gene makes has a higher binding affinity to the human ACE2 receptor than that of any other animal.

The question then is, what does this all mean? Does this circumstantial and scientific evidence amount to an overwhelming case that Covid-19 leaked from a laboratory? To answer this question, former intelligence agency leaders at the CIA, NSA, MI6 and Five Eyes intelligence network offer their unparalleled insights. Former head of British spy agency MI6 Sir Richard Dearlove said in an interview for this book that the evidence supports a laboratory leak. "The weight of evidence is actually on the escapee side and it's strongly on the escapee side. If you look at the evidence coldly, the likelihood is this is an escape from a laboratory, and it's up to the

Chinese to demonstrate conclusively to us that it isn't, not to just tell us."

Sir Richard says if you look at the "biochemistry of the virus, it's more likely it's a result of gain-of-function experiments and not zoonotic. The weight of scientific evidence actually tells us that this is an escapee from a laboratory. What the Chinese have managed to do is to turn the story onto its head. What we've got to do now is to turn it back so that people really understand what we're dealing with. I'm not saying they deliberately released it, I'm saying this is a Chinese accident but there was a cover-up from day one."

Mike Rogers is a highly decorated former US Navy admiral who served as the Commander of the Tenth Fleet and Commander of the US Fleet Cyber Command. He was a member of the military's Joint Staff, the most senior uniformed leaders within the Department of Defense, during the first stage of the Iraq war. He was director of the NSA, which specialises in signals intelligence, from 2014, when Obama was President, and through to 2018, under Trump.

Rogers, in an interview for this book, says the circumstantial evidence could point to a laboratory origin for Covid-19. "You can certainly point to lots of different data points. The fact they [the Chinese] haven't been open; the fact that in the October timeframe there certainly seems to be some unusual activity in the vicinity of the national lab there. What does that mean? It would also appear based on all the information in the public domain this clearly started well before the Chinese government initially acknowledged it. There was clearly activity ongoing for weeks, if not months, before this, and you can tell that because they were cutting down, restricting travel, they were restricting movement in the city. They were clearly taking visible steps. They were directing members of the media and health authorities to not speak to the outside world. There's some emails where the researchers talk about, 'Hey I'm going to get into trouble if I raise this with anybody.' And 'We've been told to be quiet.' That is on the public record.

"So I think clearly this happened well before the timeline that the Chinese government has officially acknowledged. Why? What are you trying to hide, that it came from you and not from the marketplace? It is a testament that there is still so much uncertainty. Part of me would be saying to the Chinese, it's in your best interest to show documentation that puts this issue to bed. They are clearly not thinking along those lines, or they don't want to think along those lines, because the documentation and the evidence in fact would reveal that it did come from the lab."

If you take the laboratory leak as a premise, Rogers says it is likely a worker was infected. "If you accept the origin was the lab, the most common scenario I've heard speculated, and we don't have definitive proof, is an employee in the lab inadvertently becomes infected who then in the course of interaction with the market comes into contact and the disease ends up shifting from the individual," he says. "I don't think we definitely know who patient zero is. The key to this always is finding patient zero. You're always trying to get to the point of origin. I don't think there's agreement that we've identified patient zero yet."

A high-level Five Eyes intelligence source describes the evidence that the virus came from the laboratory as "compelling" and says there had been "active Chinese disinformation".

Former CIA Director Mike Pompeo had access to the top-secret intelligence on the origins of the virus during his time as US Secretary of State. "My sense is that if you said you have to weigh the possibilities, I would say the most likely probability is that it was a worker who infected either someone through the wet market or some place through there or family members through a secondary transmission," he says. Pompeo believes the Wuhan Institute of Virology, over and above other Wuhan virology labs, is the most likely source of the outbreak. "I haven't seen any avenues that would support a leak from any of their other sites," he said.

Pompeo stresses the significance of the cover-up and the active effort by China to direct attention away from the laboratories. "I'm going to let you piece something together. We've walked through the main elements of the things we know; they cumulatively lead me to conclude that by far and away the most enormous weight of evidence leads one to believe that this was a leak that came from the Wuhan Institute of Virology," he says. "The other hypotheses that have been raised have either been knocked down or have been unable to be substantiated. If you add to that the source for the virus that the CCP would least like to see become the global story, would be that it came from one of their laboratories, that this [Covid-19] is something they could have controlled and they permitted it to be promulgated around the world.

"You launch a full-scale cover-up only when there is something you very much want to make sure doesn't become the factual narrative. I must say this was a comprehensive well-thought-out, Beijing-centred, constant ongoing effort to obfuscate any capacity for the WHO, any Western country or any scientist to determine patient zero and the origination of this virus. And it's ongoing. This is one of the things that people don't realise, the cover-up continues. It would still be most useful for scientists [to have access]. You saw what the WHO was able to do when they went in there, it was silly. It was embarrassingly silly. It's incomprehensible that any scientist would stare at even the questions that were presented to the Chinese as part of the WHO investigation and not laugh at its ineptitude. It was stunning."

Former Deputy Secretary of Australia's Defence Department Peter Jennings says there is a huge amount of evidence pointing to China's interest in biological weapons and the Wuhan Institute of Virology's classified research program, and that their "biosecurity standards were sloppy". "If you put those together that creates a compelling case to say the possibility of a lab accident is actually very high," he said. "Finally, of course, you have the almost hysterical way in which Xi Jinping and the Communist Party sought to cover this up, to prevent investigations and to furiously deny that there was a problem. To me that is a sign of culpability, that the Party realises what happened and they understand the risk that presents them internationally and at home. Taking all of those things into account, I think the chance of this being a leak from the WIV is actually very substantial."

Trump's former National Security Advisor Robert O'Brien says "the circumstantial evidence pretty strongly suggests that the virus came out of the lab". "But I always thought whether it was the wet market or the lab was somewhat immaterial given the history of past health crises; they keep coming out of China and affecting the entire globe," he said. "What amazes me is the whole world hasn't banded together and just said, enough is enough, you guys need international supervision. China has released these four or five plagues on the world in just 21 years and its government can't control the problem. It's really a big issue."

America's former top diplomat in East Asia David Stilwell says the demand for "perfect evidence" of a laboratory leak before the West demands answers from China is nonsensical. "People are for some reason bent on insisting on having a slam-dunk, air-tight case that China produced this virus," he says. "Of course the PRC is not going to let you in there to see their labs, but so many people have used that problem to stop further inquiry. This isn't a legal case, we are not looking for indisputable evidence; there is enough circumstantial evidence." Of the failure by the United States government and intelligence agencies to properly investigate a lab leak, Stilwell is ropeable. "This is the cover-up of the century. This makes Watergate look easy," he tells me.

While Beijing was secretive during SARS, its commitment to subterfuge escalated to another level in the Covid-19 pandemic. The Chinese regime of 2003 is vastly different from the China under Xi Jinping. So was this a cover-up to hide culpability for a virus leak from a laboratory or just evidence of the new world order? And was all the activity – the blackouts and mysterious illnesses – of late 2019 simply a coincidence, or is it a sign of something more sinister, albeit accidental?

The likes of Peter Daszak, Anthony Fauci and Shi Zhengli would have us believe the Covid-19 pandemic has no connection whatsoever to the contentious laboratory experiments at the Wuhan Institute of Virology, located near the epicentre of the first outbreak that has swept the globe. This pandemic, they contend, like others, was a natural event, Gods' work, not the work of those playing God in white coats. It's a reasonable case, given previous breakouts were linked to animals in the wild. But why Beijing's determination to so quickly, and with all the force and trickery of a formidable propaganda operation, shut down any suggestion of a link to a lab accident? Of course, scientists could have feared regulation and international scrutiny of their dangerous experiments. This secrecy shrouding the Wuhan Institute of Virology's radical research and their tightly held virus databases might very well point to a cover-up of a laboratory leak.

The answer lies in the star of this horror show itself: SARS-CoV-2. The coronavirus's genome holds all the secrets and is a guide to the answers the world demands. Its unique properties reveal so much about its likely origins as scientists, investigators and intelligence analysts seek to unravel its moment of inception. This incredibly devastating virus is like no other, despite sharing properties with its SARS cousins. In character and behaviour it gives the impression it is purpose built to infect humans. It is neither entirely a bat virus nor a pangolin virus. It acts as if it's tailor made for human carnage, almost unstoppable in its capacity to ravage the human respiratory system. The millions dead all over the world attest to that.

The world knows China's Communist regime could have done more to save millions of lives. Was it caught off guard covering up a conspiracy and then cashing in on the chaos that ensued? There is virtually no evidence that this virus started in the wild. That's not to say it didn't. There is just no evidence to prove it, while persuasive circumstantial evidence points to a likely laboratory leak.

We could have had more definitive answers by now were it not for the scandal-plagued response from international health and US authorities. Eminent US scientists with plenty to lose – millions of dollars in funding and their reputations on the line – insisted with no evidence to support their claim that this was a natural virus. Riddled with conflicts of interest, not only because of their relationships with China, but also owing to their intimate involvement in coronavirus research, some US scientists and bureaucrats ran serious interference in favour of the Communist regime and its compromised scientists. Not just publicly but in the corridors of power, advising US government intelligence and health officials at the highest level, and then, breathtakingly, as World Health Organization investigators who determined there was nothing to see; it was a natural virus – or even, absurdly, came from imported frozen food.

Other scientists, without direct vested interests, forgot their decades of Ivy-league training that taught them to look at evidence-based information and instead were blinded by their hatred of Trump and followed the consensus, insisting that something they couldn't possibly know – that hadn't been proven – was true. They said this virus could only have arisen naturally.

Even after China's extensive and deliberate cover-up of Covid-19 was exposed – with the CCP objecting to international travel bans while imposing strict ones internally – scientists still gave the Communist Party the benefit of the doubt. Western scientists poured cold water on the notion that Xi Jinping would have covered up an accidental laboratory leak, saying this was a debunked conspiracy theory. And the scientists who did query the unusual features of SARS-CoV-2 – the infectious furin cleavage site and its binding affinity with human cells above all others – were rejected by prestigious scientific journals. Even pre-print servers refused to publish their work – in an unprecedented censorship of science usually reserved for the authoritarian regimes that sadly became a hallmark of Western civilisation in 2020.

Scientific journals claiming the moral high ground, insisting they would only publish science of the greatest academic rigour, then published unscientific 'letters' that claimed, without evidence, that Covid-19 could not have a laboratory origin.

Free speech was censored still by tech giants, with Facebook wiping any content that questioned whether the virus was lab-created.

Then, the US intelligence community, perhaps fearful of antagonising China in a delicate moment in Sino–American relations, or unwilling to be seen as supporting Trump, was complicit in failing to properly explore the origins when it should have.

It's hard to separate this failure from the US election cycle and the unique challenges presented by the Trump administration. The intelligence agencies, worried about a repeat of their false advice on weapons of mass destruction in Iraq, ended up repeating the same grave mistakes, issuing false information that stated the virus could not have been genetically modified. That must have made Chinese scientists engaging in gain-of-function research laugh. Not only did the national security apparatus fail to anticipate the threat from Chinese laboratories developing synthetic viruses that even China's official government documents had warned pose a "latent threat to mankind", but they then declined to probe whether a global pandemic, the worst of its kind in a century, had in fact resulted from such research undertaken in lax laboratories. It was 16 months before the US government even officially asked the intelligence community to properly look at the untapped signals data and intercepts just sitting on their classified computers.

Lastly, the media is complicit in all of this, by and large failing to question or interrogate the narrative and spin that a laboratory leak was a debunked conspiracy theory. Journalists went along with what became the politically correct view – that the virus emerged naturally – rather than being genuinely objective and inquisitive and deciding to look at what was going on in the Wuhan labs. Mainstream media outlets treated those who *did* investigate with ridicule and contempt. The febrile political environment in the US and globally contributed to an incurious and inconceivably hostile space for anyone questioning the orthodoxy.

The unforgivable failures on so many levels mean the world is still in the dark about the precise turn of events that sparked this pandemic, and this of course leaves the world vulnerable to whatever comes next. There is still no evidence that the United States and other Western nations are any more prepared for a future pandemic than we were before this global catastrophe, with gain-of-function experiments still largely left unchecked. The failures of the scientific community, intelligence agencies, international bodies and large sections of the media have all left the world a less secure and less safe place to live.

Author's Note

On the night of March 12, 2020, as the calamity unfolding in Italy gripped our attention and the virus began to ravage the globe, I texted a trusted source tapped in to Australia's foreign secret intelligence agency.

"What do you think about the theory the virus came from a virology lab in China? Does that have credibility? I know it's officially a conspiracy theory but China is not exactly a picture of transparency so I thought it's possible," I ventured.

His reply came an hour later. "I actually think it is now accepted that it was developed within the Wuhan biological warfare laboratory. I know someone that had been very involved in the observation of that lab and its activities. The conjecture around deliberate versus inadvertent is less settled."

It was a perplexing response because, at the time, this view directly contradicted every utterance by scientists – who insisted the virus had a natural origin – and world leaders, who led calls for the closure of unhygienic wet markets they blamed for the outbreak.

The intel from my contact would ultimately put me on the path of investigating the origins of Covid-19, inquiring whether it was possible the virus wreaking havoc around the world had its genesis in a laboratory, and why the West had turned a blind eye to the risky research by Chinese and American scientists.

I raised the possibility of a laboratory leak in my newspaper columns in March 2020, reporting that advice to the Australian Government suggested this was a possible source of SARS-CoV-2, but I was mocked for it. My newspaper editor at the time, Ben English, and another editorial executive Kathy Lipari then asked me to lead coverage of a national series examining China's culpability for the global spread of the virus. Investigating China's cover-up half a world away would have been a daunting prospect at the best of times, but I was at home in lockdown in Australia, looking after my one-year-old full-time while doing as much cooking and cleaning as a 1950s housewife. As every working parent can relate, taking on new challenges in this environment is testing to say the least. Still, I reluctantly agreed.

My research quickly took me from China's cover-up of the virus to its origins. A confidential source told me intelligence agencies were focusing in on the Wuhan Institute of Virology and its scientists Shi Zhengli and her number two, Peng Zhou. This led to a major front-page story on April 28, 2020, which exposed Australia's role in training the Wuhan scientists and co-funding research with them involving live bats. Critically, this story revealed a laboratory leak was being seriously examined by the Five Eyes intelligence network of America, the United Kingdom, Canada, Australia and New Zealand. At this point, there had been no official confirmation that intelligence was even looking at this possibility. The lab leak was considered a conspiracy theory.

Just days later, on April 30, 2020, the US Office of the Director of National Intelligence effectively confirmed my revelation when it issued a statement saying the Intelligence Community was rigorously examining whether the outbreak began through contact with infected animals or was the result of an inadvertent laboratory leak.

The majority of mainstream media outlets chose to ignore this rare statement and continued to treat the possibility of an accidental lab escape as a debunked conspiracy theory. My reporting came under ferocious attack from supposedly objective journalists at Australia's public broadcaster, the ABC, as well as Nine Network newspapers and *The Guardian*.

Leading the charge was the ABC's *Media Watch* host Paul Barry, who, in a tone dripping with disdain, dedicated multiple segments on prime-time television to claiming the lab leak was very unlikely – all funded by the Australian taxpayer. The word "conspiracy" appeared five times in Barry's report on May 4, 2020, in which he assured viewers that "Scott Morrison has come down strongly against the lab theory. And since then Five Eyes intelligence agencies have dismissed it too." Neither point was accurate; the Five Eyes intelligence network was actively investigating the lab leak and the Australian Prime Minister had called for an inquiry into the origins of the virus.

In that segment, scientist Eddie Holmes was quoted as saying, "There's nothing in there at all that is a signature of laboratory manipulation. So I think you can pretty safely put that, those conspiracy theories, to bed."

By the time that episode aired, I had already spoken to enough well-placed intelligence and government sources to know I was on solid footing investigating the possibility of a lab leak. I looked into the gain-of-function research at the Wuhan laboratory, culminating in another front-page story. In that story, I also reported on the existence of a "dossier" or "research paper" by concerned Western governments that factually detailed China's cover-up of the virus, its destruction of evidence and the disappearance of whistleblowers. Astonishingly, instead of further investigating the issues my story exposed, such as the extent of the Wuhan Institute of Virology's genetic manipulation of coronaviruses in gain-of-function research, some media outlets were more interested in trying to uncover my source for the dossier. *The Guardian*, the ABC and others attacked my story by saying it was not an intelligence report – when my story claimed no such thing. (The Chinese Communist Party cover-up of Covid-19 has now been well-established and is continuing to this day as Beijing blocks access to crucial early patient blood samples, virus databases and laboratory records.)

It would be an entire year until President Joe Biden asked the intelligence community in May 2021 to take a closer look and focus on the origin question over a 90-day period. It was only then that reporting on this topic became socially acceptable.

Nevertheless, I persisted throughout that time, breaking global scoops including that Wuhan Institute of Virology scientists were hospitalised with Covid-19-like symptoms in a suspected early cluster; that China had invented a Covid-19 vaccine by February 2020; and that bats had been kept in the Wuhan Institute of Virology. Even as my stories were followed-up globally, the attacks by my media rivals continued. Being accused of peddling fringe conspiracy theories was uncomfortable and upsetting. Just for asking questions and raising the possibility of a lab leak, even senior figures like Matt Pottinger, Tom DiNanno and Sir Richard Dearlove were dubbed conspiracists. I know many journalists, scientists, researchers, government officials and concerned citizens around the world endured a similar experience. Individuals in each of these sectors braved bruising battles to play a crucial role in investigating the origins of the virus. I've tried to bring their stories to light in this book. They have each brought us one step closer to knowing what happened in Wuhan.

On this note, I am grateful to the scientists who generously gave up their time throughout the journey of writing a book to help explain scientific papers and concepts to me. A particular thank you to Nikolai Petrovsky, Gilles Demaneuf, Francisco A. de Ribera and Yuri Deigin for reviewing, editing and correcting my science chapters. I feel like I've had a snap degree in virology.

Thank you to "Billy Bostickson" from DRASTIC, who remains anonymous for security reasons, for your dedication to this topic when many others had moved on. Your detailed knowledge around every aspect of the origins of the virus is arguably unparalleled.

The bravery of Chinese whistleblowers who risked their lives to warn the world about Covid-19 must never be forgotten. I'm immensely grateful to those who have helped me expose China's culpability in the spread of the virus, especially the courageous confidential whistleblower who gave me Dr Wang's first-hand account, so that I could bring it to the world.

I appreciate Kevin Carrico's time translating complicated Chinese documents, often at breakneck speed.

There are a few who went above and beyond digging into their contact books to ensure I had the right access to tell this story. One of those is Mary Kissel, who understands the challenges of journalism and kindly supported me during this process. I am so pleased our paths crossed. Another is Dimon Liu, whose friendship I hope will continue beyond these pages, and I look forward to one day, in a Covid-free world, experiencing first-hand your wonderful cooking. David Asher, you graciously opened up your extensive contact book and research materials as I investigated this topic. I appreciate your more-than-a-dozen hours of interviews, including one long interview when you were, unbeknownst to me, in extreme agony, only to end up later in hospital. You could have postponed! And Miles Yu, thank you for your support and time. Your sense of humour lightened serious discussions and your passion for exposing the Communist Party is admirable.

Thanks to the many others who have contributed to my research on this topic and CCP infiltration more broadly including Peter Jennings, Andrew Hastie, James Paterson, Michael Danby, Luke de Pulford, Matthew Henderson, Samuel Armstrong and many others.

I'm indebted to the confidential sources I am unable to name specifically here but who have played such an important role in crucial developments on the origins of the virus and who have helped me so generously along the way. I appreciate each of you enormously and wish I could say so publicly.

A special mention to Robert Potter and Dave Robinson for sticking together in the trenches under CCP fire and *Global Times* attack, along with your incredible work on this topic and with many other stories. You guys rock.

Thank you to my very talented part-time research team, Luke McWilliams, Jack Hazlewood and Liam Mendes. Luke, at 24 years old, discovered before anyone else in the world that the Wuhan Institute of Virology's database had been taken offline, and exposed the PLA's involvement in the Institute. Jack, at just 22, located crucial documents including China's submission to the UN Convention and tracked down early conversations among dissidents on Chinese-language websites. And Liam, at 25, worked tirelessly, especially in the final stretch, helping with research and fact-checking. All three of you have a bright future in journalism or whatever endeavours you choose to pursue.

Thank you to Caroline Overington for your encouragement, confidence and speedy read-through, along with helping me write the pitch document before any book existed. You are a force of nature. To another remarkable, strong woman, Jackie Stricker-Phelps, my Year 6 English teacher, thank you for reading and editing my draft chapters; concise writing and language is in your DNA.

I'm so appreciative of the highly professional and simply wonderful team at HarperCollins Australia, especially Jim Demetriou and Helen Littleton. Helen, not only are you a joy to work with, calm and thoughtful, but you kindly guided me through the process of developing this concept and narrative. Shannon Kelly, a superstar, thank you for your tireless work on this, your careful edits, ideas and improvements. Thank you also to our copyeditor, whose background in science was particularly helpful, and to Julie Wicks, who proofread this in record time. Neil Thomas, thank you for returning to your trade to give the book a fourth set of eyes on review. Thanks to campaign manager Lara, and to designer Darren Holt for the catchy cover design that captured the mystery of this entire saga. Simon Stubbs and Richard Potter, this was not an easy book to legal, thank you. I'm incredibly grateful for the HarperCollins support internationally, especially Karen Davies and Serena Stent in the UK and the team in the US, Jean Marie Kelly and Alex Serrano – hopefully we can all meet outside of Zoom one day.

Within News Corp, a lot of people went out of their way and gave up their valuable time to make this book possible. Thank you to Michael Miller, and to Paul Whittaker and Mark Calvert at Sky News for your immense support personally and for this book. Thanks to Ben English, Gemma Jones and Kathy Lipari for putting me on this path in the first place. An enormous thank you to Chris Kenny for coming to my defence and publicly taking on my critics over and over again whenever I am under vicious attack. You are a true feminist and I am lucky to have had your support throughout my career. Thanks also to Justin Quill for your informal legal advice as a friend.

To John Lehmann, Michelle Gunn, Petra Rees, Sid Maher, Kylar Loussikian, David Tanner, Claire Harvey and the rest of the exceptional team at *The Australian* – each of you is hard-working, talented, intelligent, thoughtful and committed to producing world-class, high-quality journalism. I can't imagine a more powerhouse newspaper team, led of course by the peerless Chris Dore. Dorey, thank you for reviewing and editing the book, chapter by chapter, and for your enormous editorial support of this journalistic endeavour. You inspire me to be a better journalist, if only so I don't let you down, and I'm grateful for everything you have taught me about journalism since my mid-20s. Thanks to Liz Colman for your heart-warming friendship, the chapter edits and for finding the cover image. This book would never have happened had it not been for Siobhan McKenna. From the moment I mentioned the idea to write a book on what happened in Wuhan, you made it a reality in potentially the fastest book deal in the history of publishing. I'll be forever grateful for your support, kindness and belief in me when I doubted myself. Of course, the chance to write a book is one of many opportunities afforded to me since I first walked through the door at News Corp more than 21 years ago at the age of 16. Being a journalist is a true privilege and I'm filled with gratitude to Rupert and Lachlan Murdoch for the career I've enjoyed. Their contribution to journalism globally is unrivalled and their support in holding the powerful to account, irrespective of party affiliations, is unmatched. Their courage in backing the pursuit of unfashionable stories that are firmly in the public interest has never been more important at a time of censorship and political correctness.

On a personal note, writing a book when you have a toddler requires grandparents. Thank you to my dad, Max, for babysitting and for your eternal positivity and fun each time you bound through the door. As is the case for millions of families, the question of how the virus started is personal, with Max's mum, Stella, my grandmother, passing away from Covid-19 in January 2021 while in a UK nursing home that did not provide her access to a doctor, a hospital or even fluids. She was effectively left to fend for herself without adequate medical care in a first-world country. Thank you also to my beloved family and friends, Yaya, Rikki, Daniel and Dash, Stevie and Karen, Brian and Betsy and Nic and Laura.

I physically couldn't have written this book without my mum, Ro, the most selfless, generous, golden-hearted person. You've always been there for me, every day of my life, and instilled in me the courage to pursue difficult challenges. You selflessly put your own life on hold to babysit round the clock so I could write this. Thank you. Chaz, my best friend, I'm so lucky for your loving encouragement and your unwavering conviction in me. Even while running a start-up, you stepped in to do the heavy lifting on cooking, bath time and bedtime so I could write and conduct late-night and early-morning overseas interviews. I love you. And most of all, to my incredible child, Raphi, who knew when he woke up in the morning he would find me at the computer writing chapters and would sweetly come and snuggle on my lap while I worked. Thank you for sharing your mum for the time it took to write this. I hope one day this book's contribution to the origins question will make your sacrifice worth it. A large part of the reason I wanted to write this so quickly is so I could return to being a full-time mum to you – the greatest thing to have ever happened to me.

Notes

Chapter 1 – Dimon Liu

Varga, 'Liao Chongzhen – A bright candle of humanity', *YouTube*, November 3, 2015

'Liu Xiaoming', *China Vitae*, chinavitae.com/biography/Liu_Xiaoming/bio

Chapter 2 – Brave Whistleblowers

'Ai Fen', *Wikipedia*, en.wikipedia.org/wiki/Ai_Fen

'Anthony Ruggerio', *Washington Institute*, washingtoninstitute.org

'Wuhan doctor speaks out against authorities', *The Guardian*, March 11, 2020

'Donald Trump says China's "incompetence" on coronavirus led to "mass worldwide killing"' *ABC News*, May 21, 2020

'Donald Trump's "Chinese virus": The politics of naming', *The Conversation*, April 22, 2020

'First confirmed case of novel coronavirus in Australia', *Department of Health*, Media Release, January 25, 2020

'First Travel-related Case of 2019 Novel Coronavirus Detected in United States', *Centers for Disease Control and Prevention*

'HHS Leadership', *US Department of Health and Human Services* (online)

'Outbreak of Pneumonia of Unknown Etiology (PUE) in Wuhan, China', *Centers for Disease Control and Prevention* (online)

'The truth about "dramatic action"', *China Media Project*, January 27, 2020

'Trump angers Beijing with "Chinese virus" tweet', *BBC News*, March 17, 2020

Abby Goodnough et al, 'The lost month: How a failure to test blinded the US to COVID-19', *Seattle Times*, March 28, 2020

Alex Woodward, '"It cost the world": National Security Adviser blames spread of coronavirus on China "cover-up"', *Independent*, March 11, 2020

Angelica Snowden and Remy Varga, 'How the coronavirus pandemic unfolded in Australia from the first case on January 24', *The Australian*, January 24, 2020

Associated Press, 'Pompeo, G-7 foreign ministers spar over "Wuhan virus"', *Politico*, March 25, 2020

Tom Ball, Charlotte Wace and Chris Smyth, 'Hunt for contacts of coronavirus-stricken pair in York', *The Times*, January 31, 2020

Chaolin Huang et al, 'Clinical features of patients infected with 2019 novel coronavirus in Wuhan, China' (2020) *The Lancet*, Vol 395(10223)

CNBC Television, 'President Trump speaks at the China phase one trade deal signing', *YouTube*, January 16, 2020

CNN, 'Senator makes prediction ahead of impeachment trial', *YouTube*, January 19, 2020

Dan Mangan, 'Trump blames China for coronavirus pandemic: 'The world is paying a very big price for what they did', *CNBC*, March 19, 2020

Fox News, Facebook post, 'Fox News Morning Update', January 18, 2020

Gao Yu et al, 'In Depth: How Early Signs of a SARS-Like Virus Were Spotted, Spread, and Throttled', *Caixin*, February 29, 2020

Gong Jingqi, '"People" deleted text: the person who sent the whistle', *DW News*, March 10, 2020

House Foreign Affairs Committee, 'The origins of the COVID-19 global pandemic, including the roles of the Chinese Communist Party and the World Health Organization', September 21, 2020

Jeff Mason, Matt Spetalnick and Alexandra Alper, 'Trump ratchets up criticism of China over coronavirus', *Reuters* (online)

Jon Cohen, 'Not wearing masks to protect against coronavirus is a "big mistake", top Chinese scientist says', *Science*, March 27, 2020

Jonathan Lemire, Zeke Miller, Jill Colvin and Ricardo Alonso-Zaldivar, 'Signs missed and steps slowed in Trump's pandemic response', *Associated Press News*, April 13, 2020

Josephine Ma, 'Coronavirus: China's first confirmed Covid-19 case traced back to November 17', *South China Morning Post*, March 13, 2020

Matt Spetalnick, David Brunnstrom and Andrea Shalal, 'Trump risks blowback from war of words with China over coronavirus', *Reuters* (online)

Matthew J Belvedere, 'Trump says he trusts China's Xi on coronavirus and the US has it 'totally under control', *CNBC*, January 22, 2020

Michelle L Holshue et al, 'First Case of 2019 Novel Coronavirus in the United States' (2020) *New England Journal of Medicine*, Vol 382, 929–936

Shane Harris et al, 'US intelligence reports from January and February warned about a likely pandemic', *The Washington Post*, March 20, 2020

Sui-Lee Wee and Vivian Wang, 'China Grapples with Mystery Pneumonia-like Illness', *The New York Times*, January 21, 2020

TODAY, 'Pam Bondi: Trump's Legal Team Is "Ready to Go" for Impeachment Trial', *YouTube*, January 19, 2020

Trump White House Archived, 'President Trump Addresses the Nation', *YouTube*, March 12, 2020

WTPV News, 'President Trump arrives for fundraiser at Mar-a-Lago', *YouTube*, January 18, 2020

Yao Yuan, Ma Yujie, Zhou Jialu and Hou Wenkun, 'Xinhua Headlines: Chinese doctor recalls first encounter with mysterious virus', *Xinhuanet*, April 16, 2020

Chapter 3 – The News Breaks

'China investigates respiratory illness outbreak sickening 27', *Associated Press*, December 31, 2019

'China investigates SARS-like virus as dozens struck by pneumonia', *Deutche Welle*, December 31, 2019

'China pneumonia outbreak: Mystery virus probed in Wuhan', *BBC News*, January 3, 2020

'Chinese officials investigate cause of pneumonia outbreak in Wuhan', *Reuters*, December 31, 2019

'First Travel-related Case of 2019 Novel Coronavirus Detected in United States', *Centers for Disease Control and Prevention* (online)

'How ProMED Crowdsourced the Arrival of Covid-19 and SARS', *Wired*, March 23, 2020

'ProMED-mail Anniversary Award for Excellence in Outbreak Reporting on the Internet', *ProMED*, promedmail.org/about-promed/awards/

'Sui-Lee Wee', *The New York Times*, nytimes.com/by/sui-lee-wee

'The Doctor Whose Gut Instinct Beat AI in Spotting the Coronavirus', *Oliver Wyman Forum*, March 5, 2020

'Undiagnosed pneumonia – China (Hubei): Request for information', *ProMED*, December 30, 2019

'Unexplained pneumonia found in Wuhan, Hubei, South China Seafood Wholesale Market was closed for rectification', *CCTV*, January 2, 2020

Didi Tang, 'Chinese city admits mystery "pneumonia" virus outbreak', *The Times*, January 6, 2020

Erica Davies, 'On high alert JFK, LAX, San Fran airports to screen all passengers from infected region for deadly coronavirus that has killed two', *The Sun*, January 17, 2020

Fanfan Wang, Natasha Khan and Rachel Yeo, 'Health Officials Work to Solve China's Mystery Virus Outbreak', *The Wall Street Journal*, January 6, 2020

Gerry Shih and Lena H Sun, 'Specter of possible new virus emerging from central China raises alarms across Asia', *The Washington Post*, January 8, 2020

Gerry Shih and Lena H Sun, 'China identifies new strain of coronavirus as source of pneumonia outbreak', The *Washington Post*, January 9, 2020

Paul Farhi, 'How a blogger in Florida put out an early warning about the coronavirus crisis', *The Washington Post*, March 14, 2020

Fanfan Wang, 'Health Officials Work to Solve China's Mystery Virus Outbreak', *The Wall Street Journal*, January 6, 2020

World Health Organization, 'COVID-19 – China', January 5, 2020

World Health Organization, 'Novel Coronavirus (2019-nCoV) situation report – 1–21 January 2020', January 20, 2020

Chapter 4 – Chaos
See notes to Chapter 2 – Brave Whistleblowers

Chapter 5 – Chinese New Year
'Professor Maochun Miles Yu', *United States Naval Academy*, usna.edu/Users/history/yu/index.php

'Remarks by Deputy National Security Advisor Matt Pottinger to the Miller Center at the University of Virginia', *US Embassy in Georgia*, May 4, 2020

Bill Gertz, 'Miles Yu, Mike Pompeo adviser, helps form China policy', *Washington Times*, June 15, 2020

Fang Bing, 'Yu Maochun: CCP's Great Leap Forward Virus Research Costs the World', *Voice of America*, March 1, 2021

Shunsuke Tabeta, 'Chinese-born Pompeo adviser blasted as "traitor" in China', *Nikkei Asia*, August 25, 2020

Chapter 6 – The Last Train to Wuhan
'"Wuhan Pneumonia" high-profile "#Escape Wuhan" At least 300,000 people fled on the eve of the lockdown', *Liberty Times Net*, January 24, 2020

'Chen Qiushi has returned to his parents' home in Qingdao', *Rights Defender*, March 30, 2021

'Chen Qiushi: Chinese journalist missing since February "under state supervision"', *BBC News*, September 24, 2020

'Chen Qiushi', *Reporters Without Borders*, rsf.org/en/chen-qiushi

'Famous citizen journalist/lawyer Chen Qiushi briefing: still not released', *Rights Defender*, September 19, 2020

陈秋实, '陳秋實解除限制出境~給中國司法部的公開信', *YouTube*, January 3, 2020

@chenqiushi404, *Twitter*, February 7, 2020

Fan Jiaxun, Hou Yuezhu and Han Wei, 'Reporters' Notebook: Our 76 Days Locked Down in Wuhan', *Caixin Global*, April 7, 2020

Jeremy Page, Wenxin Fan and Natasha Khan, 'How It All Started: China's Early Coronavirus Missteps', *The Wall Street Journal*, March 6, 2020

@Xuxiaodong3, *Twitter*, February 7, 2020

Chapter 7 – The White House in Disarray

'China apologizes after envoy says Israel's travel ban reminiscent of Holocaust', *The Times of Israel*, February 2, 2020

'China opposes some countries' actions that create tension and panic', *CGTN*, February 1, 2020

'China says world "shocked" at Trump adviser Navarro's pen name for books', *Reuters*, October 22, 2019

'Chinese consul general criticises decision to bar travellers from China over coronavirus concerns', *RNZ*, February 3, 2020

'Foreign Ministry Spokesperson Hua Chunying's Remarks on Unfriendly US Comments Amid China's Fight Against Outbreak', *Ministry of Foreign Affairs of the People's Republic of China*

Caitlin Oprysko, 'Trump: Coronavirus will have "a very good ending for us"', Politico, January 1, 2020

Dian Zhang, Erin Mansfield and Dinah Voyles Pulver, 'US exported millions in masks and ventilators ahead of the coronavirus crisis', *USA Today*, April 2, 2020

Eryk Bagshaw and Anthony Galloway, 'China "not happy" with sudden Australian travel lockdown', *The Sydney Morning Herald*, February 4, 2020

Global News, 'China calls report that US is planning to ban Chinese citizens "pathetic"', *YouTube*, July 17, 2020

Jillian Kestler-D'Amours, 'Trump's expanded travel ban sows fear in communities across US', *Al Jazeera*, February 2, 2020

Jonathan Swan and Margaret Talev, 'Navarro memos warning of mass coronavirus death circulated in January', Axios, April 7, 2020

Melissa Clarke, 'Coronavirus travel ban sees Chinese students miss start of university, Australian tertiary education sector scrambling', *ABC News*, February 4, 2020

@MFA_China, *Twitter*, February 1, 2020

Miriam Valverde, 'Fact-check: Did Biden call Trump "xenophobic" for China travel restrictions?', *The Statesman*, March 3, 2020

Chapter 8 – Transparency

'8 people were dealt with in accordance with the law for disseminating false information about "Wuhan Viral Pneumonia" on the Internet', *Xinhua*, January 1, 2020

'China attempts to limit coronavirus spread by extending Lunar New Year holiday to discourage travel', *ABC News,* January 27, 2020

'China didn't warn public of likely pandemic for 6 key days', *Associated Press News*, April 15, 2020

'Li Wenliang: Coronavirus kills Chinese whistleblower doctor', *BBC News*, February 7, 2020

'New crown pneumonia another "whistleblower" appeared and was verbally educated by the police', *Caixin*, February 1, 2020

'SARS Basics Fact Sheet', *Centers for Disease Control and Prevention*, www.cdc.gov

'The third whistleblower appeared: Dr. Liu Wen is still on the front line of the fight against the epidemic', *Caixin*, February 7, 2020

'With the approval of the central government, the National Supervisory Commission decided to send an investigation team to Wuhan City, Hubei Province to conduct a comprehensive investigation on the issues reported by the masses involving Dr. Li Wenliang' *Central Commission for Discipline Inspection and State Supervision Commission*, ccdi.gov.cn

'Wuhan doctor Li Wenliang who was admonished for telling the truth about the epidemic: I want to return to the frontline of the epidemic as soon as possible', *The Paper,* February 1, 2020

'Wuhan Public Security Organs: Don't spread rumors! 8 rumors spreaders were investigated and dealt with by the police according to law', *Hubei*, January 2020

付雪洁, *Weibo*, May 30, 2020

Andrew Green, 'Li Wenliang', *The Lancet*, February 18, 2020

Associated Press, 'China exonerates doctor reprimanded for warning of virus', *Politico*, March 20, 2020

Chaolin Huang et al, 'Clinical features of patients infected with 2019 novel coronavirus in Wuhan, China' (2020) *The Lancet*, Vol 395(10223)

Chen Qingqing, 'Wife of late Wuhan "whistleblower" Dr Li Wenliang gives birth to baby boy', *Global Times*, globaltimes.cn/content/1191389.shtml

Cissy Zhou, 'Coronavirus: Whistle-blower Dr Li Wenliang confirmed dead of the disease at 34, after hours of chaotic messaging from hospital', *South China Morning Post*, February 7, 2020

Emily Feng, 'A Change In How One Chinese Province Reports Coronavirus Adds Thousands of Cases', *National Public Radio,* February 13, 2020

Erik Eckholm, 'The SARS epidemic: Epidemic; China Admits Underreporting its SARS Cases', *The New York Times*, April 21, 2003

Gong Jingqi, 'Whistleman', *Weixin* (archived), March 10, 2020

House Foreign Affairs Committee, 'The origins of the COVID-19 global pandemic, including the roles of the Chinese Communist Party and the World Health Organization', September 21, 2020

Jane McMullen, 'Covid-19: Five days that shaped the outbreak', *BBC News,* January 26, 2020

Jing-Bao Nie and Carl Elliott, 'Humiliating Whistle-Blowers: Li Wenliang, the Response to Covid-19, and the Call for a Decent Society' (2020) *Journal of Bioethical Inquiry*, Vol 17, 543–547

Jun Mai, 'Coronavirus "rumour" crackdown by Wuhan police slammed by China's top court', *South China Morning Post*, January 29, 2020

Li Liu et al, 'The Current Status and a New Approach for Chinese Doctors to Obtain Medical Knowledge Using Social Media: A Study of WeChat' (2018) *Wireless Communication and Mobile Computing*, Vol 2018

Lily Kuo, 'Coronavirus: Wuhan doctor speaks out against authorities', *The Guardian*, March 11, 2020

Lin Zehong, '"Whistleblower" of Wuhan pneumonia: I knew it could be "person-to-person" three weeks ago', *Yuanqi* (archived), January 31, 2020

Lotus Ruan, Jeffrey Knockel and Masashi Crete-Nishihata, 'Censored Contagion: How Information on the Coronavirus is Managed on Chinese Social Media', *The Citizen Lab*, March 3, 2020

Nana Dadzie Ghansah, 'The Whistleblowers', *Medium*, March 7, 2020

Natalie Winters, 'WHO COVID "Investigator" is Chinese CDC Advisor Who Accepted CCP Research Grants', *The National Pulse*, February 15, 2020

Qin Jianhang and Timmy Shen, 'Rebuked coronavirus whistleblower vindicated by top Chinese court', *Nikkei Asia*, February 5, 2020

Qin Jianhang, Wang Yanyu and Matthew Walsh, 'More Wuhan Doctors Say They Faced Official Backlash Over Virus Warnings', *Caixin Global*, February 10, 2020

Ruipeng Lei and Renzong Qiu, 'Chinese Bioethicists: Silencing Doctor Impeded Early Control of Coronavirus', *The Hastings Center*, February 13, 2020

Stephen Lee Myers and Chris Buckley, 'China Created a Fail-Safe System to Track Contagions. It Failed', *New York Times*, December 22, 2020

Wang Lianzhang, 'Gone but Not Soon Forgotten: Li Wenliang's Online Legacy', *Sixth Tone*, February 7, 2020

WION, 'Gravitas: The interview China tried to hide', *YouTube*, April 4, 2020

World Health Organization, 'Mission summary: WHO Field Visit to Wuhan, China 20–21 January 2020', January 22, 2020

World Health Organization, 'Novel coronavirus press conference at United Nations of Geneva', January 29, 2020

World Health Organization, 'Press briefing on WHO Mission to China and novel coronavirus outbreak', January 29, 2020

xiaolwl, *Weibo*, November 15, 2018

Yanzhong Huang, 'The SARS Epidemic and Its Aftermath in China: A Political Perspective', *NCBI*

Zhuang Pinghui, 'China confirms unauthorised labs were told to destroy early coronavirus samples', *South China Morning Post*, May 15, 2020

Zhu Andy, '8名散布谣言者被依法查处 武汉肺炎', *YouTube*, January 23, 2020

Chapter 9 – Don't Panic the Markets

Council on Foreign Relations, 'A Conversation with Robert Redfield', *YouTube*, December 12, 2020

Dan Mangan, 'Trump dismissed coronavirus pandemic worry in January – now claims he long warned about it', *CNBC*, March 17, 2020

Jonathon Lemire et al, 'Signs missed and steps slowed in Trump's pandemic response', *Associated Press News*, April 13, 2020

Josh Margolin and James Gordon Meek, 'Intelligence report warned of coronavirus crisis as early as November: Sources', *ABC News*, April 9, 2020

Thomas Francke, 'Trump says the coronavirus is the Democrats' "new hoax"', *CNBC*, February 28, 2020

Chapter 10 – Pompeo

'Mike Pompeo warns UK over Huawei "security risks"', *BBC News*, May 8, 2019

'Secretary Pompeo's Meeting with Hong Kong Businessman and Publisher Jimmy Lai', *US Consulate General Hong Kong & Macau*, July 8, 2019

'Three Minute Squiz with Mary Kissel', *The Squiz*, November 2017

'Transcript of Attorney General Barr's Remarks on China Policy at the Gerald R. Ford Presidential Museum', *United States Department of Justice*, July 17, 2020

'Zizi Azah Binte Abdul Majid', *Women Leaders of New Asia*, sites.asiasociety.org/womenleaders/events/2010/summit-2010/delegate-bios

Alex Ward, 'Pompeo slammed China for covering up the Tiananmen Square massacre … And China is pissed', *Vox*, June 4, 2019

@benedictrogers, *Twitter*, January 10, 2020

Christopher Wray, 'The Threat Posed by the Chinese Government and the Chinese Communist Party to the Economic and National Security of the United States', *Federal Bureau of Investigation*, July 7, 2020

Darla Mercado, 'Treasury and IRS to delay tax payment deadline by 90 days', *CNBC*, March 17, 2020

Factbase Videos, 'Press Conference: Donald Trump Holds the Daily Coronavirus Pandemic Briefing', *YouTube*, April 16, 2020

John Wagner et al, 'Sen. Burr asks Senate Ethics Committee for review of his stock sales amid uproar over possible influence of coronavirus briefings', *The Washington Post*, March 20, 2020

Jonathon Swan, 'Scoop: Inside the epic White House fight over hydroxychloroquine', *Axios*, Updated April 5, 2020

Karen DeYoung, 'Senior adviser to Pompeo resigns', *The Washington Post*, October 10, 2019

Kate Prengel, 'Mary Kissel: 5 Fast Facts You Need to Know', *Heavy*, November 2018

@lukedepulford, *Twitter*, November 9, 2020

@lukedepulford, *Twitter*, January 10, 2021

Robert O'Brien, 'The Chinese Communist Party's Ideology and Global Ambitions', *USC US–China Institute*, June 24, 2020

Shane Harris et al, 'US intelligence reports from January and February warned about a likely pandemic', *The Washington Post*, March 20, 2020

Stephen Castle, 'Pompeo Attacks China and Warns Britain Over Huawei Security Risks', *The New York Times*, May 8, 2019

Chapter 11 – The Cables

'Matthew Turpin', *Hoover Institution Fellows*, hoover.org/profiles/matthew-turpin

'National Security Council', *The White House*, www.whitehouse.gov/nsc/

David Cyranoski, 'Inside the Chinese lab poised to study world's most dangerous pathogens' (2017) *Nature*, Vol 542, 399–40

Grace Niewijk, 'Controversy Aside, Why the Source of COVID-19 Matters', *Genetic Engineering and Biology News*, September 21, 2020

Josh Rogin, 'Opinion: State Department cables warned of safety issues at Wuhan lab studying bat coronaviruses', *The Washington Post*, April 14, 2020

Violet Law, 'Coronavirus origin: Few leads, many theories in hunt for source', *Al Jazeera*, April 8, 2020

Chapter 12 – A Failure to Investigate

'Chinese Foreign Ministry Spokesperson's Remarks', *Embassy of the People's Republic of China in the Commonwealth of Australia*, au.china-embassy.org

'Come clean: US presses China on coronavirus after lab reports', *Al Jazeera*, April 16, 2020

'Coronavirus: China rejects call for probe into origins of disease', *BBC News*, April 24, 2020

'France's Macron says now not the time for pandemic probe', *Reuters*, April 22, 2020

'Interview with David Speers, ABC Insiders', *Senator the Hon Marise Payne*, April 19, 2020

'Morrison backs inquiry into virus origins', *Australian Associated Press*, April 21, 2020

'The United States and ASEAN are Partnering to Defeat COVID-19, Build Long-Term Resilience, and Support Economic Recovery', *US Embassy and Consulates in Indonesia*, April 22, 2020

@Ayjchan, *Twitter*, October 25, 2020

Aylin Woodward, 'Chinese CDC Now Says the Wuhan Wet Market Wasn't the Origin of the Virus', *Science Alert*, May 29, 2020

Brett Worthington, 'Marise Payne calls for global inquiry into China's handling of the coronavirus outbreak', *ABC News*, April 19, 2020

Chaolin Huang et al, 'Clinical features of patients infected with 2019 novel coronavirus in Wuhan, China' (2020) *The Lancet*, Vol 395(10223), 497–506

Daniel Hurst, 'Top Chinese diplomat says Australia's call for coronavirus inquiry was "shocking"', *The Guardian*, August 26, 2020

Julian Borger, 'Peter Navarro: what Trump's Covid-19 tsar lacks in expertise, he makes up', *The Guardian*, April 10, 2020

Kirsty Needham and Stephanie Nebehay, 'Australia seeks probe into coronavirus spread, France and UK say now not the time', *Reuters*, April 22, 2020

Marise Payne, 'Coronavirus: Australia can lead the way for a global response', *The Australian*, April 22, 2020

Qun Li et al, 'Early Transmission Dynamics in Wuhan, China, of Novel Coronavirus–Infected Pneumonia', *The New England Journal of Medicine*, Vol 382, 1199–1207

Rebecca Falconer, 'Australian journalists flown back from China after "diplomatic standoff"', *Axios*, September 8, 2020

Richard Ferguson, 'Coronavirus: Morrison, Payne lobby for review of Chinese behaviour', *The Australian*, April 22, 2020

Roland Wiesendanger, 'Studie zum Ursprung der Coronavirus-Pandemie', trans: 'Study on the origin of the coronavirus pandemic', *University of Hamburg*, February 2021

Teddy Ng, 'No link with seafood market in first case of China coronavirus, Chinese scientists revealed', *South China Morning Post*, January 25, 2020

Chapter 13 – Nikolai Petrovsky

'Intelligence Community Statement on Origins of Covid-19', *Office of the Director of National Intelligence*, April 30, 2020

Charles Schmidt, 'Did the coronavirus leak from a lab? These scientists say we shouldn't rule it out', *Technology Review*, March 18, 2021

Jaime Metzl, 'How to Hold Beijing Accountable for the Coronavirus', *The Wall Street Journal*, July 28, 2020

Nicholson Baker, 'The Lab-Leak Hypothesis', *New York Magazine* (archived), archive.vn/rd6mC#selection-1189.0-1189.23

Sakshi Piplani et al, 'In silico comparison of spike protein-ACE2 binding affinities across species; Significance for the possible origin of the SARS-CoV-2 virus', Unpublished, *Research Gate*

Chapter 14 – Scientists Speak Out

'Coronavirus Leaked Accidentally From a Lab in August or September 2019, Claims Norwegian Virologist', *Yahoo! News*, December 17, 2020

'Is it possible to create a virus in the laboratory without a trace? The expert's answer', *HuffPost* (archived), archive.is/zlrR8#selection-509.0-513.19

'Roles and functions of Chinese People's Political Consultative Conference', *The National Committee of the Chinese People's Political Consultative Conference*, March 17, 2020

'Statement from Prof Edward Holmes on the SARS-CoV-2 virus', *The University of Sydney*, April 2016, 2020

'The Wuhan lab at the heart of the US–China virus spat', *Bangkok Post*, May 6, 2020

Charles Schmidt, 'Lab Leak: A Scientific Debate Mired in Politics – and Unresolved', *Undark*, March 17, 2021

David A. Relman, 'Opinion: To stop the next pandemic, we need to unravel the origins of COVID-19', *PNAS*, pnas.org/content/117/47/29246

Donald G. McNeil Jr, 'Sigma Phi-ing Monkeyshines at the WHO', *Medium*, May 17, 2020

Francis Collins, 'Genomic Study Points to Natural Origin of COVID-19', *NIH Director's Blog*, March 26, 2020

Kailang Wu et al, 'A Virus-Binding Hot Spot on Human Angiotensin-Converting Enzyme 2 Is Critical for Binding of Two Different Coronaviruses', *Journal of Virology*, Vol 85(11)

@K_G_Andersen, *Twitter* (profile now deleted)

Kristian G. Andersen et al, 'The proximal origin of SARS-CoV-2' (2020) *Nature Medicine*, Vol 26, 450–452

Matt Ridley, 'So Where Did the Virus Come From?', *The Wall Street Journal*, May 29, 2020

Peng Zhou et al, 'A pneumonia outbreak associated with a new coronavirus of probable bat origin' *Nature*, Vol 579, 270–273

Sharri Markson, 'Scientists and intelligence experts back coronavirus laboratory theory', *The Daily Telegraph*, June 5, 2020

Tommy Tsan-Yuk Lam et al, 'Identifying SARS-CoV-2-related coronaviruses in Malayan pangolins' (2020) *Nature*, Vol 583, 282–285

Xiaoxu Lin and Shizong Chen, 'Major Concerns on the Identification of Bat Coronavirus Strain RaTG13 and Quality of Related Nature Paper', Unpublished, *Preprints*

Yuxuan Hou et al, 'Angiotensin-converting enzyme 2 (ACE2) proteins of different bat species confer variable susceptibility to SARS-CoV entry' (2020) *Archives of Virology*, Vol 155,1563–1569

Chapter 15 – The Scientists Who Knew

'Cambridge Working Group Consensus Statement on the Creation of Potential Pandemic Pathogens (PPPs)', *Cambridge Working Group*, cambridgeworkinggroup.org/

'Exploring the "frozen storage" of more than 1500 virus strains in Wuhan, Asia's largest virus repository', *Chinese Academy of Sciences* (archived), web.archive.org/web/20200318091607/http:/www.whb.cas.cn/xw/mtjj/201811/t20181122_5191208.html

'Fact Sheet: Activity at the Wuhan Institute of Virology', *US Department of State* (archived), web.archive.org/web/20210116020654/https://www.state.gov/fact-sheet-activity-at-the-wuhan-institute-of-virology/

Bill Gertz, 'Wuhan laboratory "most likely" coronavirus source, US government analysis finds', *Washington Times*, April 28, 2020

Billy Bostickson and Yvette Ghannam, 'Wuhan laboratories, bat research and biosafety', Unpublished, *Research Gate*

Carlos S. Moreno, 'Written comments for NSABB meeting Jan 7–8, 2016', January 3, 2016

Declan Butler, 'Engineered bat virus stirs debate over risky research', *Nature*, November 12, 2015

Jocelyn Kaiser, 'Controversial experiments that could make bird flu more risky poised to resume', *Science*, February 8, 2019

Joint Report, *WHO–China Study*, 'WHO-convened Global Study of Origins of SARS-CoV-2: China Part', January 14–February 10, 2021

Lynn C. Klotz and Edward J. Sylvester, 'The unacceptable risks of a man-made pandemic', *The Bulletin*, August 7, 2012

Marc Lipsitch and Thomas V. Inglesby, 'Moratorium on Research Intended To Create Novel Potential Pandemic Pathogens', *ASM Journals*

@PeterDaszak, *Twitter*, January 1, 2020

Ralph S Baric, 'Synthetic Viral Genomics: Risks and Benefits for Science and Society', *Working Papers for Synthetic Genomics: Risks and Benefits for Science and Society*, 35–81

Shi-Hui Sun et al, 'A Mouse Model of SARS-CoV-2 Infection and Pathogenesis', *Cell Host & Microbe*, Vol 28(1), 124–133

Steven Mosher, 'Renowned European scientist: COVID-19 was engineered in China lab, effective vaccine "unlikely"', *LifeSite News*, August 10, 2020

Steven Salzberg, letter to NSABB, cambridgeworkinggroup.org/documents/salzberg.pdf

@TheSeeker268, *Twitter*, May 13, 2021

Vineet D. Menachery, 'A SARS-like cluster of circulating bat coronaviruses shows potential for human emergence', *Nature Medicine*, Vol 21, 1508–1513

@WhoWuhan, *Twitter* (profile now deleted)

Wuze Ren et al, 'Difference in Receptor Usage between Severe Acute Respiratory Syndrome (SARS) Coronavirus and SARS-Like Coronavirus of Bat Origin' (2008) *Journal of Virology*, Vol 82(4), 1899–1907

Chapter 16 – America's Doctor

'Editorial Board', *Virologica Sinica* (archived), web.archive.org/web/20200205233521/https://www.virosin.org/news/EditorialBoard.htm

'Grant to Regents of the University of Minnesota from Department of Health and Human Services', *USA Spending*, FAIN R01AI089728, www.usaspending.gov/award/ASST_NON_R01AI089728_7529

'Grants to EcoHealth Alliance Inc', *USA Spending*, www.usaspending.gov/search/?hash=77699a9921379a9ef25abe891c383718

'Researcher Zeng Xiankun of the US Army Institute of Infectious Diseases was invited to "Ge Hong Forum"', *Wuhan Institute of Virology*, archive.is/daAGl

Amanda Andre to Ralph Baric, Email, 'EcoHealth Alliance W9', January 24, 2018, usrtk.org/wp-content/uploads/2020/12/EHAfunds_2017_Baric-Files.pdf

Dany Shoham, 'China's Biological Warfare Programme and the Curious Case of Dr. Xiangguo Qiu' (2019) *CBW Magazine*, Vol 12(4)

Ian Birrell, 'China tried to patent potential coronavirus drug Remsvidir the DAY AFTER Beijing confirmed virus was transmissible between humans', *Daily Mail*, April 26, 2020

Jennifer M. Brannan et al, 'Post-exposure immunotherapy for two ebolaviruses and Marburg virus in nonhuman primates', *Nature Communications*, Vol 10

Meeting Report, 'Second China–US Workshop on the Challenges of Emerging Infections, Laboratory Safety and Global Health Security' (archived), May 17–19, 2017, web.archive.org/web/20200516011404/ http://english.whiov.cas.cn/News/Int_Cooperation_News/201707/ W020170718313905257748.pdf

Michael S. Lauer, NIH Deputy Director for Extramural Research, letter to Aleksei Chmura and Peter Daszak, July 8, 2020, nlcampaigns.org/ Daszak_7_8_20_Reactivation_and_Suspension.pdf

Michael S. Lauer, NIH Deputy Director for Extramural Research, letter to Aleksei Chmura and Peter Daszak, October 23, 2020, nlcampaigns. org/NIH_Response_10_23_20_further_demands.pdf

@NIHDirector, *Twitter*, June 24, 2015

Shi Zhengli to Ralph Baric, Emails, 'Re: RE: Nice meeting you in Galveston and invitation to Wuhan meeting in October 2018', February 7, 2018, usrtk.org/wp-content/uploads/2020/12/NAS_Galveston_ZLS_ Emails_2017_Baric-Files.pdf

Chapter 17   USAMRIID

'USAMRIID: Biodefense Solutions to Protect our Nation', *Medical Research Institute of Infectious Diseases*, usamriid.army.mil

Heather Mongilio, 'CDC inspection findings reveal more about USAMRIID research suspension', *The Frederick News-Post*, November 23, 2019

Sylvia Carignan, 'Army report says science director creating "environment of fear" at USAMRIID', *The Frederick News-Post*, August 13, 2016

USAMRIID, Press Release, 'Antiviral Compound Provides Full Protection from Ebola Virus in Nonhuman Primates', October 9, 2015

Chapter 18 – 0.3 Per Cent

David Cyranoski, 'Chinese institutes investigate pathogen outbreaks in lab workers', *Nature*, December 17, 2019

@ggreenwald, *Twitter*, May 12, 2021

Mara Hvistendahl, 'Chinese University Fires Administrators, Offers Compensation after Lab Accident', *Science*, September 13, 2011

Natalie Rahhal, 'China built a lab to study SARS and Ebola in Wuhan – and US biosafety experts warned in 2017 that a virus could "escape" the facility that's become key in fighting the outbreak', *Daily Mail*, January 24, 2020

Robert Walgate, 'SARS escaped Beijing lab twice', *NCBI*, April 27, 2004

Stephen Moyes, 'Wuhan lab blamed for coronavirus lied about safety precautions it took during controversial bat tests', *The Sun*, April 29, 2020

William J. Broad and Judith Miller, 'Soviet Defector Says China Had Accident at a Germ Plant', *The New York Times*, April 5, 1999

Yang Xu et al, 'Thoughts on Strengthening the Planning of my country's High-level Biosafety Laboratory System', *Bulletin of Chinese Academy of Sciences*, October 16, 2016

Zhang Feng, 'Officials punished for SARS virus leak', *China Daily*, February 7, 2004

Chapter 19 – The Cave of Death

Antoni G Wrobel et al, 'SARS-CoV-2 and bat RaTG13 spike glycoprotein structures inform on virus evolution and furin-cleavage effects' (2020) *Nature Structural & Molecular Biology*, Vol 27, 763–767

Jane Qiu, 'How China's "Bat Woman" Hunted Down Viruses from SARS to the New Coronavirus', *Scientific American*, June 1, 2020

Dake Kang, Maria Cheng and Sam McNeil, 'China clamps down in hidden hunt for coronavirus origins', *Associated Press* (archived), archive.is/QBUrV

George Arbuthnott, Jonathan Calvert and Philip Sherwell, 'Revealed: Seven year coronavirus trail from mine deaths to a Wuhan lab', *The Sunday Times* (archived), archive.ph/CUiQv

Jackson Ryan, 'How the coronavirus origin story is being rewritten by a guerrilla Twitter group', *CNet*, April 15, 2021

Kangpeng Xiao et al, 'Isolation of SARS-CoV-2-related coronavirus from Malayan pangolins' (2020) *Nature*, Vol 583, 286–289

Li Xu, 'The Analysis of Six Patients with Severe Pneumonia Caused by Unknown Viruses', Unpublished, www.documentcloud.org/documents/6981198-Analysis-of-Six-Patients-With-Unknown-Viruses.html

Liangjun Chen et al, 'RNA based mNGS approach identifies a novel human coronavirus from two individual pneumonia cases in 2019 Wuhan outbreak' (2020) *Emerging Microbes and Infections,* Vol 9(1), 313–319

Liji Thomas, 'Research sheds doubt on the Pangolin link to SARS-CoV 2', *News Medical*, July 8, 2020

Monali C. Rahalkar and Rahul A. Bahulikar, 'Lethal Pneumonia Cases in Mojiang Miners (2012) and the Mineshaft Could Provide Important Clues to the Origin of SARS-CoV-2' (2020) *Frontiers in Public Health*, October 20, 2020

Monali C. Rahalkar and Rahul A. Bahulikar, 'Understanding the Origin of "BatCoVRaTG13", a Virus Closest to SARS-CoV-2', Unpublished, *Preprints*

Peng Zhou et al, 'A pneumonia outbreak associated with a new coronavirus of probable bat origin' (2020) *Nature*, Vol 579, 270–273

Richard Stone, 'A New Killer Virus in China?', *Science*, sciencemag.org/news/2014/03/new-killer-virus-china

Sharri Markson and Ashleigh Gleeson, 'The Covid Files: How the Red Army oversaw coronavirus research', *The Daily Telegraph*, May 11, 2020

Tomislav Meštrović, 'Did SARS-CoV-2 adapt to humans long before the index case?', *News Medical*, May 19, 2020

Tommy Tsan-Yuk Lam et al, 'Identifying SARS-CoV-2-related coronaviruses in Malayan pangolins' (2020) *Nature*, Vol 583

Xiaobing Li et al, 'Pathogenicity, tissue tropism and potential vertical transmission of SARSr-CoV-2 in Malayan pangolins', Unpublished, *BioRxiv*

Xing-Yi Ge et al, 'Coexistence of multiple coronaviruses in several bat colonies in an abandoned mineshaft' (2016) *Virologica Sinica*, Vol 31(1), 31–40

Yujia Alina Chan and Shing Hei Zhan, 'Single source of pangolin CoVs with a near identical Spike RBD to SARS-CoV-2', Unpublished, *BioRxiv*

Zhiqiang Wu et al, 'Novel Henipa-like Virus, Mojiang Paramyxovirus, in Rats, China, 2012' (2014) *Emerging Infectious Diseases*, Vol 20(6)

Chapter 20 – Conflicted

'Australian broadcaster slams NZ Govt for not supporting concern over World Health Organization's Covid-19 origin report', *New Zealand Herald*, April 2, 2021

'Hogan top COVID adviser Redfield tosses viral kindling on anti-Asian fires', *Baltimore Sun*, March 30, 2021

'New Zealand defends absence from joint statement on World Health Organization coronavirus report', *ABC News,* April 1, 2021

Alexander Nazaryan, 'WHO's "not credible" coronavirus report angers scientists and politicians alike', *Yahoo! News*, April 1, 2021

Ben Sasse, 'Sasse Statement on WHO Report', *US Senator for Nebraska Ben Sasse*, March 29, 2021

Carey Gillam, 'Validity of key studies on origin of coronavirus in doubt; science journals investigating', *US Right to Know*, November 9, 2020

Charles Calisher et al, 'Statement in support of the scientists, public health professionals, and medical professionals of China combatting COVID-19' (2020) *The Lancet*, Vol 395(10226)

@CharlesRixey, *Twitter*, May 13, 2021

Colin D Butler et al, 'Open Letter: Call for a Full and Unrestricted International Forensic Investigation into the Origins of COVID-19', March 4, 2021, int.nyt.com/data/documenttools/covid-origins-letter/5c9743168205f926/full.pdf

Daniel Payne, 'Emails show scientists scrubbed early warning of potential lab origin of COVID-19', *Just the News*, March 15, 2021

Harshit Sabarwal, 'Japan demands further probe into Covid-19 origins after WHO releases report', *Hindustan Times*, March 31, 2021

Josh Rogin, 'Opinion: What if the former CDC Director is right about the Wuhan labs?', *The Washington Post*, April 1, 2021

@MarionKoopmans, *Twitter*, February 10, 2021

@McWLuke, *Twitter* (profile now deleted)

Nell Greenfieldboyce, 'How a Tilt Toward Safety Stopped a Scientist's Virus Research', *National Public Radio* (archived), archive.vn/32NT4

Nidhi Subbaraman, '"Heinous!": Coronavirus researcher shut down for Wuhan-lab link slams new funding restrictions', *Nature*, August 21, 2020

@PeterDaszak, *Twitter*, August 20, 2020

@PeterDaszak, *Twitter*, February 9–10, 2021

@PeterDaszak, *Twitter*, February 14, 2021

Peter Daszak Emails, 'A Statement in support of the scientists, public health and medical professionals of China', usrtk.org/wp-content/uploads/2020/11/Biohazard_FOIA_Maryland_Emails_11.6.20.pdf

@TheSeeker268, *Twitter*, April 4, 2021

Ping Liu et al, 'Are pangolins the intermediate host of the 2019 novel coronavirus (SARS-CoV-2)?' (2020) *PLOS Pathogens*, Vol 17(6)

Sainath Suryanarayanan, 'Chinese-linked journal editor sought help to rebut Covid-19 lab origin hypothesis', *US Right to Know*, April 7, 2021

Sainath Suryanarayanan, 'EcoHealth Alliance orchestrated key scientists' statement on "natural origin" of SARS-CoV-2', *US Right to Know*, November 18, 2020

Sainath Suryanarayanan to Jinping Chen, Bcc Gary Ruskin, Emails, 'Questions regarding Liu et al. (2020) in PLoS Pathogens', October 28, 2020, usrtk.org/wp-content/uploads/2020/11/Pangolin_Papers_Emails_JPChen_PLoS.pdf

Stanley Perlman to Sainath Suryanarayanan, Emails, 'Questions regarding Liu et al. (2020) in PLoS Pathogens', October 27, 2020, usrtk.org/wp-content/uploads/2020/11/Pangolin_Papers_Perlman_Emails.pdf

US Department of State, 'Joint Statement on the WHO-Convened COVID-19 Origins Study', March 30, 2021

Vineet D Menachery et al, 'A SARS-like cluster of circulating bat coronaviruses shows potential for human emergence' (2015) *Nature Medicine*, Vol 21, 1508–1513

Chapter 21 – Military Games

'China Rights Lawyer Dies in "Mysterious" Circumstances, Supporters Say', *News Channel 2*, wktv.com/content/national/475238643.html

'Chinese People's Liberation Army Academy of Military Medical Sciences', *Souky* (archived), archive.is/4IXEC

'Murder allegations spur secondary autopsy of Chinese dissident', *ChinaAid*, May 2019

'Updated: Human rights defender mysteriously dies', *ChinaAid*, May 2019

Cao Yunyi, 'Tales of China's first nuclear bomb project', *Shanghai Daily*, September 18, 2018

CGTN, 'Grand opening ceremony of the 7th Military World Games', *YouTube*, October 18, 2019

Chris Buckley, 'China dissidents bide time against Party', *Reuters*, May 29, 2009

Christian Shepherd, 'Death of Chinese rights lawyer raises suspicions', *Yahoo! Entertainment*, February 26, 2018

Han Jie and Wen Yuqing, 'Veteran of 1989 Democracy Movement in Tiananmen Square Dies Suddenly', *Radio Free Asia*, April 24, 2019

Hans Moritz, 'Mysteriöser Tod nach Notlandung am Münchner Flughafen – handelt es sich um einen Auftrags-Mord?' (trans: 'Mysterious death after an emergency landing at Munich Airport – is it a contract murder?'), *Frankfurter Rundschau*, May 17, 2019

Jill Levine, 'Deng Xiaoping, Dazibao and Dissent: A Critical Analysis of the Xidan Democracy Wall Movement' (2013) *Senior Capstone Projects*, Paper 163

Nancy Pelosi, 'Pelosi Remarks at Virtual Hearing on China, Genocide and the Olympics', *Speaker of the House*, May 18, 2021

Chapter 22 – A Latent Threat to Mankind

'2020 Reviewer Acknowledgment', *Virologica Sinica* (archived), web. archive.org/web/20210303152158/https://virosin.org/news/lianjie/ eaea826d-722c-418f-b517-34168c64d2c4_en.htm

'Fact Sheet: Activity at the Wuhan Institute of Virology', *US Department of State*, January 15, 2021

'Prof Cao Wuchun (Executive Director)', *Center for Applications of Spatial Information Technologies in Public Health*, archive.is/ KrkGu#selection-247.0-415.71

'Tong Yigang', College of Life Science and Technology, Beijing University of Chemical Technology, tongyigang.tripod.com/

Bill Gertz, 'Coronavirus link to China biowarfare program possible, analyst says', *Washington Times*, January 26, 2020

Guo Jiwei, *War of the Right to Live*, Xinhua Publishing House

Hong-Lei Zhang et al, 'Visualization of chikungunya virus infection in vitro and in vivo' (2019) *Emerg Microbes Infect*, Vol 8(1)

Jonathan Epstein to Ralph Baric, Email, 'dual use safety language', March 23, 2018, usrtk.org/wp-content/uploads/2020/12/EHA_Epstein_2018_ Baric-Files.pdf

Lu Beibei He Fuchu, 'Biotechnology will become the new strategic commanding heights of the future military revolution', *People's Liberation Army Daily* (archived), web.archive.org/web/20190813042422/http://www.81.cn/jwgz/2015-10/06/content_6709533.htm

Mike Pompeo and Miles Yu, 'China's Reckless Labs Put the World at Risk, *Wall Street Journal*, February 23, 2021

Richard D. Fisher, 'SARS Crisis: Don't Rule Out Linkages to China's Biowarfare' (2003) *China Brief*, Vol 3(8)

Rodolphe de Maistre et al, 'Wuhan Institute of Biological Products Co', Unpublished, *Research Gate*

Simon Whitby (ed) et al, 'Preventing Biological Threats: What You Can Do', *University of Bradford*

United Nations Biological Weapons Convention, 'Eighth Review Conference of the States Parties to the Convention on the Prohibition of the Development, Production and Stockpiling of Bacteriological (Biological) and Toxin Weapons and on Their Destruction', BWC/CONF.VIII/INF.2, October 21, 2016, undocs.org/BWC/CONF.VIII/INF.2

Yan-Peng Xu et al, 'Zika virus infection induces RNAi-mediated antiviral immunity in human neural progenitors and brain organoids', *National Library of Medicine* (2019) *Cell Res.*, Vol 29(4)

Chapter 23 – A Can of Worms
See notes to Chapter 22 – A Latent Threat to Mankind

Chapter 24 – The Window for an Outbreak

'2019 International Training Course on Biosafety Laboratory Management and Technology Held in Wuhan', *Wuhan Institute of Virology* (archived), web.archive.org/web/20191229215242/http:/www.whiov.ac.cn/xwdt_105286/zhxw/201912/t20191206_5450147.html

'Announcement on the purchase of fluorescent quantitative PCR instrument project by Wuhan Institute of Virology, Chinese Academy of Sciences', *Hubei Guohua Project Management*, archive.is/zRqj8

'Behind the verdict in the case of Li Ning, academician of the Chinese Academy of Engineering', *The Paper*, January 13, 2020, m.thepaper.cn/yidian_promDetail.jsp?contid=5506443

'Chen Quanjiao', *Wuhan Institute of Virology*, www.whiov.cas.cn/yjsjy/zsxxyjs/dsjs/bssds/202012/t20201221_5831045.html

'COVID-19 Coronavirus Real Time PCR Kit', bioPerfectus technologies, fda.gov/media/139279/download

'Director of Wuhan Institute of Virology says "let science speak"', *CGTN*, May 25, 2020

'Fact Sheet: Activity at the Wuhan Institute of Virology', *US Department of State* (archived), web.archive.org/web/20210116020654/https://www.state.gov/fact-sheet-activity-at-the-wuhan-institute-of-virology/

'In the post-SARS era, staged the largest emergency drill', *Chinese Center for Disease Control and Prevention*, archive.is/WXZGf

'Statement by Chen Quanjiao, Wuhan Institute of Virology, Chinese Academy of Sciences', *Wuhan Institute of Virology*, whiov.cas.cn/tzgg_160286/202005/t20200511_5577842.html

'The opening test of the special passage for the military sports meeting airport', *Xinhua*, September 26, 2019

'The research group currently has 6 researchers and 13 students', *Lab of Diagnostic Microbiology* (archived), archive.vn/Uwlii

'Vaccine pursuer dedicated to finding bio shield against possible germ warfare', *Global Times*, March 26, 2020

'Xi Focus: Xi signs order to award 4 persons for outstanding contribution in COVID-19 fight', *Xinhua*, August 11, 2020

黄燕玲赵浩瀚,郭鹏, 徐雨 (2017), Patent CN107703314B, 'A kind of corticotropin solution and its application', China

Andrew Kerr, '"Bat Lady" Denial of Chinese Military Involvement In Wuhan Lab Has Put China On Collision Course With US Intelligence', *Daily Caller*, March 23, 2021

Anna Fifield, 'Wolf Warrior strives to make China first with coronavirus vaccine', *The Washington Post*, March 22, 2020

Anthony Klan, 'Pakistan, handling "anthrax-like" pathogens', *The Klaxon*, July 23, 2020

Betsy McKay, 'NIH Presses US Nonprofit for Information on Wuhan Virology Lab', *Wall Street Journal*, August 19, 2020

Bill Gertz, 'Wuhan laboratory "most likely" coronavirus source, US government analysis finds', *Washington Times*, April 28, 2020

Elaine Okanyene Nsoesie, 'Analysis of hospital traffic and search engine data in Wuhan China indicates early disease activity in the Fall of 2019', *Harvard Library*, dash.harvard.edu/handle/1/42669767

George Arbuthnott, Jonathan Calvert and Philip Sherwell, 'Revealed: Seven year coronavirus trail from mine deaths to a Wuhan lab', *The Times* (archived), archive.ph/CUiQv#selection-1229.0-1233.145

Guli, '中国首席生化武器专家陈薇少将接管武汉P4病毒实验室' (trans: 'Major General Chen Wei, China's Chief Biochemical Weapons Expert, Takes Over Wuhan P4 Virus Laboratory'), *RFI*, February 8, 2020

@Harvard2TheBigHouse, 'DRASTIC Research 2020: Origins', *Sutori*, www.sutori.com/story/d-r-a-s-t-i-c-2020-origins--xCvdWonoJTx4TYVtAC4EhQ1b

Ian Birrell, 'Worrying new clues about the origins of Covid: How scientists at Wuhan lab helped Chinese army in secret project to find animal viruses', *Daily Mail*, April 25, 2021

James S Brady, 'Press Briefing by Press Secretary Jen Psaki, May 24, 2021', *The White House*

@JamieMetzl, *Twitter*, March 4, 2021

Jerry Dunleavy, 'Wuhan lab's "Bat Lady" denies US intel on collaboration with Chinese military', *Washington Examiner*, March 24, 2021

Jonathon Pekar, 'Timing the SARS-CoV-2 index case in Hubei province' (2021) *Science*, Vol 372(6540), 412–417

Josh Rogin, 'In 2018, Diplomats Warned of Risky Coronavirus Experiments in a Wuhan Lab. No One Listened', *Politico*, March 8, 2021

laowhy86, 'Found the Source of the Coronavirus', *YouTube*, April 2, 2020

Liang Xianrui, '好消息! "四川造" 新冠病毒检测试剂盒月底投入量产' (trans: 'Good news! "Made in Sichuan" new coronavirus detection kit put into mass production at the end of the month'), *Qianlong*, January 29, 2020

Liu Caiyu and Leng Shumei, 'Biosafety guideline issued to fix chronic management loopholes at virus labs', *Global Times*, February 16, 2020

Lu Beibei He Fuchu, 'Biotechnology will become the new strategic commanding heights of the future military revolution', *People's Liberation Army Daily* (archived), web.archive.org/web/20190813042422/http:/www.81.cn/jwgz/2015-10/06/content_6709533.htm

Meredith Wadman, 'NIH imposes "outrageous" conditions on resuming coronavirus grant targeted by Trump', *Science*, August 19, 2020

Milton Leitenberg, 'Did the SARS-CoV-2 virus arise from a bat coronavirus research program in a Chinese laboratory? Very possibly', *The Bulletin*, June 4, 2020

Minnie Chan and William Zheng, 'Meet the major general on China's coronavirus scientific front line', *South China Morning Post*, March 3, 2020

Minnie Chan, 'How China's military took a frontline role in the coronavirus crisis', *South China Morning Post*, March 17, 2020

@Perseus852, *Twitter*, February 18, 2020

Peter C. Taylor et al, 'Neutralizing monoclonal antibodies for treatment of COVID-19', *Nature Reviews Immunology*, Vol 21, 382–393

Phoebe Zhang and Simone McCarthy, 'Coronavirus: Xi Jinping calls for overhaul of China's health crisis response system', *South China Morning Post*, February 14, 2020

US Department of State, 'Fact Sheet: Activity at the Wuhan Institute of Virology', January 15, 2021

Xie Bin, '寻找黄燕玲' (trans: 'Looking for Huang Yanling'), *CReaders*, blog.creaders.net/u/3027/202002/366239.html

Yushun Wan et al, 'Molecular Mechanism for Antibody-Dependent Enhancement of Coronavirus Entry', *Journal of Virology*, Vol 94(5)

Chapter 25 – The Missing

@榮德居士, *Weibo*, March 10, 2020

@饺子就酒999, '武汉病毒所的黄燕玲真的失踪了吗?' (trans: 'Is Huang Yanling of Wuhan Virus Institute really missing?'), *Weibo*, February 16, 2020

'Disappearance of Huang Yanling', *MeetHackers*, April 22, 2020

'Li Zehua: Journalist who "disappeared" after Wuhan chase reappears', *BBC News*, April 23, 2020

'不是黄燕玲？那新型冠状病毒第一个病人是谁' (trans: 'Not Huang Yanling? Who is the first patient of the new coronavirus?'), *Antpedia*, February 18, 2020

'Wuhan Institute of Virology denies patient zero of COVID-19 came from institute', *Global Times*, February 16, 2020

'Wuhan Institute of Virology responded to the online transmission of "Patient Zero": The information transmitted online is not true, and she has not returned to Wuhan after graduation', *Interface News* (archived), web.archive.org/web/20210421111349/https://www.sohu.com/a/373454525_313745

'Yanling Huang's research while affiliated with Wuhan Institute of Virology and other places', *Research Gate*, researchgate.net/scientific-contributions/Yanling-Huang-2035568207

Chen Xing, '网传"零号病人"为谣言！黄燕玲所在公司研发总监：其目前正常上下班、身体正常' (trans: '"Patient Zero" is spread on the Internet as a rumor! Huang Yanling's R&D director of the company: She is currently commuting to and from work and her body is normal'), *NBD*, February 16, 2020, nbd.com.cn/articles/2020-02-16/1408726.html

Xiao Zhenchun, 'Refutes rumors under the name of the patent Huang Yanling', *Weixin*, weixin.qq.com/s/h6DBBQKNGJt528lwdOMpnA

Chapter 26 – The Case for a Lab Leak

'Rampant Repression: A data analysis of China's use of residential surveillance at a designated location 2013–2020', Safeguard Defenders

Alice Su, 'A migrant worker tries to save his village from the coronavirus — and gets arrested', *Los Angeles Times*, January 31, 2020

Guo Rui and Teddy Ng, '"I am just exhausted": Chinese doctors press on after coronavirus whistle-blower died', *Inkstone*, February 10, 2020